SPEAKING
OF HEALTH

Assessing Health Communication
Strategies for Diverse Populations

Committee on Communication for
Behavior Change in the 21st Century:
Improving the Health of Diverse Populations

Board on Neuroscience and Behavioral Health

INSTITUTE OF MEDICINE
OF THE NATIONAL ACADEMIES

THE NATIONAL ACADEMIES PRESS
Washington, D.C.
www.nap.edu

THE NATIONAL ACADEMIES PRESS • 500 Fifth Street, N.W. • Washington, DC 20001

NOTICE: The project that is the subject of this report was approved by the Governing Board of the National Research Council, whose members are drawn from the councils of the National Academy of Sciences, the National Academy of Engineering, and the Institute of Medicine. The members of the committee responsible for the report were chosen for their special competences and with regard for appropriate balance.

Support for this project was provided by the Institute of Medicine. The views presented in this report are those of the Institute of Medicine Committee on Communication for Behavior Change in the 21st Century: Improving the Health of Diverse Populations and are not necessarily those of the funding agencies.

Library of Congress Cataloging-in-Publication Data

Institute of Medicine (U.S.). Committee on Communication for Behavior Change in the 21st Century: Improving the Health of Diverse Populations.
  Speaking of health : assessing health communication strategies for diverse populations / Committee on Communication for Behavior Change in the 21st Century: Improving the Health of Diverse Populations, Board on Neuroscience and Behavioral Health, Institute of Medicine.
    p. ; cm.
Includes bibliographical references and index.
  ISBN 0-309-07271-9 (alk. paper)
  1. Communication in medicine. 2. Health promotion.
  [DNLM: 1. Health Promotion—methods. 2. Communication. 3. Cultural Diversity. 4. Health Services Accessibility. WA 590 I59s 2002] I.
Title.
  R118 .I575 2002
  613—dc21
                                    2002012033

Additional copies of this report are available for sale from the National Academies Press, 500 Fifth Street, N.W., Box 285, Washington, DC 20055. Call (800) 624-6242 or (202) 334-3313 (in the Washington metropolitan area); Internet, http://www.nap.edu.

For more information about the Institute of Medicine, visit the IOM home page at: www.iom.edu.

Printed in the United States of America.

COVER: Cindy Friedman, Susan Bershad, Mary Ivory, and Leslie Sullivan, *Volunteers: The Stars of the House*, 1997. 72" × 72". Textile. Philadelphia Ronald McDonald House.

The serpent has been a symbol of long life, healing, and knowledge among almost all cultures and religions since the beginning of recorded history. The serpent adopted as a logotype by the Institute of Medicine is a relief carving from ancient Greece, now held by the Staatliche Museen in Berlin.

*"Knowing is not enough; we must apply.
Willing is not enough; we must do."*
—Goethe

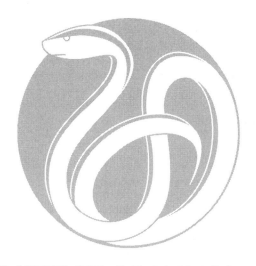

INSTITUTE OF MEDICINE
OF THE NATIONAL ACADEMIES

Shaping the Future for Health

THE NATIONAL ACADEMIES
Advisers to the Nation on Science, Engineering, and Medicine

The **National Academy of Sciences** is a private, nonprofit, self-perpetuating society of distinguished scholars engaged in scientific and engineering research, dedicated to the furtherance of science and technology and to their use for the general welfare. Upon the authority of the charter granted to it by the Congress in 1863, the Academy has a mandate that requires it to advise the federal government on scientific and technical matters. Dr. Bruce M. Alberts is president of the National Academy of Sciences.

The **National Academy of Engineering** was established in 1964, under the charter of the National Academy of Sciences, as a parallel organization of outstanding engineers. It is autonomous in its administration and in the selection of its members, sharing with the National Academy of Sciences the responsibility for advising the federal government. The National Academy of Engineering also sponsors engineering programs aimed at meeting national needs, encourages education and research, and recognizes the superior achievements of engineers. Dr. Wm. A. Wulf is president of the National Academy of Engineering.

The **Institute of Medicine** was established in 1970 by the National Academy of Sciences to secure the services of eminent members of appropriate professions in the examination of policy matters pertaining to the health of the public. The Institute acts under the responsibility given to the National Academy of Sciences by its congressional charter to be an adviser to the federal government and, upon its own initiative, to identify issues of medical care, research, and education. Dr. Harvey V. Fineberg is president of the Institute of Medicine.

The **National Research Council** was organized by the National Academy of Sciences in 1916 to associate the broad community of science and technology with the Academy's purposes of furthering knowledge and advising the federal government. Functioning in accordance with general policies determined by the Academy, the Council has become the principal operating agency of both the National Academy of Sciences and the National Academy of Engineering in providing services to the government, the public, and the scientific and engineering communities. The Council is administered jointly by both Academies and the Institute of Medicine. Dr. Bruce M. Alberts and Dr. Wm. A. Wulf are chair and vice chair, respectively, of the National Research Council.

www.national-academies.org

Staff

ANNE S. MAVOR, *Study Director* (since September 2001),
Division of Behavioral and Social Sciences and Education
(DBSSE), NRC

CAROLE A. CHRVALA, *Senior Program Officer* (until April 2001),
NBH, IOM

TERRY C. PELLMAR, *Director*, Board on Neuroscience and
Behavioral Health, IOM

ALLISON L. FRIEDMAN, *Research Assistant* (until August 2001),
NBH, IOM

SUSAN R. MCCUTCHEN, *Research Associate* (since September
2001) DBSSE, NRC

WENDY E. KEENAN, *Senior Project Assistant* (since September
2001), DBSSE, NRC

WENDY BLANPIED, *Project Assistant* (between September 2000
and May 2001), NBH, IOM

AMELIA MATHIS, *Project Assistant* (until May 2001), NBH, IOM

LINDA V. LEONARD, *Administrative Assistant* (until September
2000), NBH, IOM

LORA K. TAYLOR, *Administrative Assistant* (between October
2000 and June 2001), NBH, IOM

CATHERINE PAIGE, *Administrative Assistant* (since October 2001),
NBH, IOM

Staff

TERRY C. PELLMAR, Director
MICHAEL ABRAMS, Program Officer
ADRIENNE STITH-BUTLER, Program Officer
MILAP NOWRANGI, Research Assistant
BRIAN McQUILLAN, Senior Project Assistant
ALLISON M. PANZER, Senior Project Assistant
CATHERINE A. PAIGE, Administrative Assistant

Reviewers

This report has been reviewed in draft form by individuals chosen for their diverse perspectives and technical expertise, in accordance with procedures approved by the NRC's Report Review Committee. The purpose of this independent review is to provide candid and critical comments that will assist the institution in making its published report as sound as possible and to ensure that the report meets institutional standards for objectivity, evidence, and responsiveness to the study charge. The review comments and draft manuscript remain confidential to protect the integrity of the deliberative process. We wish to thank the following individuals for their review of this report:

Noreen M. Clark, University of Michigan
Karen Glanz, University of Hawaii
Russell E. Glasgow, AMC Cancer Research Center
Lawrence W. Green, Centers for Disease Control and
    Prevention
Helen P. Hazuda, University of Texas Health Science Center
    at San Antonio
Matthew Kreuter, Saint Louis University

Thomas R. Prohaska, University of Illinois at Chicago
William A. Smith, Academy for Educational Development

Although the reviewers listed above have provided many constructive comments and suggestions, they were not asked to endorse the conclusions or recommendations nor did they see the final draft of the report before its release. The review of this report was overseen by S. Leonard Syme, University of California, Berkeley. Appointed by the Institute of Medicine, he was responsible for making certain that an independent examination of this report was carried out in accordance with institutional procedures and that all review comments were carefully considered. Responsibility for the final content of this report rests entirely with the authoring committee and the institution.

Chair's Preface

In 1993, McGinnis and Foege published a landmark article that reviewed the causes of death in the United States in 1990 in terms of both the listed causes (e.g., heart attack, homicide) and the "actual causes" or underlying factors (e.g., obesity, violence). Behavioral factors were implicated in 50 percent of all deaths for that year (McGinnis and Foege, 1993). The importance of behavior for health has long been emphasized by behavioral scientists, such as anthropologists, psychologists, and sociologists; by public health researchers and practitioners; and by clinicians in areas such as preventative medicine and maternal and child health. Until recently, however, the importance of behavior for health was minimized in favor of the dramatic impact of biomedical innovations, and perhaps their perceived ease of administration as well. In fact, many in the health care delivery field deemed behavior intractable, or at least very difficult to change, and thus they preferred to look for what Rene Dubos (1959) called the "magic bullets" of medicine.

Usually, it is less costly both financially and in human terms to prevent than it is to treat. Type 2 diabetes provides an example. Both primary (prevention of onset) and secondary (prevention of complications) prevention are preferable to the costs of treatment and the burden of the disease. Both types of prevention involve behavior change around smoking, diet, and exercise, and secondary prevention involves complex monitoring and medication behaviors as well. In some cases, behavioral interventions are the only option for prevention, with treatment very costly, and not always successful. An example is HIV/AIDS, where vaccines are still in the developmental stage, and the only prevention involves sometimes complex and difficult behaviors. Even where vaccines exist, such as for hepatitis B, behavioral interventions can be crucial in controlling the spread of the disease and in limiting the consequences of an infection.

Technology alone is not enough. Despite the existence of a measles vaccine for the last 40 years of the 20th century, U.S. cities continued to experience occasional epidemics and some measles deaths into the 1990s. Even if there were "magic bullets" for all conditions, behavioral interventions would be needed to help motivate people to utilize them.

Unfortunately, knowledge is rarely sufficient to change behavior, although knowledge is important. The risks of smoking and other tobacco use are well known, but that knowledge is seldom enough to get people to stop smoking or to keep people from initiating the behavior. There is evidence that smoking prevention and cessation programs work (Wasserman, 2001; Fiore et al., 2000), but they must be funded and applied.

On one hand, human behavior is difficult to change, but on the other hand, it is constantly changing. One has only to witness the changing trends in food, clothing, and music in U.S. society, as well as the rapid increase in Internet use, to see behavioral change. Nor are those changes random. They are influenced by concerted efforts on the part of advertisers—and their investment of billions of dollars. During the past 20 years in particular, the health community began to work with the advertising community to develop behavior change strategies. Some of these were mass media campaigns, which will be discussed in this volume. Behavioral scientists working in public health also developed effective health communication strategies that ranged from interventions for individuals to school- and work-based programs, to programs delivered through health care providers, to mass media and community-based campaigns. Most often, programs that used multiple interventions were found to have greatest effectiveness. As new media such as the Internet and computer games emerged, so did communication strategies that employed these media.

Public health workers began to recognize the need to look at cultural factors when demographic and epidemiological data uncovered differences in risks of disease and death for various population subgroups. This came into sharper focus in the 1990s, as more attention was brought to bear on the disparities in health and illness among different ethnic, age, socioeconomic, gender, and other groups. The existence of these disparities meant that prevention and treatment efforts needed to be focused on those populations in most need, and questions had to be asked about the appropriateness and acceptability of these interventions.

The categories of "race" and ethnicity, which permitted the identification of health disparities, are considered crude and inaccurate by anthropologists and others focusing on variations in groups. This volume critically examines how culture and ethnicity are defined and operationalized, and suggests more recent ways of describing identity, such as cultural processes and life experiences that shape both individuals and groups and lead to variations within groups that may affect health behaviors. Modifications to permit a more accurate understanding of the relationships among cultural processes, life experiences, and health behaviors, especially as these might relate to communication for health behavior change, are also discussed.

Relevant behaviors vary from individual to individual, and are influenced by factors such as age, gender, economic options, social class, sexual orientation, life experiences, and cultural processes. Given this, a key question that this volume asks is: Will the same message content, medium, and format be received and understood equally by all? If not, how, when, and in what format should messages be focused for particular individuals or groups? To put it another way, does it matter more for planning interventions that two women have never had mammograms or that these women are of two different ethnicities or ages?

The committee charged with preparing this volume grappled with many related issues as well. From the start, the committee recognized that ethical issues arise when behavior change is involved, especially when strategies are modified to be culturally attractive and when persuasion strategies are used. This led to a consideration of ethical issues surrounding communication strategies. The committee struggled with theory. There are many behavior change theories, and no single theory explains all health behaviors. Many communication programs are designed and tested in the absence of theory. The challenge was to encourage use of theory, discuss aspects of the existing theories that best inform behavior change interventions for diverse populations, and identify gaps in theories. However, the committee did not produce a summary of existing theories because there are already many good sources for such reviews.

Three exemplars were chosen to illustrate the issues and approaches as they relate to communication and diverse populations. Mammography was selected as an exemplar because having a mammogram is an occasional behavior—yearly, at most, for screening purposes—and one that has been the subject of hundreds of communication interventions, including many for diverse populations. There is a strong foundation of evidence-based interventions. Diabetes was chosen because it involves primary and secondary preventive behaviors that are complex and difficult and must be practiced daily to achieve benefit. The evidence base is much less robust than for mammography. For both mammography and diabetes, the committee assumed that attitudes and behaviors might vary both across and within populations. The third exemplar, mass communication, was chosen because of its ubiquity as a public health strategy. As a result, the committee deemed it important to examine the success of mass communication campaigns for diverse populations.

The committee also chose to examine the new and emerging technologies that are dramatically changing the way we communicate about health and the way people obtain health information.

The breadth of the topic assigned to the committee for consideration is remarkable. Thus, conscious choices had to be made to limit the scope of this volume. Time and space precluded further attention to many important questions raised about each topic. At the same time, many areas for future investigation are identified. In particular, the lack of theory in the design of many communications and the lack of research and evaluation related to costly interventions were a surprise. The fact that shaping interventions to conform to specific cultures is often done in the absence of evidence and with no evaluation is of concern. These findings emerged in part because the committee included disciplines that seldom converge on this topic. It was extremely valuable to have the range of disciplines and experiences represented on the committee.

Many people contributed to this report. It was begun under the leadership of Carole Chrvala as study director, and Allison Friedman as research assistant. Wendy Keenan provided administrative support in the final project phase. Background papers by Nurit Guttman, David Gustafson, Michael McDonald, Tim Murphy, Charles Salmon, and Leslie Snyder provided very helpful ideas and materials. Terry Pellmar provided steady oversight and guidance, and key support at times when the task seemed overwhelming. Suzanne Stoiber believed in the importance of the topic, and was supportive throughout. Anne Mavor provided extraordinary leadership, support and very hard work. She stepped in as the second study director, and this report would not exist without her efforts.

Finally, the committee members are grateful to the Institute of Medicine, and to the leadership and support of outgoing IOM President Ken Shine for the opportunity to begin the dialogue about communication for health behavior change in diverse populations.

Susan C. Scrimshaw, Ph.D.

Contents

xvii

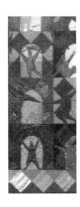

Executive Summary

Clear evidence from the Centers for Disease Control and Prevention, the National Institutes of Health, the Institute of Medicine, and other agencies that collect data on health behaviors and outcomes shows that significant health disparities continue to exist across diverse populations, despite efforts to reduce or eliminate those disparities. This problem is likely to grow if predictions of increasing social and cultural diversity in the United States over the next 50 years are correct. If effective actions are not taken, this increasing diversity could lead to a disproportionate rise in populations who have poorer health outcomes.

Given the likely growth in diversity, communication interventions to affect health behavior are an increasingly important strategy for improving the health of the American people. Constructing such interventions to effectively influence individuals in diverse populations to engage in healthy behavior, however, relies on an understanding of the social and cultural contexts that shape the behavior of individuals, families, and communities. Belief systems, religious and cultural values, and group identity are all powerful filters through which information is received and processed. Although many communication programs address diversity in their development and implementation, there is little evidence of the differential effects of these programs according to diversity subgroups. As a result, money and time are spent without knowing when a common format would suffice, or when a variety of targeted or even tailored interventions would be more appropriate. Given the likely growth in diversity, there is an urgent need now to enhance our current understanding of the dynamics of health communication to achieve the greatest impact for the most people.

This volume is the product of the Committee on Communication for Behavior Change in the 21st Century: Improving the Health of Diverse Populations, established by the Institute of Medicine in 1999. It focuses on those programs that involve some use of communication technology and have incorporated the transmission or exchange of messages within interventions designed to influence behavior to improve health. Programs exclusively involving interpersonal communication, such as between physician and patient, were not the focus; interventions that include other elements along with communication technology are considered.

The charge to the committee was to (1) review existing theory and research applications in health communication and health behavior change, especially as they relate to culturally diverse populations, and define research areas that would benefit from expanded or new research efforts; (2) consider up to three specific examples of health communication interventions to evaluate whether and how those strategies affect culturally diverse groups; and (3) recommend how health communication strategies may be designed and implemented to help achieve sustained gains in public health across cultural groups. The committee included experts in anthropology, psychology, mental health, cancer prevention and control, health behavior change and theory, communication and the media, social marketing, and public health. In the context of this charge, the committee considered the following questions:

- Is there evidence that targeting or tailoring messages for different cultural groups makes a difference in the effect of these messages on behavior change?

- What is the role of theory in the construction of communication programs, in the context of diversity? In particular, is there a need to modify theory for different subgroups of the population?
- Are there special ethical issues that arise in health communication because of diversity?
- Is the promise of communication for diverse populations different according to the health behavior(s) and disease process addressed?
- What are the implications of the rapid development of new technology-based health behavior interventions for health disparities?
- What are the most useful categories of diversity to be used in designing communication interventions?

With the issue of differential disease burden in mind, the committee chose as its exemplars the following: promotion of primary and secondary prevention strategies conveyed through mass health communication campaigns; secondary prevention of breast cancer with screening mammography; and primary, secondary, and tertiary prevention of Type 2 diabetes. These exemplars offer different communication challenges for behavior change in diverse populations.

We chose large-scale communication campaigns because they are widely used as a mechanism for affecting the behaviors of broad populations when the risk is widespread. We chose mammography because it involves a discrete behavior that should occur every year or two in a large segment of the healthy population. Diabetes was selected as a contrast to mammography; its treatment requires a complex set of continuing behaviors responsive to an evolving illness by those who have the illness as well as those around them. As noted, the focus of the committee's review and analysis of the exemplars was to examine the effects of health communication on the health behavior of diverse populations. To ensure completeness of coverage, the review included studies in which communication campaigns were combined with other interventions (such as access to health care facilities) as well as studies that examined communication strategies exclusively.

The following section provides a brief overview of the concepts contained in this volume and the committee's major recommendations. Chapter 8 presents a more detailed list of the overall findings and recommendations.

THE IMPORTANCE OF THEORY AND ETHICS IN DESIGNING HEALTH COMMUNICATION

Behavior and Communication Theory

A large body of literature exists on theories of behavior that focus on the structural, social, and psychological factors that influence behavior and on theories of communication that underlie approaches to influencing changes in these factors. Our perspective is restricted to those elements that appear to be most relevant to modifying a person's health-directed activities through communication. Theory can increase the potential effectiveness of health communication by identifying critical beliefs to target, by structuring communication, and by guiding the selection of sources and channels of communication. Important determinants of whether a person does or does not perform a given behavior are the person's beliefs about performing that behavior, the obstacles and facilitating factors in the environment, and the person's feelings about his or her ability to perform the behavior. Recognizing that these determinants may vary significantly from one population to another illustrates the importance of considering diversity in developing effective health communication. Once one or more behaviors and target populations have been identified, behavior change theory can be used to demonstrate why some members of a target population change their behavior and others do not. The proper implementation of behavior change and communication theory requires that one goes to a sample of the population to identify the outcomes, referents, and barriers that are relevant for that population.

Theories of behavior change and communication have an important place in the construction of communication programs in general and for diverse populations. The committee encourages program developers and implementers to use these theories in a more consistent and aggressive way in developing implementation plans for health communication interventions. Additional research is needed about the translational process of moving from theory to implementation. The committee recommends that more attention be given to how theories are translated into effective practice and implemented in health communication interventions; that is, how the theoretical principles are applied in practice. One approach might employ case studies that document specific interventions and include discussions of the operational difficulties of translating theory into practice.

Ethics

Respecting an individual's autonomy to make choices, maximizing benefit, avoiding harm, and treating groups and individuals justly and equitably are core ethical principles. These principles are easily endorsed, but not always easily achieved. Implementing ethical principles can be complicated by the developers' needs to consider tradeoffs among efficiency, cost, and improving the health of the most in need versus benefiting a broader range of persons. Sometimes these choices have to be made under conditions of uncertainty, either in terms of uncertainty about the scientific support for an intervention or uncertainty about the effect of the intervention. Some communication strategies come into conflict when trying to secure benefit for one segment of the population versus another. This risk may be heightened in the context of reaching heterogeneous audiences with a common message. There is always the opportunity for unintended consequences to occur (e.g., confusion, unwarranted anxiety), even with the most well-intentioned and well-executed health communication interventions. Some of these concerns can be minimized through close cooperation with the groups whose health care one hopes to improve. This recommendation may be complex to implement in practice, given the need to choose among potential representatives and the possible tension between technical "expertise" and preferences of intended beneficiaries. However, the committee believes that health communication program managers should not only explicitly consider ethical guidelines in their decisions about implementation, but also should involve affected individuals and communities as active participants in decision making about each campaign.

COMMUNICATION INTERVENTIONS FOR DIVERSE POPULATIONS

The State of the Evidence

The committee's review of the literature makes it clear that researchers, program planners, and managers quite often take diversity into account when they construct their communication programs. This is true both for communication interventions that addressed mammography and for those that were examined in the review of large-scale campaigns. However, we found few examples of communication programs that addressed diabetes. Nevertheless, three broad diversity-respecting strategies emerged from the rich variety of approaches described in the literature. They are:

• The construction of a unified communication program with a common denominator message that will be relevant across most populations.
• The construction of a unified communication program with systematic variations of message executions to make them appeal to different segments, while retaining the same fundamental message strategy.
• The development of distinct message strategies and/or distinct interventions for each target segment.

However, the evidence base is quite thin about differential effects of interventions according to diversity subgroups. Some of those programs have been successful in changing behavior, including that of the diversity subgroups of particular interest in this volume. However, the available data do not effectively address whether there is added benefit in addressing health disparities by using communication that takes diversity into account. That is, there are few studies that address the relative effectiveness of communication interventions across relevant diverse groups, and none were found that systematically compare the various approaches to addressing diversity or that compare those approaches with efforts that ignore diversity altogether. This is not to say there are no diversity-respecting programs. Rather, where such programs exist, they do not provide direct evidence about the interaction of communication programs and subgroup status. In general, the evidence does not indicate whether the efforts to consider diversity were worthwhile, or which approaches were worthwhile and under what circumstances. Based on these findings, the committee believes the following:

- There is a need to undertake comparative effectiveness research in each of the following areas: secondary analysis of evidence already collected from existing communication programs, effectiveness evaluation of new and ongoing programs, and field testing of alternative diversity strategies.
- Until more convincing evidence is available pro or con, it is sensible for many existing programs to continue to pay attention to diversity, particularly when diversity is associated with substantial disparities in health status and outcomes. This recommendation is subject to the following limitations: (1) the most important categories of diversity may not be the conventional ones, and (2) communication interventions should be targeted to specific subgroups only when the evidence from program research suggests that important differences exist in health behavior or the antecedents of health behavior or when there is a strong hypothesis for such differences.

Components of a Successful Program

Many successful communication programs have been reported in the literature. A review of these can be found in Chapters 3 and 4. The committee finds that these programs have met certain conditions, and that these conditions should serve as a guide for future program development. These conditions include a strong science base for recommended behaviors, a realistic possibility that recommendations can be implemented by the population, coordination with other programs addressing related issues, enough resources available for the development and particularly the transmission of messages so that the intended audience sees them at needed frequency, and often the resources to maintain the campaign over time if the pace of change is slow.

The Promise of New Technology

New uses of current and widely accessible communication media, such as print and telephone, have been possible because of computer applications that have permitted content to be tailored to individuals, thus allowing people to use older tools in new ways. Among the most important of these innovative uses are tailored print communication and telephone-delivered interventions. The potential of these media for reaching people with and without Internet access, and people with highly diverse linguistic and cultural requirements, should not be underestimated, nor should the challenge of harnessing the new media for reaching diverse audiences.

Achieving the potential of new technologies for diverse populations requires attention to access, as well as to the acceptability, availability, appropriateness, and applicability of content. Without deliberate action, new computer technologies may exacerbate inequities in health and health care. To improve the health care of diverse populations, the committee believes that investments are needed in research, training, and delivery of technology-based communication interventions. In many cases, new technology should be combined with established communication strategies, such as face-to-face contact and telephone counseling. Research methods are needed to estimate untapped potential and costs of communication technology used to improve health care for diverse populations.

TOWARD A NEW DEFINITION OF DIVERSITY

Diversity is frequently defined for policy and research purposes by broad social and demographic categories such as race, ethnicity, socioeconomic status, age, and gender. Although these categories may have important political relevance, there is usually as much heterogeneity with regard to behavior and its determinants within a specified group as between groups. The committee argues that communication programs need to focus on other, more meaningful ways of describing heterogeneity. Specifically, they should focus on cultural process, on understanding the life experiences of the communities and individuals being served, and on the sociocultural environment of individuals within the populations to be reached. There are multiple dimensions to be considered, ranging from economic contexts and community resources such as access to health services to commonly held attitudes, norms, efficacy beliefs, and practices pertinent to the health issue in question.

The committee recommends that policy makers and program planners continue to use demographic factors to understand whether health benefits are equally distributed and to identify intergroup differences. Where there are existing disparities, it will be important to monitor trends in gap opening and closing according to these categories. At the same time, program planners need to recognize that other measures such as life experiences and cultural processes are needed to understand within-group variations and to understand their association with health behaviors. Actual planning of health communication programs rarely will be well served by an assumption of homogeneity within any of these categories. This may also require efforts to more systematically educate policy makers about the relevant domains of diversity for purposes of communication interventions.

INFRASTRUCTURE NEEDS

The field of public health communication relies on contributions of many disciplines. Skilled communicators and intervention developers are central to successful communication programs, but they depend on expertise from many other fields. Public health communication requires theories about behavior and behavior change; deep understanding of audiences, their cultural experience, and their social and structural circumstances; and understanding of the health infrastructure around the health concern and its medical nature. Increasingly, public health communication requires technical expertise with new technologies and medical knowledge about health problems. Some programs also need the expertise of marketers, and others need informatics expertise. If advances are to be made in communication for diverse populations, the field of public health communication should be strengthened. This requires not only investment in research and training, but the active participation and collaboration of people from many disciplines. Interdisciplinary teams to design and implement communication strategies in diverse populations should be encouraged by funding agencies.

National campaigns to address major health priorities require the mustering of substantial resources and, often, coordinated efforts of multiple agencies, if national audiences are to be reached and effects are to be sustained over time. They cannot be undertaken successfully without such commitment. A national strategy and infrastructure for prioritizing and implementing such large-scale campaigns are needed.

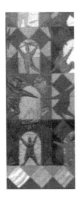

1

Introduction

As the 21st century begins, the nation is facing increasing concern about health problems, particularly chronic diseases such as diabetes, and escalating health care costs. Our society is becoming more diverse in every conceivable way, and diversity is often, though not always, associated with health disparities. On the other hand, we have available increasingly robust theories about health behavior and exciting new opportunities for expanded health communication strategies through enhanced technologies. These offer the potential for interactive approaches that can be tailored more precisely to individual and small group needs.

Many broad social, economic, and political forces affect the health status of populations (e.g., Institute of Medicine, 2000), and these forces ultimately must be addressed. Yet health communication, in its various applications, offers a potentially important approach to a better informed and presumably healthier population by focusing on the behavioral aspects of risk factors, such as diet, smoking, alcohol use, sedentary lifestyle, and sexual behavior (McGinnis and Foege, 1993).

In 1999, the Institute of Medicine convened the Committee on Communication for Behavior Change in the 21st Century: Improving the Health of Diverse Populations, in response to requests from the Board on Neuroscience and Behavioral Health and the Board on Health Sciences Policy to examine the potential of health communication strategies to improve public health behaviors, especially among demographically and socioculturally diverse populations. Health communication strategies, for purposes of this volume, are defined as approaches that seek to persuade or motivate people to change their behavior in order to improve their health. This volume is concerned primarily with communication strategies that are designed for larger groups or the public, rather than individual persuasion strategies such as doctor-patient communication. However, the committee recognized that health communication can be initiated by a variety of sources, including health care providers, campaign developers, and individuals seeking health information.

The salience and timeliness of examining how communication strategies relate to diversity within the U.S. population are emphasized by recent federal initiatives on disparities in health. Examples include the Eliminating Racial and Ethnic Disparities in Health campaign, Healthy People 2010, and the Minority Health and Health Disparities Research and Education Act of 2000. Although informed by the concerns about disparities raised by these initiatives, this volume adopts a considerably broader view of social and cultural differences that will be addressed briefly here and in detail in Chapter 7.

Substantial evidence exists on the relationship of diversity—mostly categorized by race/ethnicity, socioeconomic status, age, and gender—and health status (Centers for Disease Control and Prevention, 2001). The less socially or politically advantaged a population group is, the more compromised its health status. There is also reasonably good evidence that health communication campaigns can influence health behavior (e.g., Hornik, 2002). However, there is little evidence on the enhanced impact of health campaigns that are planned with special attention to addressing the needs of diverse audiences. This does not mean that health communication campaigns have not taken diversity into account.

Most campaigns are concerned about diversity and shape their message and placement based on age, gender, ethnicity, race, sexual preference, or other relevant personal variables. However, there is a striking lack of data available to answer essential questions about diversity—for example, does a health communication effort that takes extra care in understanding and responding to the needs of a diverse audience show effects that are greater than if such efforts are not made? In other words, it is not possible now to answer the question of whether added value, defined as better health outcomes, results from incorporating a focus on diversity compared to an intervention designed for a more general audience.

The challenge for those involved in the design, implementation, evaluation, and research concerning health communication is to influence behaviors with the greatest potential to significantly improve health outcomes across demographically and culturally diverse population groups. This volume addresses the challenge of improving health communication in a racially and culturally diverse society. Although targeting messages to specific audiences should increase effectiveness, this volume describes the difficulty and complexity of categorizing audiences in a meaningful way. Many of the "markers" that are used to describe groups are of little relevance and utility in crafting communication—or must be considered in a subtle way. Belief systems, religious and cultural values, life experiences, and group identity are all powerful filters through which information is received and processed. We need to know more about these in order to understand how to frame messages that will be understood and lead to action. A major goal of this volume is to clarify and evaluate the potential of health communication strategies to meet this challenge.

The committee that was formed to explore this fundamental question of the value of integrating diversity factors more scientifically into health communication approaches includes experts in anthropology, psychology, mental health, cancer prevention and control, health behavior change and theory, communication and the media, social marketing, and public health. This expertise was supplemented by consultants in communication technology and ethics. The committee's specific charges were as follows:

- Review existing theory and research applications in health communication and health behavior change, especially as they relate to culturally diverse populations, and define research areas that would benefit from expanded or new research efforts;
- Consider up to three specific examples of health communication interventions to evaluate whether and how those strategies affect culturally diverse groups; and
- Recommend how health communication strategies may be designed and implemented to achieve sustained gains in public health across cultural groups.

The results of this effort are intended to inform policy makers, researchers, funders/sponsors, advocacy organizations, practitioners, and others in developing, implementing, evaluating, and conducting research on communication strategies to improve the public's health.

CONTEXT

Health and Diversity

The importance of understanding diversity for public health is clearly evident. Yet current categories, which use arbitrary groupings of "race" and ethnicity, are not useful enough and do not contribute to necessary knowledge on the relationship between diversity and health behavior. New ways of understanding diversity will be required to develop more appropriate, and presumably more successful, approaches for health communication efforts. Yet jettisoning current categories of diversity as a means for identifying need and targeting programs will likely be controversial. Many political organizations, constituency groups, the U.S. Congress, and major administrative agencies of the government are organized around current definitions and categories. If the definition of diversity is changed, then the basis for funding decisions will change. This uncertainty could result in considerable argument, which happened during efforts to change the census categories for racial/ ethnic identification. Making diversity scientifically and programmatically meaningful undoubtedly will cause political conflict.

Categories for Describing Diversity

Discussions of disparities and health outcome differences across cultural groups contrast broad ethnic or racial categories that, although they have some utility for simplifying and focusing public discussion, relate little, if at all, to variation in socioculturally based beliefs and behaviors that have specific implications for health outcomes. The widely used broad ethnic categories, in particular, are simply not valid indicators of meaningful variation in health-related beliefs and behaviors. The most useful information for framing this volume—data that provide a much deeper and more sophisticated understanding of how specific beliefs and behaviors and health status covary across the U.S. population and of how health behavior is shaped by sociocultural processes—is not available, and one of the committee's recommendations is to develop this exact information. For example, how individuals come to think about and make sense of the world is mediated, to a large extent, by their social group identification and participation and by their life experiences. The term "cultural processes" is used to refer to these socially grounded ways of learning that contribute to how an individual thinks, feels, and acts.

Part of the challenge in addressing health behavior change for diverse populations is determining the circumstances under which diversity matters. The categorical comparisons that are available, and that are used throughout this volume, emphasize the importance of attending to cultural differences, even if presenting information in this way risks misguiding the reader into thinking these categories are relevant to the committee's charge.

Economic status and social class are considered dimensions of diversity for this volume because there are differences in health outcomes, and presumably in health risks, for these groupings (Lynch and Kaplan 2000; House and Williams, 2000). Although economic status and social class can be considered separately, they are most often grouped. Socioeconomic status (SES) commonly includes education, occupation, and income, but other factors such as net worth may be considered. The measurement of socioeconomic status has been discussed at length in the literature, and is clearly summarized in Lynch and Kaplan (2000). Similarly, the relationship between socioeconomic status and health has been discussed in detail in a recent Institute of Medicine report, *Promoting Health* (2000).

In discussing the relationship between SES and race/ethnicity, House and Williams (2000:97) note: "Although not useful as biological markers, current racial/ethnic categories capture an important part of the inequality and injustice in American society. . . . There are important power and status differences between groups." In fact, as they document, these power and status differences relate directly to the health disparities through factors such as environmental conditions and access to preventative and curative health care. They also note that SES alone does not explain health disparities. Furthermore, caution must be applied to the measurement of SES, and to assumptions about relationships between poverty and culture. As just mentioned, poor health outcomes are not confined to people with low SES, nor does low SES mean inevitably poorer outcomes.

Age and gender also show differences in health outcomes. These are partly because of biological factors, but also because of other kinds of factors underlying health disparities such as access to care, education, and environmental contexts, as well as health beliefs and behaviors. Both age and gender affect how people are treated in U.S. society. The very old and the very young are likely to have fewer rights and be subjected to more discrimination, as are women, regardless of ethnicity.

The committee members acknowledge that sexual orientation is a relevant and important parameter of diversity for the development, implementation, and evaluation of effective health communication interventions. Indeed, significant differences have been reported on various health measures for women and men, depending on sexual orientation (Institute of Medicine, 1999a; Dean et al., 2000). Many of the differences in health outcomes are related to differential risk behaviors, such as higher risk of sexually transmitted diseases and AIDS from unsafe sexual behavior in gay men, higher rates of poor diet and being overweight among lesbian women, and higher rates of smoking, alcohol use, and substance abuse among lesbian, gay, and bisexual persons.

Unlike the other defining constructs of diversity in this volume, however, sexual orientation is not routinely used as a demographic grouping to assess or report differences in health behaviors or health outcomes. In fact, the collection of reliable information about gay and lesbian populations has been constrained by political obstacles and methodological challenges (Dean et al., 2000; Institute of Medicine, 1999a).

Similarly, other dimensions of diversity are highly relevant to communication, but we cannot focus on them in an examination of existing studies. For example, the issue of an individual's primary language is minimally addressed in this volume, although it is clearly an important topic. For the decade starting in 1990, the "most recent wave of immigration is composed largely of non-European, non-English speaking 'people of color' arriving in unprecedented numbers from Asia, the Caribbean, and Latin America" (Suárez-Orozco, 2000:5). Significant numbers of U.S. residents also communicate primarily using languages other than standard English. Literacy and education are additional dimensions of diversity that are not closely examined. The lack of attention to such factors should not be viewed as a measure of their importance, but rather reflect constraints in terms of what reasonably could be examined within the scope of the committee's time frame and available data.

The U.S. Population and Categorical Demographic Diversity

The U.S. population now has more than 281 million residents. The number of persons in the United States has tripled over the past century among persons under age 65, and increased by a factor of 11 among those age 65 and over (U.S. Census Bureau, 2000). Ethnic diversity has increased among all age categories in the population, particularly among younger populations. By the year 2050, the percentage of non-Hispanic whites in the United States is expected to decrease to 53 percent overall. As many as 56 percent of adolescents are projected to represent ethnic minority groups; that is, groups other than non-Hispanic whites or EuroAmericans (National Center for Health Statistics, 2000; Brown et al., 1996). More people are completing formal education, poverty rates have reached their lowest levels since 1979, and real median household income has reached a record high, increasing for all types of households in all regions of the United States in 1998 (U.S. Census Bureau, 1998, 2000; Dalaker and Proctor, 2000).

All of these changes in demographics suggest that the cultural landscape of the U.S. population is changing toward a larger, older, more ethnically diverse, and more educated population. For example, Hispanics constitute a relatively younger population lagging in education and income, while whites are older and have higher accumulated wealth. Among populations age 15 and older, non-Hispanic whites (83 percent) were most likely to have at least a high school education in 2000, followed by Asian Americans/ Pacific Islanders (78 percent), non-Hispanic African-Americans (72 percent), and Hispanics (53 percent) (Bennett and Martin, 1995).

The income gap between rich and poor remains considerable (U.S. Census Bureau, 1998). In 2000, Asian Americans/ Pacific Islanders had the highest median income ($55,500) and Hispanics and African-Americans had the lowest ($33,400 and $30,400, respectively). The poverty rate across all groups is approximately 11 percent, with African-Americans and Hispanics well above the mean and non-Hispanic whites well below the mean (U.S. Census Bureau, 2001).

In 1995, approximately 49 million people (20 percent) in the United States lived in a household that had at least one difficulty in meeting basic needs, such as the inability to meet essential living expenses (e.g., pay utility bills, mortgage, or rent), buy food, or seek medical or dental care when needed (Bauman, 1995). Approximately 5 percent of American households reported that members sometimes did not have enough food to eat, while nearly 20 percent reported either not having enough food or the kind of food they wanted to eat (Bauman, 1995). Income, ethnicity, age, gender of householder, health insurance coverage, and Hispanic origin were among the major risk factors for not having enough food to eat.

The burden of death and disease frequently falls most heavily on some ethnic groups and on those with lower levels of education and income. The age-adjusted rates for the leading causes of death among men and women in the three largest ethnic groups (non-Hispanic whites, non-Hispanic Blacks, and Hispanics) are shown in Tables 1-1 and 1-2 (Centers for Disease Control and Prevention, 2001).[1] These tables show that the highest rates among all groups are for heart disease and cancer. However, significant variations exist. Non-Hispanic white and Black males and females have significantly higher rates for these two diseases than Hispanics. For the most part, Hispanics have significantly lower rates across all leading causes of death. Male non-Hispanic Blacks have the highest rates of death for several diseases, including heart disease, cancer, cerebrovascular disease, and diabetes. Furthermore, the disparities among these groups increase with age; for example, the difference in mortality rate between Black and white males is three times greater at age 65 than at age 45.

Table 1-3 shows the age-adjusted death rates for four major causes of death from cancer for whites, African-Americans, Hispanics, Asian Americans/Pacific Islanders, and Native American

---

[1]Age-adjusted data were not available for Asian Americans/Pacific Islanders and Native Americans, perhaps because these groups are small and the data are judged to be unstable.

TABLE 1-1 Age-Adjusted Rates for 10 Leading Causes of Death by Ethnic Group—Males (rate per 100,000)

Disease	All	Non-Hispanic White	Non-Hispanic Black	Hispanic
Heart	328.1	329.5	344.3	212.7
All cancer	251.6	251.4	350.1	151.4
Cerebrovascular diseases	62.4	60.5	89.7	44.6
Chronic obstructive pulmonary disease	58.1	61.3	51.4	27.3
Unintentional accidents	50.6	49.1	64.2	47.2
Pneumonia and influenza	28.0	28.0	33.0	18.6
Diabetes mellitus	27.7	25.0	50.1	34.5
Suicide	18.2	20.3	10.8	10.7
Kidney infections	16.2	14.8	33.8	12.9
Chronic liver disease and cirrhosis	13.7	12.7	15.6	23.0

SOURCE: Centers for Disease Control and Prevention (2001).

TABLE 1-2 Age-Adjusted Rates for 10 Leading Causes of Death by Ethnic Group—Females (rate per 100,000)

Disease	All	Non-Hispanic White	Non-Hispanic Black	Hispanic
Heart	220.9	218.1	297.0	146.5
All cancer	169.9	172.1	205.6	101.4
Cerebrovascular diseases	60.5	59.6	80.0	36.6
Chronic obstructive pulmonary disease	38.2	41.5	24.5	15.3
Diabetes mellitus	23.3	19.5	51.7	32.6
Unintentional accidents	22.7	23.1	24.4	15.5
Pneumonia and influenza	20.8	21.1	21.7	13.5
Alzheimer's disease	17.6	18.8	12.4	8.4
Kidney infections	11.2	9.7	26.6	8.8
Septicemia	10.5	9.5	23.0	6.8

SOURCE: Centers for Disease Control and Prevention (2001).

TABLE 1-3 Age-Adjusted Rates for Four Major Causes of
Death from Cancer by Ethnic Group[a] (rate per 100,000)[b]

Cancer	White	African-American	Asian American/ Pacific Islander	Native American	Hispanic[c]
Lung and bronchus					
Males	69.5	99.5	34.2	40.9	31.6
Females	34.0	33.0	14.9	19.8	11.0
Colon and rectum					
Males	21.3	27.7	13.1	11.6	13.1
Females	14.3	19.9	8.9	8.9	8.3
Prostate (males)	23.3	54.1	10.4	14.2	16.2
Breast (females)	25.3	31.4	11.2	12.1	15.1

[a]Data are from the American Cancer Society, Surveillance Research (2001). SOURCE: Surveillance, Epidemiology, and End Results Program, Division of Cancer Control and Population Science, National Cancer Institute (2000). Mortality derived from data originating from the National Center for Health Statistics, Centers for Disease Control and Prevention (2000).

[b]Per 100,000, age adjusted to the 1970 U.S. standard population.

[c]Hispanic is not mutually exclusive from white, African-American, Asian American/ Pacific Islander, and Native American.

for both males and females based on data from the Surveillance, Epidemiology, and End Results Program of the National Cancer Institute (Centers for Disease Control and Prevention, 2000). Black males have the highest death rates for lung, colon, and prostate cancer; Black women have the highest death rates for colon and breast cancer. Asian Americans/Pacific Islanders have the lowest rates of breast and prostate cancer; Hispanics have the lowest rates of lung cancer. Several factors may contribute to these disparities, including health behaviors, access to and availability of prevention and treatment services, patterns of service utilization, environmental and occupational risks, community support and cohesion, differences in insurance coverage, and underlying biological risk factors.

The Role of Communication

Recognizing the potential of verbal and nonverbal messages to modify beliefs and behavior, the public health community has been working with communication and media experts for more than 30 years to develop mass media campaigns to change health behavior. At the same time, behavioral scientists working in public health have developed communication strategies, including materials for individuals, programs at school and at work, programs delivered through health care providers, and large-scale campaigns.

The design and development of effective health communication strategies has become increasingly important with the development of new, but untested, technologies that could have potential for disseminating health communication across diverse cultural groups. This potential power to affect public health through communication, however, is attended by concerns that not all groups benefit equally from communication or social innovation, as exemplified by the "digital divide" in access to and use of the Internet (Rogers, 1995). Communication technologies may fundamentally change who has access to health information, and therefore shift the distribution of health-behavioral risk factors and health status. Would this shift increase or reduce health disparities as defined by conventional cultural categories? Would groups that differ in health-related beliefs and behaviors respond differently to health communication strategies? Are there options for optimizing health improvement from health communication programs? The answers to these questions may depend on whether disparities are malleable to communication strategies, and whether these strategies can be designed adequately to be effective for persons with different culturally based beliefs and behaviors.

Many of the basic benefits of communication strategies may be obtained across diverse cultural groups through a generic strategy that capitalizes on their similarities in beliefs and behaviors. Alternatively, it may be that the communication intervention or delivery strategy must be targeted to particular groups to have similar effects across groups, or tailored to the beliefs and values of the group members to optimize the impacts. In this regard, it is of particular policy interest to know whether targeting and tailoring communication interventions is especially useful in improving the health of populations with historical or current health or health care disadvantages. Thus, the question of the marginal benefit of special attention in communication interventions to subgroups may depend on the goals of interventions and, specifically, how much attention should be focused on vulnerable populations—a societal ethical question. Furthermore, whether communication strategies or their implementation must be modified to be effective for different cultural groups will be a function of the particular health problem and subpopulation.

In setting the scope, we purposely attempted to include public health strategies, such as campaigns, and medical practice strategies, such as pamphlets or Internet-based communication by providers to larger groups of patients.

Ethical Considerations

A number of ethical principles need to be considered in the development and implementation of health communication for diverse populations, including avoidance of harm, providing benefit, respecting an individual's autonomy to make a rational choice, and treating groups and individuals justly and equitably. These principles are not always easy to achieve. First, implementing ethical principles can be complicated by the developers' need to consider tradeoffs among efficiency, cost, and improving the health of the most in need versus a broader range of persons. Second, a communication strategy that incorporates ethical principles may function effectively and appropriately for one segment of the population, but not for another. Third, unintended consequences may occur even with the most well-intentioned and well-executed health communication interventions. Such outcomes for diverse populations include confusion about the meaning of a message, unwarranted anxiety resulting from implying individual culpability, or the stigmatizing of certain cultural practices.

One method for dealing with these kinds of concerns is to seek and maintain mutual collaboration with the community during all phases of the communication intervention process. This method will increase the likelihood that the messages and strategies of the intervention will unfold in a manner that is appropriate for the intended audience.

APPROACH AND SCOPE

Given the important role that communication campaigns are likely to play in the coming years, the field of public health communication should be strengthened and become more science based. This means supporting research that improves our understanding of the values and context that determine how information will be received, supporting evaluation of campaigns to measure their effectiveness, and paying more attention to the ethical and social concerns that must be appreciated and respected in the design of communication campaigns.

In our review and analysis, we draw on several disciplines. First, we rely on communication sciences and fields such as social marketing to define the essential components and issues in communication strategies and to review the contributions of technological advances to those strategies in the near future.

Second, we rely on theories of culture and cultural process to help define the scope of inquiry into culturally based beliefs and behaviors and cultural comparisons. We begin with a broad view of sociocultural and demographic diversity, considering ethnic groups, gender differences, and differences in factors such as socioeconomic status and sexual orientation. Awareness of culture and the concepts of culture as shared understanding within a community is essential to improving our understanding of the dynamic factors that influence the process of health communication. Many potential sources of shared understanding, such as ethnicity, training for a specific occupation, education, age, religion, language, gender, and generation, may provide a basis for social groupings within which cultural processes unfold and contribute to intracultural variation because individuals participate in or are exposed to different cultural processes.

Third, we focus on key social science theoretical contributions to communication interventions and their dissemination. Social cognitive and behavioral theories have brought an important conceptual and structural integrity to communication intervention design and evaluation. Rather than reviewing individual theories, we describe how health behavior is determined by underlying beliefs and how these beliefs are shaped by communication. We discuss the contributions of behavioral and communication theories to conceptualize the relevant beliefs and behaviors and to hypothesize which interventions will affect them. In addition, we call on theories of diffusion of innovations (1) to understand which communication-based interventions might be disseminated and what might happen to those interventions and their impacts in the process of dissemination, and (2) to understand better the process of dissemination itself.

Fourth, we broaden the context for our main questions by considering the equity of benefits of communication interventions across diverse groups and the role of communication in reducing the disparities among these groups. Furthermore, because communication interventions often use persuasive techniques, we must examine the ethical issues involved in attempting to persuade diverse populations that include vulnerable groups to change their behaviors in the interest of public health goals.

We believe exciting new opportunities are present to achieve the goal of maximizing health benefits of communication strategies for a wide range of socioculturally diverse groups. Pursuing this goal involves understanding basic principles of communication interventions, such as how messages are constructed for targeted audiences and how they are effectively conveyed. Messages can be made more coherent and powerful and can be evaluated more effectively by organizing communication interventions around well-constructed, extensively studied social science theories. However, doing so requires consideration of what the specific beliefs and behaviors are for populations of interest and how sociocultural groups that differ in their beliefs and behaviors may respond to or be affected differently by communication interventions.

The committee's strategy in preparing this volume was to use an interdisciplinary approach to examine the current state of health communication to diverse populations and to suggest fruitful approaches for developing improved interventions in the future. More specifically, by drawing on the relevant disciplines, we explore two questions: (1) Can we improve our ability to optimize public health in the context of diversity through communication? (2) Can we improve the science base in this area?

Conducting a comprehensive evaluation of health communication is a challenging task given the size and complexity of the activities in this area. To make the task more manageable, we developed an approach to analyze the field through a broad examination of three exemplars. One exemplar is national or large-scale regional public health campaigns. The second is communication to improve mammography or breast cancer screening rates. The third area is the management of and outcomes for diabetes mellitus. These three exemplars offer our analysis a focus on a communication method (public health campaign), a public health problem (mammography screening), and disease management that spans public health and medical practice concerns (diabetes mellitus). For all three cases, a prime object of intervention is changing beliefs, intentions to act, or behaviors themselves, such as modifying personal health practices, accessing health care, or adhering to treatment recommendations.

All three involve areas of public health and medicine. For national campaigns and screening mammography, there has been extensive development of health communication strategies for large groups of people; for diabetes mellitus, few systematic communication efforts have been implemented. This area offers an important opportunity for the future development and testing of communication interventions to change behavior. There are surely other health conditions or types of communication intervention strategies in which the benefits of communication strategies for improving health across diverse groups differ from what we observe for these three areas. However, our selected cases represent major areas of national attention and provide the opportunity to examine different methodological, theoretical, and research approaches to the design and conduct of communication strategies to change health behavior. We note that communication strategies are sometimes only one part of multicomponent interventions (e.g., to improve health) that combine communication and resources or that intervene both at group and individual levels. In reviewing the literature, we attended to interventions that use communication strategies exclusively as well as to those that include such strategies as a major component.

ORGANIZATION OF THE VOLUME

The volume is intended to inform policy makers, researchers, funders/sponsors, advocacy organizations, practitioners, and others in providing and evaluating communication interventions to improve public health. It is organized into eight chapters. Chapter 2 provides a framework for the committee's review and analysis by examining the contributions of behavior and communication theory to the design, development, implementation, and evaluation of health communication to diverse populations. Chapters 3 through 5 present the three exemplars—national campaigns, mammography, and diabetes mellitus. As noted, our review of the diabetes literature resulted in the conclusion that little systematic work has been done on communication campaigns to change behavior in this area. As a result, the committee presents a discussion of diabetes as a challenge for health communication developers in the future. Chapter 6 reviews the state of technology and assesses its potential. Chapter 7 discusses the problems associated with developing appropriate definitions of diversity and provides guidance for a new direction. Chapter 8 presents the committee's findings and recommendations.

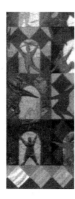

2

Theory

T his chapter synthesizes the main theories of communication and behavior change, including media advocacy and the diffusion of innovations, as they apply to health behavior change by diverse populations in the United States. Our perspective is restricted to those elements that appear to be most relevant to modifying a person's health-directed activities through communication.

WHAT DOES THEORY DO?

Behavioral theories are defined by constructs, their relationships, and guidance for their implementation in applied settings. In health communication intervention programs, behavioral theories provide a framework for identifying the critical factors underlying the performance (or nonperformance) of specific health-related behaviors. The more one knows about the determinants of a given behavior, the more likely it is that one can develop an effective communication intervention to reinforce or change that behavior.

Perhaps the most critical determinant of whether a person does or does not perform a given behavior is the person's beliefs about performing that behavior. Thus, behavioral theory, when properly applied, allows one to identify the beliefs that should be changed or reinforced to influence a given behavior change in a given population. Changing a person's beliefs can be a precursor to changing a person's behavior. Thus, behavior change can be said to be mediated by belief change. By recognizing that the critical beliefs in one population may be different from those in another population, behavioral theory helps in understanding the importance of diversity in developing effective health communications. However, knowing which beliefs to address does not tell us how to go about designing messages or interventions that can effectively reinforce or change those beliefs. Theories of communication and persuasion guide the selection of communication sources and channels and the preparation of the content of messages. For example, data about women's beliefs regarding the value of mammography are important in creating interventions to enhance mammography use. However, finding out that many women in a given population do not believe that getting a mammogram will lead to early detection of breast cancer does not reveal how to design messages to convince them otherwise, or how to achieve social and environmental changes to influence this belief and therefore influence behavior change. By recognizing that different sources, channels, and message executions may be necessary for different populations, communication theories also point to the importance of considering diversity in developing effective health communication interventions.

We also recognize that communication interventions influence beliefs (and behavior) in different ways. Sometimes people exposed to a message learn the information that it contains, and this knowledge has a "direct" effect on their beliefs. But the context in which one receives the message also may influence how the message is received. For example, if a person is exposed to a message in the company of friends, their reactions to the message may strongly influence whether the person learns or accepts the message content. If one's friends respond to an antismoking or a dental hygiene message with anger or derision, the context may be converted into one of resistance rather than careful processing and possible acceptance of the message content. Theories of media effects provide a framework for understanding how mass communication messages ultimately influence beliefs and behavior.

In this chapter, we first consider behavioral theories and their implementation. We then consider theories of communication and persuasion, and theories of media effects. Rather than summarizing and describing the various theories in each of these areas, our focus is on identifying the critical concepts in these theories and on their theoretical integration. Many good reviews of theories have been conducted (e.g., Glanz, Lewis, and Rimer, 1997), but far fewer attempts have been made to synthesize constructs and achieve integration among behavioral theories or between behavioral and communication theories. Finally, we consider the implications of these theories for developing health messages for diverse audiences. "Good" theories not only recognize the role of diversity, but, when implemented properly, are specific to both the behavior of interest and to the population involved.

FACTORS INFLUENCING BEHAVIORAL PERFORMANCE: KEY CONSTRUCTS FROM BEHAVIORAL THEORIES

This volume shows that health disparities may reflect variations in biological risk factors, differences in access to diagnostic or treatment facilities, or behavioral differences. These latter differences (in health behaviors) are amenable to change via communication interventions. In order to develop health communication messages to eliminate or reduce the behavioral differences, it is essential to understand factors influencing the performance (or nonperformance) of a given health behavior. There are many theories of behavioral prediction, including:

• Theory of Planned Behavior (e.g., Ajzen, 1985, 1991; Ajzen and Madden, 1986);

• Theory of Subjective Culture and Interpersonal Relations (e.g., Triandis, 1972);

• Transtheoretical Model of Behavior Change (Prochaska and DiClemente, 1983, 1986, 1992; Prochaska, DiClemente, and Norcross, 1992; Prochaska et al., 1994);

• Information/Motivation/Behavioral-Skills Model (Fisher and Fisher, 1992);

• Health Belief Model (Becker, 1974, 1988; Rosenstock, 1974; Rosenstock, Strecher, and Becker, 1994);

• Social Cognitive Theory (Bandura, 1977, 1986, 1991, 1994);

• Theory of Reasoned Action (Fishbein and Ajzen, 1975; Ajzen and Fishbein, 1980; Fishbein, Middlestadt, and Hitchcock, 1991).

However, there is a growing academic consensus that only a limited number of variables need to be considered in predicting and understanding any given behavior (see, e.g., Petraitis, Flay, and Miller, 1995; Fishbein, 2000). The variables come primarily from three theories that have been widely used in, and have a major influence on, current behavioral health research: the Health Belief Model, Social Cognitive Theory, and the Theory of Reasoned Action. (See Annex A at the end of this chapter for a brief description of each of these theories.)

One way to predict whether or not a given person will engage in a given health behavior is to ask. People are remarkably accurate predictors of their own behaviors, and appropriate measures of *intention* (one's subjective probability that he or she will or will not engage in a given behavior) consistently have been shown to be the best single predictors of the likelihood that one will (or will not) perform the behavior in question (see, e.g., Sheppard, Hartwick, and Warshaw, 1988; Van den Putte, 1991). However, people do not always act on their intentions. One may intend to perform a given health behavior, but discover that he or she does not have the necessary skills and abilities to carry out the behavior. In addition, one may encounter unanticipated environmental con-

straints (or barriers) that impede or prevent behavioral performance. At the same time, it is important to recognize that environmental (or ecological) factors may also facilitate acting on one's
intentions as well as behavioral performance per se.

Nevertheless, if a person has made a strong commitment (or
formed a strong intention) to perform a given behavior, and if he
or she has the necessary skills and abilities required to perform
that behavior, and if there are no environmental constraints or
barriers to prevent performance of that behavior (i.e., if a context
of opportunity exists for performing the behavior), the probability
is very high that he or she will perform that behavior.

Thus, if one has formed a strong intention (or made a strong
commitment) to perform a given behavior, but is unable to act on
that intention, a communication intervention should be directed at
"skills training," or at removing or helping people to overcome
barriers or environmental constraints. Such interventions often
increase a person's sense of personal agency or self-efficacy, a concept discussed later. On the other hand, if people are not engaging
in a behavior because they have little or no intention to do so, the
intervention should be directed at developing or strengthening intentions. Note that intention is viewed as a continuous, rather
than as a dichotomous, variable. People do not simply "have" or
"not have" an intention to perform a given behavior, but rather,
people have stronger or weaker intentions to perform (or not perform) the health behavior in question. People may tell us that they
"definitely will" versus "probably will" perform a given health
behavior, such as obtaining a mammogram. Similarly, there is a
difference between saying that it is "slightly probable," "quite
probable," or "extremely probable" that one will engage (or not
engage) in some health behavior. Although it could be argued that
many health-related behaviors are performed automatically, without reflection on or awareness of intention, when asked, people
can tell us whether they will or will not perform a given behavior,
and these measures of intention (or self-prediction) are highly related to actual behavioral performance. Thus, from a communica-

tion perspective, it is important to know whether and why people do or do not hold a given intention.

Behavioral change theories suggest that only a limited number of variables directly influence *the strength of* intentions. Some theorists view these determinants of intention as also having a direct influence on behavior—an influence that goes beyond their indirect influence through intention.

Although different theories use different terminology, three major factors appear to influence intention (and thus behavior): (1) one's attitude toward performing the behavior; (2) one's perception of the norms governing performance or nonperformance of the behavior; and (3) one's sense of personal agency or self-efficacy regarding personally performing the behavior.

Attitude

The attitude concept refers to the extent to which one "likes" or "dislikes" a given object, institution, event, or behavior, and is often defined as an overall feeling of favorableness or unfavorableness toward that object, institution, event, or behavior (Eagley and Chaiken, 1993). For the purpose of behavioral prediction, the critical attitude is the attitude toward one's own performance of the behavior in question. The more favorable one is to personally performing a given behavior, the more likely it is that one will intend to perform that behavior. The attitude toward performing a given behavior is assumed to be based on a person's beliefs about performing that behavior (Fishbein and Ajzen, 1975; Ajzen and Fishbein, 1980). The more a person believes that performing a given behavior will lead to positive consequences (e.g., "My performing this behavior will make me feel better"; "will show my partner that I care"; "is the responsible thing to do") and/or prevent negative consequences (e.g., "will protect me from disease Y"; "will reduce the probability of an amputation"), the more favorable the person's attitude is toward performing that behavior. Similarly, the more a person believes that performing the behavior will lead to negative consequences (e.g., "My performing this be-

havior will be painful"; "will be expensive"; "will make my partner angry") or prevent positive consequences (e.g., "will not make
me feel better"; "will not make me healthy"), the more unfavor-
able the attitude. Although many theories do not use the attitude
construct, nearly all agree that intention (or behavior) is a function
of one's beliefs that performing the behavior will lead to various
outcomes and the evaluation of those outcomes. It is assumed that
a person will not form an intention (or perform a behavior) if the
costs of performing that behavior outweigh the benefits. These
underlying beliefs are called "outcome expectancies" or "behavioral beliefs."

Perceived Norms

Perceived norms are the degree to which a person perceives
that a given behavior is viewed as appropriate or inappropriate by
members of the person's social network or society at large. Norms
reflect the amount of social pressure one feels about performing or
not performing a specific behavior. Generally speaking, there are
two types of normative pressure. On one hand, a person may
believe that particular individuals or groups that are important to
the person think that he or she should (or should not) perform the
behavior in question. On the other hand, a person may believe
these important others are, or are not, performing that behavior.
Although it is likely that we have all been told to "do what I say,
not what I do," it is clear that both types of normative pressure
ultimately influence behavior and intention. Although the notion
of normative pressure seeks to capture an overall perception about
what most "important" others are saying or doing concerning the
behavior, this overall judgment must somehow incorporate and
integrate the desires and/or actions of specific others. Indeed, these
underlying normative beliefs (about the expectations or behaviors
of specific others) are assumed to influence (or determine) a
person's overall perception of social pressure.

Personal Agency

Agency is a belief that one has the necessary skills and abilities to perform the behavior in question. Two types of considerations underlie a person's sense of personal agency. First, there is the notion of *self-efficacy,* the belief that one can perform the behavior even under a number of difficult challenges. Second, there are beliefs that performance of the behavior is "up to me" and "under my control." Both self-efficacy and perceived behavioral control are seen as a function of beliefs concerning specific barriers or impediments to behavioral performance.

Influence of Attitudes, Norms, and Personal Agency on Behavior

Although there seems to be general agreement among behavioral theorists that attitudes (or the outcome expectancies underlying attitude), perceived norms, and personal agency are critical to understanding why people do or do not engage in any given behavior, there is considerably less agreement concerning the ways in which these variables influence behavior. Some theorists view these variables as having only an indirect influence on behavior or behavior change through their influence on intentions, while others would argue that their influence is direct. This is particularly true with respect to personal agency, and considerable evidence shows that personal agency (or self-efficacy) directly influences the likelihood that one will or will not perform a given health behavior (for a comprehensive review, see Bandura, 2001). For example, the stronger one's feeling of self-efficacy, the greater the probability that one will persist in attempts to perform a behavior, even after an initial failure (Bandura, 1997a).

Another disagreement among theoreticians concerns the role of social norms. Some theorists argue that perceived normative pressure directly influences intentions (and/or behavior) (e.g., Ajzen and Fishbein, 1980); others argue that normative pressure influences intentions (and/or behavior) only indirectly, by influencing outcome expectancies (Bandura, 1997). For example, from this perspective, knowledge that another person "X" thinks one should not perform a given behavior will only influence performance of that behavior if this normative belief leads to an outcome expectancy, such as "My performing this behavior will make person X angry."

Despite these differences, and regardless of the exact theoretical model one adopts, communication interventions to change health behavior should increase skills, remove or help individuals overcome environmental constraints, or change intention (by changing attitudes, norms, or a sense of personal agency; i.e., by changing the factors that directly or indirectly influence intention and behavior). The relative importance of these variables as determinants of behavior and behavior change will vary as a function of both the health behavior and the population being considered. Thus, a given health-protective behavior may not be performed because of a lack of skills, while another health-protective behavior may not be performed because people have no intention to do so. Similarly, the same behavior may not be performed in one population because of environmental constraints, while the failure of behavioral performance may be because of a lack of skills or abilities in another population.

The relative importance of attitudes, norms, and personal agency as determinants of intention (and behavior) also varies from behavior to behavior and from population to population. For example, intentions to perform one behavior (or the actual performance of that behavior) may be primarily under attitudinal control, while the intention to perform another behavior may be largely under normative control or be primarily influenced by beliefs about personal agency. Similarly, members of one population may intend to not perform a given behavior because they have negative attitudes toward performing that behavior, while members of another population may have decided not to perform the behavior because their important others think they should not perform the behavior or because they do not believe they have the necessary skills and abilities required to perform that behavior (i.e., they do not have a sense of personal agency or self-efficacy with respect to performing that behavior).

One immediate implication is that health communication interventions should be directed at changing those variables that are important determinants of health behavior change in the population being considered. Communication interventions that address an "unimportant" variable are unlikely to be successful. Thus, prior to developing a communication intervention, it is important to determine whether people have or have not formed an appropriate intention, and, if not, to determine whether that intention is influenced primarily by attitudes, norms, and/or issues of personal agency.

Once the critical determinants of a specific behavior change in a particular population have been identified, one should be able to develop health communication interventions to change those determinants. Ultimately, this process involves changing a person's underlying beliefs about the consequences of performing the health behavior, about the expectations or behaviors of others, or about one's ability to perform the behavior under a variety of challenging circumstances. For example, in order to change an attitude, it is often necessary to change outcome expectancies, that is, beliefs that performing the behavior will lead to certain positively or negatively valued outcomes. Clearly, the more that one believes that performing the behavior in question will lead to "good" outcomes and prevent "bad" outcomes, the more favorable the person's attitude will be toward performing that behavior. Similarly, the more one believes that specific relevant others think he or she should perform the behavior and the more one believes these others are performing the behaviors themselves, the more one will experience social pressure to perform the behavior change. Finally, the more one believes he or she can perform the health behavior, even when specific impediments are present, the stronger that person's sense of self-efficacy or personal agency will be.

The substantive uniqueness of each behavior comes into play at this level of underlying beliefs. For example, the barriers to obtaining a mammogram and/or the outcomes (or consequences) of getting a mammogram may be very different from those associated with taking a PSA test (a blood test for detecting prostate cancer), or getting genetic screening. These specific health beliefs must be addressed in a communication intervention if one wishes to change intentions and behavior. Although an investigator or a practitioner can sit in his or her office and develop measures of attitudes, perceived norms, and self-efficacy, he or she cannot know what a given population (or a given person) believes about performing a given behavior without interacting with that population. Thus, one must go to members of a target population to identify salient outcome, normative, and efficacy beliefs; one must understand the health behavior change from the population's perspective. Although behavioral theory suggests that a common set of variables is relevant to all populations, it recognizes that the relative importance and substantive meaning of these variables depends on the specific population being considered. By appropriately implementing a theory, one can identify the behavioral, normative, and/or efficacy beliefs that discriminate between people, in any given population, who do and do not perform a specific behavior. Theories of communication and behavior change inherently recognize the role and importance of diversity. Program planners should act on this knowledge.

The above discussion focuses attention on a limited set of variables that have consistently been found to be among the strongest predictors of any given behavior (see, e.g., Petraitis, Flay, and Miller, 1995). Although focusing on behavior-specific variables may provide the best prediction of any given behavior, this approach does little to explain the genesis of the beliefs that underlie attitudes, norms, and self-efficacy. Clearly, the beliefs that one holds concerning his or her performance of a given behavior are likely to be influenced by a large number of other variables. For example, one's life experience will influence what one believes about performing a given behavior, and thus one often finds relations among demographic variables such as gender, ethnicity, age, education, socioeconomic status, and behavioral performance. Similarly, women who perceive they are at high risk for, and/or are afraid that they may have, breast cancer, may have beliefs about "My getting a mammogram" that are very different from women who do not believe they are at risk. Thus, factors that may influence one's beliefs include perceived risk; moods and emotions as well as personality, culture, knowledge, and attitudes toward objects or institutions; and stigma. In addition, ecological and social factors such as availability of health services, types of interpersonal networks, and media exposure and/or exposure to various interventions may all serve to shape and influence one's behavioral, normative, and efficacy beliefs.

Although these are all important variables, and although they may help us to understand why people hold a given belief, they are perhaps best seen as "distal" variables that exert their influence over specific behaviors by affecting the more "proximal" determinants of those behaviors. However, there is no necessary relationship between any of these variables and behavior-specific beliefs. That is, these distal variables may or may not affect people's underlying behavioral, normative, or control beliefs about a given behavior. For example, rich and poor, old and young, those who do or do not perceive they are at risk for a given illness, those who do or do not have knowledge of a disease and how it is transmitted, and those who do or do not feel stigmatized may have different behavioral, normative, and control beliefs with respect to one behavior, but may have similar beliefs with respect to another.

When one or more of these distal variables leads to different beliefs, it is possible that the variable also will be related to behavior change. However, even though a given distal variable may influence outcome expectancies, that variable may still be unrelated to behavior if attitudinal considerations are not important determinants of that behavior change. Thus, rather than focusing on distal variables, to be most effective, health communication interventions should focus on the behavioral, normative, or control beliefs that underlie attitudes, perceived norms, and/or a person's sense of personal agency.

For example, let us assume that a behavioral analysis indicated that whether or not one intended to (or actually did) get a flu vaccination is determined primarily by the outcome expectancy (or behavioral belief) that "My getting a flu shot will protect me from getting the flu." Assume that those who intended to get (or who actually got) a flu vaccination believed that getting the flu shot would protect them from the flu, while those who did not intend to get (or who did not get) the vaccination believed that "My getting a flu shot will *not* protect me from getting the flu." If this scenario were the case, an appropriate communication to increase the likelihood that people will intend to and will actually get a flu vaccination would be one that tried to change this latter belief. The more we understand about why some people do or do not hold this belief, the more likely we are to be able to develop an effective communication intervention to change that belief.

However, there are many reasons why people may believe a flu vaccination will *not* protect them from getting the flu. Some may believe that they are not "at risk" for getting the flu, and, thus, they may not believe that "Getting a flu shot will protect me from getting the flu." Others may believe that "Whether I get the flu or not is God's will" and, therefore, they too might believe that getting a flu vaccination will not protect them. Still others may believe "There are too many different types of flu viruses out there and a vaccination can't protect me from all of them" and thus, they also might not believe that "My getting a flu shot will protect me from getting the flu." Although this type of information may be useful when one is dealing with a person via interpersonal communication, it is only helpful for developing health communication messages under certain circumstances.

More specifically, if within a given population a distal variable is consistently related to the "target belief," and if it is possible to affect that distal variable through a communication intervention, then it may be reasonable to focus communication messages on that variable. For example, if the distal variable is "perceived risk" and if perceived risk is significantly related to the target belief (e.g., to the belief that "My getting a flu shot will protect me from getting the flu"), then a communication intervention directed at increasing one's perception of personal risk may be appropriate.

However, one must ask whether one should try to increase perceived risk, or if one should use the information that perceived risk is related to the target belief to develop a message directed at changing the target belief per se. From a behavior theory perspective, if the distal variable cannot be shown to be causally related to the target belief, this latter strategy is more likely to increase the likelihood that members of the target audience will intend to get (and actually will get) a flu vaccination.

Even when a distal variable is not amenable to change through communication, it may provide important insights for designing health communication interventions. For example, we might find that women are more likely to believe that "Getting a flu shot will protect me from getting the flu" than are men, or that those with a college degree are more likely to hold this belief than are those with less education. Data such as these should influence the development of communication interventions under the following circumstances:

1. If the distal variable defines population segments that hold different beliefs, or that show different association of beliefs to intentions or behaviors, communication interventions may need to address different beliefs for different population segments. For example, if men and women hold different beliefs about the expected outcomes of "dieting," the communication messages directed to each group should be correspondingly different.

2. If the distal variable defines population segments that are likely to be differentially exposed to a communication, different approaches may be necessary to reach different population segments. For example, assume that older and younger people differ on the target belief. Given that older and younger people use different media, a communication intervention should use different channels to reach these two population segments.

Figure 2-1 summarizes the preceding discussion. Intentions, skills and abilities, environmental constraints, and personal agency (or self-efficacy) are viewed as the immediate determinants of be-

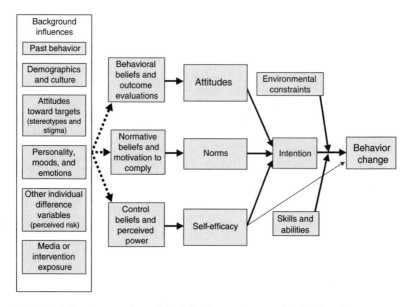

FIGURE 2-1   A general model of the determinants of behavior change.

havior, while attitudes, norms, and self-efficacy are viewed as the primary determinants of intention. These three determinants of intention are themselves determined by underlying behavioral, normative, and efficacy beliefs. Finally, Figure 2-1 shows that there are a large number of distal variables that may influence these underlying beliefs. Not all behavioral change theorists would agree with this general diagram. Some would delete certain variables; some scholars would treat what we called distal variables as more proximal determinants of intention (and/or behavior); others might rearrange the causal ordering of the variables. For ease of presentation, Figure 2-1 does not include feedback loops. Behavioral performance may lead to changes in a person's behavioral, normative, or control beliefs, and these changes may, in turn, lead to changes in attitudes, perceived norms, or self-efficacy. We suggest that the variables connected by solid lines in Figure 2-1 are critical to an understanding of health behavior change and must be considered in developing health communication interventions. The distal variables also may be important, but these variables have, at best, an indirect influence on behavior change, depending on whether they do or do not influence underlying beliefs. Figure 2-1 implies that changing health behavior ultimately will depend on changing behavioral, normative, or efficacy beliefs.

APPLYING BEHAVIOR CHANGE THEORY

The first step in applying any behavioral prediction or behavioral change model is to identify the specific behavior of interest. This task is not as straightforward as it seems. First, it is important to distinguish among behaviors, behavioral categories, and goals. The most effective health communication interventions are directed at changing specific behaviors (e.g., walking for 20 minutes three times a week) rather than behavioral categories (e.g., exercise) or goals (e.g., lose weight) (see, e.g., Fishbein, 1995, 2000).

The definition of a behavior involves several elements: the action (getting/using/buying/doing), the target (a mammogram/a condom), and the context (at the women's clinic/for vaginal sex with spouse). A change in any one of the elements changes the behavior under consideration. For example, getting a mammogram is a different behavior than getting a PSA test (a change in target). Similarly, getting a mammogram at a women's clinic is different from getting a mammogram at a university hospital (a change in context). Moreover, it is also important to include an additional element—time. This element is particularly important when one is developing a communication or other type of intervention. For example, getting a mammogram in the next 3 months or always using a condom are different behaviors than getting a mammogram in the next 2 weeks or occasionally using a condom. Clearly, a change in any one element in the behavioral definition usually will lead to very different beliefs about the consequences of performing that behavior, about the expectations and behaviors of relevant others, and about the barriers that may impede behavioral performance.

The selection of a target behavior depends on many factors. First and foremost, sound epidemiological evidence should link that behavior to a given health outcome. Second, the recommended behavior must be feasible; that is, it must be one that members of the target population can perform. For example, trying to get members of a given population to eat fruits and vegetables that are not available or are too expensive for most members of the population would be inappropriate. Thus, it is necessary to work with members of the target population to identify the behavior change that one wishes to influence. These considerations are addressed more fully in Chapter 3, which discusses mass media campaigns.

The second step in applying a behavior change theory is to identify the specific population. For any given behavior change, both the relative importance of attitudes, norms, and self-efficacy as determinants of intention (and/or behavior change) and the substantive content of the behavioral, normative, and control beliefs underlying these determinants may vary as a function of the population under consideration. Thus, it is imperative to define the population (or populations) to be considered. Because the "audience" is one of the critical constructs in theories of communication and behavior change, it will be considered in more detail in this chapter and in Chapter 3.

Once one or more behaviors and target populations have been identified, theory can be used to understand why some members of a target population are performing the behavior change and others are not. That is, by obtaining measures of each of the central variables in Figure 2-1 (i.e., beliefs, attitudes, norms, self-efficacy, intentions, and behavior), one can determine whether a given behavior or behavior change (e.g., getting a colonoscopy) is not being performed because people have not formed intentions to get a colonoscopy or because they are unable to act on their intentions. Similarly, one can determine, for the population under consideration, whether intention is influenced primarily by attitudes, norms, or self-efficacy. Finally, one can identify the specific beliefs (whether behavioral, normative, or control) that discriminate between those who do or do not (intend to) perform the behavior. It is important to recognize that behavioral theory focuses on the behavior of interest, and thus its primary focus is on beliefs about the performance of the behavior.

These discriminating beliefs need to be addressed in theory-based communication interventions. As discussed previously, although the ultimate goal of health communication should be to reinforce or change a given health behavior, communication creates, changes, or reinforces specific beliefs. When the beliefs are selected appropriately, these changes should, in turn, influence attitudes, perceived norms, or self-efficacy—the proximal determinants of one's intentions to engage in (and often their actual performance of) that behavior change.

Identification of these beliefs requires understanding the behavior from the perspective of the population in question. Proper implementation of communication and behavior change theory requires that one goes to a sample of that population to identify the outcomes, referents, and barriers that are relevant for that population (see Middlestadt et al., 1996). Survey data can identify those beliefs that discriminate between those who do or do not (intend to) perform the behavior change in question (see, e.g., Hornik and Woolf, 1999). Once one has identified a set of "discriminating" beliefs, theories of communication and behavior change become important to develop messages and other interventions.

THEORIES OF COMMUNICATION AND BEHAVIOR CHANGE: KEY CONSTRUCTS

Because of our central concern about health communication for diverse audiences, the remainder of this chapter focuses primarily on factors that should be considered in order to develop effective communication campaigns and other interventions. Although messages and campaigns comprise only one type of behavior change intervention, most of these factors are also relevant for the development of other types of interventions. Theories of communication, directly or indirectly, address the question of "*Who* says *what* to *whom, through what channel, with what effect*?" This single framework, suggested by Harold Lasswell in 1939, often has been criticized because it has been interpreted as focusing all attention on the efforts of the communicator. In recognition of this concern, *effects* in the current view of much communication theory also are defined by how audiences process the messages. It is important to consider how prior beliefs and social and institutional affiliations affect how people make sense of, and respond to, messages. Thus, in attempting to develop effective health communication interventions, one must consider the *communicator*, the *audience*, the *message*, and the *medium*.

The Audience

To effectively implement behavioral theory and to develop effective health communication interventions, a precise description of the intended audience is needed first. The *intended audience* is the segment of the population whose behavior a health communication intervention attempts to change.

Communication campaigns select and define their intended audiences in very different ways. Some campaigns divide the prospective audience into segments according to characteristics of social diversity such as age, income, gender, or education. Even a single segment characterized by one demographic variable may comprise multiple diverse audiences. For example, the intended audience for a mammography campaign for older women will include women varying in ethnicity, income, education, age, family history, sexual orientation, and beliefs.

Information about intended audiences can be obtained through existing national or local survey data or by conducting formative research. These procedures involve data collection on an audience's sociodemographic characteristics (e.g., age, education, gender, employment, ethnicity, marital status, sexual orientation), behavioral predictors or antecedents (e.g., audience beliefs, values, skills, attitudes), and current behaviors.

For example, a nutrition campaign intended for Hispanics and non-Hispanic whites from the Southwestern United States may choose to further segment by age, but select the age groupings differently for the two ethnic groups, based on differences in lifestyle factors. Young, single whites not living with their parents may be a separate segment requiring specific health communication messages, while young Hispanics, who are more likely to live with their parents, may receive a nutrition message that is similar to the one developed for their parents. In this case, it may be more useful to segment based on variables such as living conditions, social values, or language in the development of a culturally specific campaign.

Campaigns may have single or multiple intended audiences; campaign planners should first know as much as possible about the audience in order to develop appropriate and effective campaign goals and strategies. This need is amplified when the intended audience represents diverse population segments with which the campaign implementers are initially unfamiliar. For a more complete discussion of segmentation, see Chapter 3. Once an audience segment(s) is identified, the campaign intervention is designed and altered to communicate effectively with the target segment and change their health behavior.

The Message

A message is a specific statement of limited scope that usually contains only one main idea and relates to the *communication objectives* specified by a given health communication intervention (Ferguson, 1999). Ideally, message content is developed based on carefully planned communication strategies, which are derived from a knowledge of behavior change and communication theories as well as data collected through formative audience research (Weinreich, 1999). Although messages may be designed for different purposes (e.g., to increase awareness or knowledge, to increase self-efficacy, or to change attitudes and perceived norms), we will focus on communication messages designed to change health behavior. As indicated earlier, the most effective messages are those designed to change one or more well-defined behaviors.

Health campaigns are refined for diverse audiences by adapting behavior change goals so that they are relevant, appropriate, and appealing to the audience being addressed. Health campaigns must specify, as precisely as possible, the health behavior change that is desired from a specific audience when its members are exposed to the messages. The action behaviors promoted by the message should be within a range of what realistically can be accomplished by the target audience (Weinreich, 1999). This strategy may involve promoting adoption of a new health-enhancing behavior or the cessation of a risk behavior. The desired action ideally is determined from a thorough analysis of the audience's current behavior. Appropriate implementation of behavioral theories then can serve to identify factors that can influence the desired behavior change in relation to the current behavior.

As already indicated, proper use of theory should help one to identify whether a given health behavior change is determined primarily by attitudinal, normative, and/or efficacy considerations, and should lead to the identification of a number of behavioral, normative, and/or control beliefs that clearly discriminate between members of any given population who do, or do not, engage in the behavior in question (i.e., that are highly correlated with the intention or behavior change). In addition, proper application of theory also should help to identify beliefs that are supportive of the behavior change and that are already held by most members of the population, but that have only moderate correlations with the intention or behavior. Which of these beliefs should a communication intervention address?

Beliefs

Belief Change

Hornik and Woolf (1999) described three factors to consider in identifying beliefs to target (i.e., try to change) in a communication (or other type of intervention). First, in the population under consideration, the belief should be strongly related to the intention or health behavior to be changed. Second, there should be enough people who do not already hold the targeted belief to warrant trying to change it. An example would be the belief that "My smoking is harmful to my health." Because this belief is widely held by smokers as well as nonsmokers, little will be accomplished by trying to change it. Thus one must consider whether a communication intervention designed to change a given belief has the potential of moving enough people to make the intervention worthwhile. Finally, one must consider whether changing the belief is even possible. That is, can one support the targeted belief with a plausible argument based on strong evidence?

Relationship with Intentions and Behaviors

Clearly, with respect to the first criterion, theory-based survey data can identify beliefs that discriminate between intenders and nonintenders or that are highly related to the intention or behavior one wishes to change.

How Many People Already Hold the Targeted Belief?

Even though a belief may be highly related to the intention and behavior one wishes to change, little will be accomplished if most people already strongly hold the belief in question. It is important to recognize, however, that beliefs are not "held" versus "not held," but vary in degree of strength. For example, people may "strongly agree" (think it is "extremely likely") or "agree" (think it is "quite likely") that a given behavior will lead to a given outcome. Clearly, if 80 percent of those who "strongly agree" but only 20 percent of those who "agree" have strong intentions to perform the behavior in question, then strengthening this belief is an appropriate target for an intervention. Thus, it is important to consider "belief strength" and to determine whether strengthening existing beliefs (i.e., moving people from "quite likely" to "extremely likely") could influence their intentions (and behavior). Messages that can move people from "quite" to "extremely" likely can significantly affect the likelihood that these people will form strong intentions to perform the behavior in question.

Can the Belief Be Changed?

In stark contrast to the first two criteria, which are empirically based, the third criterion suggested by Hornik and Woolf (1999) is largely a subjective judgment. Clearly, not all beliefs are equally amenable to change, and relatively little will be accomplished by attacking a belief that is very difficult, if not impossible, to change. For example, if a woman's regular partner tells her that "I hate condoms and will not use them," it is extremely unlikely that one will be able to develop a message that would increase her belief that "My regular partner thinks we should always use condoms for vaginal sex." Similarly, if a man has used a condom and, as a result, strongly believes that "using a condom decreases my sexual sensation," it may not be possible to change this belief with a communication message. Beliefs based on direct experience are more difficult to change than are those based on information provided by others. Similarly, it seems reasonable to assume that people will find it more difficult to accept beliefs that may produce dissonance (i.e., that are inconsistent with their beliefs, attitudes, intentions, and behaviors) than to accept beliefs that are consonant with one or more of these psychosocial variables (Festinger, 1957).

Priming

In addition to changing behavior by changing beliefs, it is also assumed that behavior can be changed by changing the strength of the association between proximal variables. For example, by raising the accessibility or "salience" of certain beliefs, one may strengthen the association between those beliefs and attitudes, perceived norms, or personal agency. Similarly, by increasing the salience or accessibility of attitudes, norms, or self-efficacy, one may strengthen the association between these variables and intentions (or behavior). When such increases in the association between variables occur, it is often referred to as "priming." Thus, rather than focusing exclusively on beliefs that clearly discriminate between intenders and nonintenders (or actors and nonactors), it often may be useful to identify beliefs that support a given behavior, that are held (at least to some extent) by most of the population, and that have only a low or moderate relationship to the intention or behavior in question. Targeting these beliefs could strengthen their association with attitudes, perceived norms, or self-efficacy. It is important to recognize that priming (i.e., the strengthening of the association between two variables) may also involve some belief change, although not necessarily a change in mean belief strength. That is, the size of a correlation is a function of the covariance between two variables, as well as the total variance of each of the two variables, and changes in variance are due to changes in belief.

Message Content and Delivery

Although appropriate application of a theory of behavioral prediction can identify the critical determinants of a given intention (or behavior) as well as the critical beliefs underlying these determinants, the theory does not tell one how to best change these beliefs or whether these beliefs are amenable to change. Consistent with this view, Hornik and Woolf (1999) distinguished between message strategy and the message per se. According to these authors, message strategy is "the essential belief(s) that a message will be designed to impart," while the message per se is "the product of a creative process that will turn the strategy into a specific realization."

Although there are no empirically supported theories to guide the convergence of a given strategy into a specific realization, communication research identified a number of message factors that can influence the likelihood that a given message will be accepted. For example, two-sided messages (i.e., those that recognize and refute counterarguments) are usually more effective than one-sided messages (Hovland, Janis, and Kelley, 1953; Hovland, Lumsdaine, and Sheffield, 1949; Allen, 1998), and messages that explicitly state a conclusion are often more effective than those that leave the conclusion implicit (McGuire, 1969; Cruz, 1998). By contrast, there is considerably less agreement concerning the role of fear or humor in developing effective messages (Mongeau, 1998). For example, considerable debate continues about the use and misuse of fear appeals (or threat), with some scholars and health professionals regarding "fear" as a central factor in motivating behavioral change (Rogers, 1983; Leventhal, Singer, and Jones, 1965; Leventhal, 1970),[1] and others viewing it as a source of defensiveness and resistance to change (Janis, 1967; Rippletoe and Rogers, 1987).

Messages should be appropriate for, and relevant to, the population being considered. Very different messages will be needed if, for example, one is trying to increase the condom use of a person who says "I hate condoms and I'm never going to use them" or "I've thought about using condoms, but I don't know how to introduce their use to my partner." This simple illustration has two important implications. First, it suggests that behavior is not an "all or none" event, but that people may go through a number of steps or stages in adopting a behavior. One attempt to formalize this process has been proposed by Prochaska and associates (Prochaska, DiClemente, and Norcross, 1992). They proposed a stages of change or transtheoretical model that suggests that people move through the following stages:

1. Precontemplation, where the individual has no intention to perform the health behavior change and may not have even considered it.

---

[1]Annex B provides a description of self-regulation models in which fear is considered as a central factor.

2. Contemplation, where the individual has formed an intention to perform the new behavior sometime in the future, but has not yet done so.

3. Preparation, where the individual has a positive intention and makes some initial or occasional attempts to perform the behavior change.

4. Action, where the behavior is being performed consistently.

5. Maintenance, where the individual persists in performing the behavior change consistently for a long enough time period (usually defined as 6 months) that it becomes a regular part of one's routine and where the probability of relapse is greatly reduced.

Stage models do not assume that the process of change is necessarily linear. That is, people may skip certain stages and/or go back to previous stages. For example, if in the preparation stage the individual is negatively reinforced for trying to perform the behavior change, the individual may go back to either the contemplation or precontemplation stage. Similarly, circumstances or events may lead to a "relapse," sending those in the action or maintenance stage back to the preparation or contemplation stage. Perhaps the most important feature of stage-related models is that they suggest that attempts to evaluate the effectiveness of health communication interventions by looking solely at whether or not the target audience is consistently performing the recommended behavior change may be missing important campaign effects. For example, a campaign that moves people from precontemplation to contemplation may be an important first step in a behavior change process, especially for complex behaviors that are difficult to adopt.

A second implication of stage-based models is that a message that may be effective in moving people from preparation to action, for example, may be completely ineffective in moving people from the precontemplation to the contemplation stage. Communication interventions that may help people act on their intentions may have little or no effect on those individuals who have yet to form strong intentions. Thus, it becomes important to design messages that take into account what stage people are in during the process of change. Very different communication interventions are required for audiences that have formed an intention to engage in some recommended behavior change, compared with interventions for audiences that have not formed an intention. (Chapter 6 discusses how new communication technologies may facilitate this process.)

Finally, it is important to recognize that message production values (e.g., black and white printing versus color printing; multiple versus few scene changes; hard rock versus rap music) also can influence the likelihood that people will accept a given health behavior change. For example, Palmgreen and associates (Palmgreen et al., 1991; Stephenson, 1999) showed that changes in these types of production values substantially affect the extent to which "high-sensation seekers" attend to, and learn the contents of, a given drug abuse prevention message. Thus, many of the variables that are viewed as "external" to theories of behavior change (e.g., personality, demographics, and culture) may directly influence the likelihood that a given message will lead to health behavior change. However, other important variables also may influence the outcome of behavior change.

The Communicator or Source

The source of health communication messages may be someone whom the intended audience relates to or knows, someone who represents the target audience, someone who is a recognizable celebrity or public figure, someone whom the intended audience regards as an influential role model, or someone who is friendly and anonymous, such as a fictional/animated character (Weinreich, 1999).

The source that delivers health communication campaign messages can have an important impact on whether messages are perceived as meaningful, credible, and/or relevant to target audiences. The selection of a source may be particularly important for health communication messages to diverse populations. Different populations will relate to, and be more or less influenced by, different messengers. The appropriate messenger may vary with the health issue of focus, the characteristics of the intended audience, and the purpose and style of the message. Furthermore, different subgroups within an audience may find different types of information supportive of the desired action. For example, scientific findings from an expert source may be the most important and credible basis for health behavior change for one audience segment, while information about social norms from a peer may be most important to another audience segment.

In the selection of appropriate, effective sources of communication messages, it is important to understand various characteristics of the intended audience, such as: Who influences the relevant behaviors of the target audience? Who are the most important role models? Who does the audience trust for credible information? What kind of person does the audience turn to for information related to the health topic at hand (i.e., authority figures, health professionals, peers, parents, celebrity role models) (Weinreich, 1999)? This information can be obtained through formative research. The most influential sources of communication may vary with the specific health behavior change and with the characteristics of the intended audience; formative research is necessary to identify the most relevant, appropriate sources of social influence for specific groups.

For example, formative research revealed that health providers are commonly identified as an important source of health communication messages relevant to health behavior change (Snell and Buck, 1996; Rimer, 1994). Promotion of health behaviors that are largely mediated by social influences and norms may be communicated more effectively through peer groups or by family or community members, celebrity role models, or religious leaders (Cruz and Mickalide, 2000; National Safe Kids Campaign, 2000). Messages that attempt to achieve health behavior change in environmental issues or politically mediated public health problems, such as traffic safety or the sale of alcohol and cigarettes to minors, may

be communicated most effectively by authority figures or representatives of law enforcement agencies.

Generally speaking, the most effective communication sources
are those that are viewed as trustworthy and as having expertise in
the relevant behavioral domain (Eagley and Chaiken, 1993). In
some cases, however, the similarity of the source with the audience
is critical. For example, Bandura (1997) identified four sources
for the development of self-efficacy beliefs: enactive mastery experiences, vicarious learning, persuasion, and one's own physiological and affective states. Particularly in the case of vicarious learning
(i.e., learning through seeing others perform or attempt to perform
the behavior in question), the selection of the other (or "model") is
critical. The more one can "identify" with the model (i.e., see the
model as similar to one's self), the more one is likely to view the
model's attainments as diagnostic of one's own capabilities.

Although a complete discussion of vicarious learning and modeling is beyond the scope of this chapter, our previous discussion
shows that, in order to maximize the potential impact of a given
message, the selection of a communication source is a complex
process involving knowledge of the audience and of the health behavior change message. However, the influence of a source depends, in part, on the nature of the message per se. The "stronger"
the message, the less important the source. Credible sources can
increase the likelihood that a "weak" message will be accepted,
but the credibility of the source has relatively little influence on the
likelihood that an audience will accept a "strong" message
(McCroskey, 1970).

The Channel of Communication

The wide range of channels through which health communication messages are disseminated includes the mass media (television, radio, magazines, newspapers, and advertising); outdoor
advertising; brochures, posters, and newsletters; comic books and
fotonovellas; direct mail; interpersonal communications (such as
in-person and telephone counseling); music and other videos;

songs; dramatic presentations; community events; point-of-purchase materials; and the Internet (Weinreich, 1999). Different age, gender, ethnic, and socioeconomic categories tend to favor different media, so it is prudent when targeting by these individual characteristics to investigate which media are best for each group. For example, a health communication campaign may use billboards and store displays to reach lower-income, inner-city dwellers, and newspapers to reach suburban households. Efforts to reach gay, lesbian, and bisexual populations often supplement mainstream media with specialized publications geared toward these groups, such as gay newspapers.

Generally speaking, in considering choice of channels, three questions should be addressed: (1) What messages can be sent through a particular channel? (2) How is each channel perceived by the audience? (3) When multiple channels are present, how do they interact in their effects?

What messages can be sent through a particular channel? The answer can be divided into two parts: First, the choice of a channel may impose limitations on what message content can be communicated. Radio provides no visuals, but may encourage the imagination; television provides information through sight and sound dynamically, but can only simulate interaction; online media provide opportunities for structured interaction, but may not be able to control individual paths of such interaction; outreach workers may be able to respond to the concerns and questions raised by individuals, but the health messages they transmit may lack consistency or fidelity. The effects of modes (e.g., visual and audio) incorporated in a channel, the effects of static versus continuing motion, and the effects of lesser and greater opportunities for interaction with audience individuals are all important exemplars.

The choice of channel may affect the fidelity of a health communication. For example, health communication that depends on interpersonal networks or on the voluntary involvement of institutions may provide less control over the exact content of a health message. A campaign may target the audience of a daytime talk show program for a message about domestic violence, but the nature of the talk show, which may be sympathetic to the message but whose primary purpose is attracting audiences, will affect the final shape of the message. A health communication campaign that depends on "free" exposure is forced to use channels over which it has less control.

How is each channel perceived by the audience? A continuing issue in the literature compares mass media versus interpersonal channels with regard to their role at various stages in the diffusion of a new idea (Rogers, 1995). People often rely more heavily on mass media channels when they are first learning about an idea, but use interpersonal channels as they move toward making a decision (Rogers, 1995). Depending on the nature of the health behavior change and its context, either mass media or interpersonal communication channels can play an important role at either stage (Chaffee, 1982; Hornik, 1989; Schooler et al., 1998; Hornik, 1997). Audience individuals may not view messages from various channels as equally credible. Some communication channels and sources may be perceived by certain individuals as credible when they address health behavior change, while other channels (such as salespeople or Web sites on the Internet) may engender skepticism. These perceptions of communication channels may vary at different stages in the diffusion process.

When multiple channels are present, how do they interact in their effects? There are three possibilities. Channels may be additive—an exposure achieved through one channel is the same as exposure through any other channel. Alternatively, channels may positively interact or reinforce one another, such that the effects of exposure through any one channel increase when other channels are present. For example, the effect of an antismoking television message may be greater when a complementary school-based antismoking program reaches some audience individuals. Finally, channels may interact negatively, if additional exposures through one channel add nothing to the already available message exposures provided by another channel. Here, channels may substitute for one another. In addition, messages coming from different channels (and sources) may also be in conflict. For example, messages about antismoking conveyed by a school-based intervention may disagree with tobacco company advertising.

Media Effects

Assuming that behavior change theory was used to identify the critical beliefs to target in a given population, to develop an appropriate message, and to select an appropriate source and channel, two additional questions must be addressed. First is the question of audience exposure. Will enough members of the target audience be exposed to the message, either directly or indirectly? Second, given sufficient exposure, how does the message influence beliefs (and behavior change)?

No matter how well designed a health communication message may be, it is unlikely to produce belief (or behavior) change if people are not exposed to the message. Considerations of exposure address two complementary issues: (1) What influences the likelihood that a person will be exposed to a given message? (2) How do effects vary with the degree of exposure achieved?

People cannot be exposed to a message if that message is not made available to them; perhaps the primary factor influencing whether or not a message will be available is funding. Money can buy media time and space, and unfortunately for the great majority of health communication intervention messages, little money is often available for purchasing media time/space or for paying outreach agents. Thus, the practical question for most health communication interventions is what gets a message free distribution. Free distribution may involve time or space in the mass media, whether in the form of public service announcements, health messages embedded in entertainment programs, or coverage of a health topic on news programs, in newspapers or magazines, or on talk shows. Free distribution outside the mass media may involve adoption of a message by community institutions. For example, youth organizations may offer to distribute antidrug messages to their members, or schools may add antidrug components to their after-school sports programs. Some messages are distributed through social networks, generating "buzz," while other messages do not attract such social multiplication. Whether or not an individual is exposed to a message is influenced by message content, formal features of the message, or the context in which the messages are embedded.

How many exposures to a message, and what density of exposures in a given period of time, are needed before health behavior change occurs? How many exposures are needed before there are decreasing returns, such that additional exposure has little effect, or even a rejection of the message? The relationship between exposure and a given outcome effect (e.g., a change in belief) is determined by many factors, including: (1) the way humans attend to, and process, information (Zajonc, 1998; Petty and Cacioppo, 1979a; Peachmann and Stewart, 1990); (2) other characteristics of target audiences; (3) the complexities of the health problem addressed; (4) the presence of competing messages; and (5) the intrinsic character of the health message.

Repeated exposure by an individual provides more opportunities for learning the health message: Ten exposures to a message that marijuana initiation will damage parent-child relations may produce more awareness and more belief change than five exposures. Repeated exposure to a given message also may have an agenda-setting or priming effect (Dearing and Rogers, 1994; Cappella et al., 2001). Youth may already know that parents would be upset if they initiated marijuana use, but they may consider it more closely in deciding whether or not to initiate use after exposure to repeated messages on this topic. Repetition carries with it a message that the issue is important for consideration in making a decision about drug use.

Repeated exposure, particularly when a message is carried by a variety of communication channels, may carry an implicit message about what is socially expected. Repeated messages about marijuana use may address specific beliefs about the consequences of use, but they will also carry a message about the nature of societal norms for the health behavior change. Repetition through diverse channels may convey the meta-message that society cares about this health issue. Similarly, repeated exposure to a message in multiple channels may increase the probability of interpersonal discussion of the message, further multiplying exposure and diffusion of a communication message. Finally, repeated message exposure carries with it an implicit legitimization of the subject of the health message. It also may increase the likelihood of policy attention to the problem. Issues given high exposure often interest politicians.

The previous discussion sets the stage for considering media effects. It is often assumed that a portion of the target audience will be exposed to a given message, and that a portion of those exposed to the message will learn its contents and change their health behavior. For example, consider again adolescent initiation of marijuana use. A health communication message might focus on the belief that beginning marijuana use will damage relationships with parents. We might hypothesize that youth watching the marijuana use ad immediately form (or strengthen) their belief, and as a result of this belief change, some youth may reduce their intention to use or their actual use of marijuana. Communication also can affect one's beliefs (and behaviors) in other ways. For example, rather than having an immediate direct effect on beliefs, there may be a time lag between exposure to the message and belief (and/or behavior) change. In addition, rather than being directly exposed to a message, one may be indirectly exposed to the contents of the message through interpersonal interaction. Equally important, messages directed toward a specific belief or behavior may generalize to other beliefs or health behavior changes.

Five different paths through which a health communication message may have an effect on target beliefs (and behaviors) are: (1) immediate learning, (2) delayed learning, (3) generalized learning, (4) social diffusion, and (5) institutional diffusion.

1. *Immediate learning.* People can learn directly from health communication messages that enable them to make different decisions. For example, youth learn that trying marijuana has negative

consequences, so they form more negative attitudes and intentions and therefore are less likely to try marijuana. This new knowledge is assumed to have immediate consequences on their beliefs and behaviors. In this way, young people may learn about the negative and positive consequences of using a particular drug, about social expectations regarding drug use, and about skills and self-efficacy in avoiding drug use.

2. *Delayed learning.* Even though a communication message is conveyed today, its impact may not be appreciated until some time in the near future. For example, antidrug messages for 12- and 13-year-old youth (who rarely use marijuana) might be expected to influence future behavior only when opportunities to engage in drug use occur.

3. *Generalized learning.* Communication interventions provide direct exposure to specific messages, but people may be persuaded about related concepts as well. Thus, an anticocaine campaign might produce messages saying that cocaine has a particular negative consequence and that medical authorities are opposed to cocaine use. People exposed to these messages may generalize these cognitions to a broad negative view of other types of drug use. Thus, although the message focused on cocaine use, beliefs about marijuana use also change. This generalized learning means that exposure effects are not message specific and will not necessarily operate through an intervening path of acceptance of the specific consequences emphasized.

4. *Social diffusion.* Messages can stimulate discussion among peers and between youth and their parents, and these discussions can affect what people believe. Such discussions may provide new information about consequences or social expectations as well as new skills or increased self-efficacy. Discussions may link individuals who have been exposed to the communication message with those who have not. Thus, the effects of a health communication intervention would not be limited only to those individuals who have been directly exposed to the health communication messages. If the messages are about drugs, discussions may produce or reinforce antidrug ideas, or they may produce prodrug ideas.

5. *Institutional diffusion.* The presence of advertisements (or other intervention messages) can produce a broad response among public institutions (such as school boards, state legislatures, and the media). In turn, these institutions may initiate health policies or programs that affect cognitions and social expectations of the targeted audience. Thus, an antidrug communication intervention may stimulate concern among school board members about drug use and lead them to allocate more school time to drug education. Religious, athletic, and other private youth organizations may increase their antidrug activities. News organizations may cover drug issues more actively, and the nature of their messages may change. Movies, music, or entertainment television may change their level of attention to, and the content of, drug-related messages. Like the social diffusion route, institutional diffusion does not require an individual-level association between message exposure and beliefs or behavior change. This path of influence can be seen at the level of community analysis. Also, institutional diffusion can be a slow process, and there might be a relatively long lag between exposure to aspects of the communication intervention and institutional response and an even longer lag until the effects on audience beliefs or behavior become apparent.

Each of the five models of communication effects described represents a complementary process through which a health communication intervention might influence underlying beliefs and behavior. Any one of these models may describe the actual path of effect, or all of them may describe paths of effect that occurred. One important implication of these models is that they suggest that very different strategies may be necessary for evaluating the effectiveness of a given health communication intervention. Models of immediate, delayed, or generalized learning suggest that evaluating message (or campaign) effectiveness by comparing individuals who have or have not been exposed is appropriate. These models differ, however, in that they suggest that the evaluation of campaign effects should focus on different outcomes or on different time frames.

The diffusion model focuses attention on the social process surrounding health communication interventions. Messages may not only persuade individuals directly, but also stimulate interpersonal discussion about health behavior change. Evaluations under this model could not rely on comparing individuals who varied in exposure to the health messages, but would need to compare social networks that were more and less likely to have diffused messages. The institutional diffusion path carries with it a different implication. The audience for the communication interventions may be decision makers who determine institutional policies, rather than individuals whose behavior(s) are of concern. Indeed, if individuals are the audience, this audience may be seen primarily as a constituency who can influence policy makers, rather than as individuals whose risk behavior is to be changed. Evaluations of health communication interventions whose major path to influence is through institutional action cannot be conducted by comparing individuals with more and less exposure to messages. The appropriate unit of analysis is the institutional catchment area, often a geographically or politically defined unit, such as a city or state.

Media Advocacy

One possible way to speed up the likelihood of an institutional response is through *media advocacy,* the strategic use of mass media in combination with community organizing to advance healthy public policies. The primary focus is on the role of news media, with secondary attention to the use of paid advertising (U.S. Department of Health and Human Services, 1988; Wallack et al., 1993; Wallack, 1994; Wallack and Dorfman, 1996; Wallack and Sciandra, 1990-91; Winett and Wallack, 1996; Wallack et al., 1999). Media advocacy seeks to raise the volume of voices for social change, and to shape the sound so that it resonates with social justice values that are the presumed basis of public health (Beauchamp, 1976; Mann, 1997). Media advocacy has been used by a wide range of grassroots community groups, public health leadership groups, public health and social advocates, and public health researchers (Wallack et al., 1993; Wallack et al., 1999).

From a theoretical perspective, media advocacy borrows from mass communication research, political science, sociology, and political psychology to develop strategy. Central to media advocacy are the concepts of agenda setting (McCoombs and Shaw, 1972; Dearing and Rogers, 1994) and framing (Iyengar, 1991; Gamson, 1989; Ryan, 1991). From a practical perspective, media advocacy borrows from community organizing, key elements of formative research (i.e., focus groups and polling), and political campaign strategy (e.g., application of selective pressure on key groups or individuals) (Wallack et al., 1993).

Media advocacy differs from traditional public health campaigns. It is most marked by an *emphasis* on:

- Linking public health and social problems to inequities in social arrangements rather than to flaws in the individual.
- Changing public policy rather than personal health behavior.
- Focusing primarily on reaching opinion leaders and policy makers, rather than on those individuals who are directly affected (the traditional audience of public health communication campaigns).
- Working with groups to increase participation and amplify their voices rather than providing health behavior change messages.
- Having a primary goal of reducing the power gap, rather than filling the information gap.

Media advocacy is generally seen as part of a broader strategy, rather than as a strategy per se. It focuses on four primary activities in support of community organizing, policy development, and advancing policy:

- *Developing overall strategy.* Media advocacy uses critical thinking to understand and respond to problems as social issues, rather than as personal problems. Following problem definition, the focus is on elaborating policy options; identifying the person, group, or organization with the power to create the necessary change; and identifying organizations that can apply pressure to advance the policy and create change. (For example, in Oakland, California, various elements of the community were organized to apply pressure on the zoning commission, mayor's office, city council, and state legislature, which were all targets at various points in the campaign.) Finally, various messages for the different targets of the campaign are developed.

• *Setting the agenda.* Getting an issue in the media can help set the agenda and provide legitimacy and credibility to the health issue. Media advocacy involves understanding how journalism works in order to increase access to the news media. This approach includes maintaining a media list, monitoring the news media, understanding the elements of newsworthiness, pitching stories, and holding news events and developing editorial page strategies for reaching key opinion leaders about a given health issue.

• *Shaping the debate.* The news media generally focus on the plight of the victim, while policy advocates emphasize social conditions that create victims. Media advocates frame policy issues using public health values that resonate with broad audiences. Some of the steps include "translate[ing] personal problems into public issues" (Mills, 1959); emphasizing social accountability as well as personal responsibility; identifying individuals and organizations who must assume a greater burden for addressing the problem; presenting a clear and concise policy solution; and packaging the story by combining key elements such as visuals, expert voices, authentic voices (those who have experience with the problem), media bites, social math (creating a context for large numbers that is interesting to the press and understandable to the public), research summaries, fact sheets, and policy papers.

• *Advancing the policy.* Policy battles are often long and contentious, and it is important to use the media effectively to keep the issue on the media agenda. The Oakland, California, effort took 4 years and now must focus media attention to ensure that the policy is properly implemented. Thus, it is important to develop strategies to maintain the media spotlight on the policy issue on a continuing basis. This effort means identifying opportunities to reintroduce the issue to the media—informing them of key anniversaries of relevant dates, publication of new reports, and significant meetings or hearings—and linking the policy solution to breaking news.

Diffusion of Innovations

When a new idea or innovation is introduced, diffusion theory (see, e.g., Rogers, 1995) suggests that the innovation has five characteristics, as perceived by members of a social system, that determine its rate of adoption: (1) relative advantage—the degree to which an innovation is perceived as being better than the idea it supersedes; (2) compatibility—the degree to which an innovation is perceived as being consistent with the existing values, past experiences, and needs of potential adopters; (3) complexity—the degree to which an innovation is perceived as being difficult to understand and use; (4) trialability—the degree to which an innovation may be experimented with on a limited basis; and (5) observability—the degree to which the results of an innovation are visible to others. In summary, innovations that are perceived by individuals as having *greater* relative advantage, compatibility, trialability, and observability and *less* complexity will be adopted more rapidly than other innovations.

In addition to the perceived characteristics of the innovation, people (or organizations and other units of adoption) vary in their innovativeness, the degree to which they are relatively earlier in adopting new ideas than other members of a social system. According to diffusion theory, there are five adopter categories: (1) innovators—the first 2.5 percent of the individuals in a system to adopt an innovation; (2) early adopters—the next 13.5 percent of the individuals in a system to adopt the innovation; (3) early majority—the next 34 percent to adopt; (4) late majority—the next

34 percent; and (5) laggards—the last 16 percent of the individuals in a system to adopt an innovation.

Generally speaking, the early adopter category, more than any other, has the greatest degree of opinion leadership in most systems, and potential adopters often look to early adopters for advice and information about the innovation. Several health communication interventions identified opinion leaders in a given community (e.g., among medical practitioners or members of the public), and then introduced innovations through these opinion leaders, in order to speed up the rate of diffusion of a health innovation (Kelly et al., 1992; Kelly, 1994).

IMPLICATIONS OF THEORY FOR HEALTH COMMUNICATION WITH DIVERSE POPULATIONS

It should be clear that theories of communication and behavior change, and theories of media effects, all recognize the importance of considering diversity in developing effective health communication interventions to produce behavior change. More specifically, behavior change theories recognize that the relative importance of the theoretical determinants of any given behavior may vary across populations. For example, a given health behavior change may be attitudinally driven in one population, normatively driven in another, and primarily under the influence of personal agency in a third population. Moreover, even if the same determinant is of primary importance for two diverse populations, the substantive content of the beliefs underlying that determinant may differ. For example, although attitude may be the most important determinant of a given health behavior in both Asian-American and African-American communities, members of one community may hold very different beliefs from members of the other community about the consequences of performing that health behavior.

Similarly, theories of communication and behavior change recognize that sources and channels that are perceived as credible by one population (i.e., for one audience) may be distrusted or not utilized by another. Moreover, production values and formats in communication messages that positively appeal to one population may be viewed as unpleasant or boring by another. Finally, a message may lead directly to immediate or delayed health behavior change in one population, but will only affect beliefs if it leads to institutional diffusion in another. Although these considerations make it clear that one should develop health communication interventions with a specific target audience in mind, it is important to recognize that in many cases, the same belief or set of beliefs may be identified as a critical target for a number of diverse populations. The same message may be equally effective for diverse audiences. Moreover, when there is a "strong" message, the source may be less important than the message per se. Indeed, there is growing evidence that the source of a message is most important with a "weak" message, but has little or no effect with a "strong" message.

Does theory matter? Theory can increase the potential effectiveness of communication interventions by identifying critical beliefs to target, by structuring the communication message, and by guiding the selection of sources and channels of communication.

Does diversity matter in developing health communication interventions? To maximize communication effectiveness, one should adapt message formats, sources, channels, and frequency of exposure for different audiences. Factors such as age, gender, race/ethnicity, and sexual orientation all draw on different interactions with the world and lead to different understandings regarding what is important and what is appropriate. Theory provides us with a roadmap to incorporate cultural differences into health communication interventions.

Do we need new behavior change theories? Existing behavioral theories need to be more fully applied in implementing health communication interventions. The main need is not for new theory, but for better application of the communication and behavior change theories that we already have. Individuals developing communication interventions need to fully understand the behavior they are trying to change or to reinforce from the perspective of the particular population with whom they are dealing. That is, they need to know whether, in that population, a given health behavior is controlled by attitudes, perceived norms, or issues of personal agency. More important, they need to identify these behavioral, normative, and/or control beliefs that most strongly discriminate between those who do and do not perform a given health behavior. Once target beliefs have been identified, one must identify the communicator, medium, and type of message that will have the greatest chance of influencing the beliefs either directly or indirectly.

Although theory is quite clear about the need to consider population differences in developing effective communication interventions, is there evidence that the appropriate use of theory helps to change health behaviors in diverse audiences? In the following chapters we examine the existing evidence and determine whether there are research gaps that need to be addressed.

In sum, communication and behavior change theories provide a powerful tool for organizing our thoughts, the existing evidence, and cultural realities so that health communication interventions can be more comprehensive, more sophisticated, and more likely to have desired effects on health behavior change. The following annex (Annex A) describes three of the behavioral theories that have had the strongest impact on health behavior interventions. Annex B describes self-regulation models.

ANNEX A:
OVERVIEW OF KEY CONCEPTS IN
THREE BEHAVIOR CHANGE THEORIES

The Health Belief Model

According to the original Health Belief Model, two major factors influence the likelihood that a person will adopt a recommended health-protective behavior change. First, the person must feel susceptible to a disease with serious or severe consequences. Second, the person must believe that the benefits of taking the recommended action outweigh the perceived barriers to (and/or costs of) performing the preventive action. In addition, the model recognized that a number of events (e.g., knowing someone who is ill, exposure to media campaigns, or other information) can serve as "cues to action." These cues sometimes have been viewed as influencing "threat" (Janz and Becker, 1984) and sometimes as influencing behavior directly (Rosenstock, Strecher, and Becker, 1994). Most recently, the concept of self-efficacy has been added to the Health Belief Model (Rosenstock, Strecher, and Becker, 1994). Finally, the Health Belief Model also recognized that a number of demographic and individual difference variables could influence health beliefs (i.e., susceptibility, severity, costs, benefits, and self-efficacy).

Social Cognitive Theory

According to Social Cognitive Theory (Bandura, 1977b, 1986, 1997a), three primary factors determine the likelihood that someone will adopt a health behavior change: (1) self-efficacy, (2) goals, and (3) outcome expectancies. To adopt a given behavior change, individuals must have a sense of personal agency or self-efficacy that they can perform the desired behavior change, even in the face of various circumstances or barriers that make the change difficult to adopt and implement. Unless people believe they can exercise some control over their health behavior, they have little incentive to act or to persevere in the face of difficulties.

Health behavior also is affected by the outcomes that people expect their actions to produce. These expected outcomes include physical effects, social costs and benefits, and positive and negative self-evaluative reactions to one's health behavior. Personal goals, rooted in a value system, provide further self-incentives and guides for health habits. Personal health behavior change would be easy if there were no impediments to surmount. The facilitators and obstacles that people perceive in changing their behavior is another determinant of health behavior change.

In effecting large-scale change, communication systems operate through two pathways (Bandura, 2002a). In the direct pathway, communication media promote change by informing, modeling, motivating, and guiding people. In the socially mediated pathway, media influences are used to link people in social networks and community settings. These places provide continued personalized guidance, as well as natural incentives and social supports for desired changes.

The Theory of Reasoned Action

According to the Theory of Reasoned Action (Fishbein and Ajzen, 1975; Ajzen and Fishbein, 1980), performance of a given behavior change is determined primarily by the strength of a person's intention to perform that behavior. The intention to perform a given behavior is, in turn, viewed as a function of two factors, namely the person's attitude toward performing the behavior (i.e., one's overall positive or negative feeling about personally performing the behavior) and/or the person's subjective norm concerning the behavior (i.e., the person's perception that his or her important others think he or she should or should not perform the behavior). Attitudes are a function of behavioral beliefs (i.e., beliefs that performing the behavior will lead to certain outcomes) and their evaluative aspects (i.e., the evaluation of these outcomes); subjective norms are viewed as a function of normative beliefs (i.e., beliefs that a specific individual or population thinks one should or should not perform the behavior in question) and motivations to comply (i.e., the degree to which, in general, one wants to do what the referent thinks one should do).

It is worth noting that an extension of the Theory of Reasoned Action, the Theory of Planned Behavior (Ajzen, 1988, 1991), includes the concept of personal agency or perceived behavioral control. More specifically, according to the Theory of Planned Behavior, perceived behavioral control is viewed as a factor that directly influences both intention and behavior.

* * * * *

Taken together, these three theories identify a limited number of variables that serve as determinants of any given health behavior change. All or some of these variables are found in nearly all other behavioral theories (e.g., the Information, Motivation, Behavioral Skills Model, Prochaska's Stages of Change Model). Although there is considerable empirical evidence for the role of attitude, perceived norms, and self-efficacy as proximal determinants of intention and behavior (e.g., Shepphard, Hartwick, and Warshaw, 1988; Sheeran, Abraham, and Orbell, 1999), there is only limited support for the role of perceived risk (e.g., Gerrard, Gibbons, and Bushman, 1996). Thus, most behavior change theories suggest three critical determinants of a person's intentions and behaviors: (1) the person's attitude toward performing the behavior, which is based on one's beliefs about the positive and negative consequences (i.e., costs and benefits) of performing that behavior; (2) perceived norms, which include the perception that those with whom the individual interacts most closely support the person's adoption of the behavior and that others in the community are performing the behavior; and (3) self-efficacy, which involves the person's perception that he or she can perform the behavior under a variety of challenging circumstances.

ANNEX B:
SELF-REGULATION MODELS

The Common Sense Model (Skelton and Croyle, 1991; Leventhal, Meyer, and Nerenz, 1980; Petrie and Weinman, 1997; Cameron and Leventhal, 2002), is a specific example of a self-regulation that adds a detailed set of constructs specific to health behaviors presented in cognitive behavioral models. The model is based on findings from studies of health communication (Leventhal, 1970), showing that health actions are a product of a cognitive system representing the individual's subjective or perceptual experience of health threats, and a system representing emotional reactions to these threats. The cognitive system is composed of 4 components: (1) the representation of the threat (e.g., the name of the disease and the symptoms identifying its presence, likely duration and time of onset, cause, consequences (physical, social, economic), and controllability); (2) procedures for avoiding and/or controlling it and how these procedures are represented (medication is necessary; medication is addictive and dangerous; see Horne, 1997); (3) action plans (Leventhal, 1970) or implementation intentions (Gollwitzer and Oettingen, 1998), which specify time and place to perform specific procedures; and (4) the appraisal of action outcomes. Appraisal or efficacy assessments are made in relation to the goals set by the representation of both the threat and the procedure. For example, an analgesic medication will be appraised for its efficacy in eliminating pain and the time it takes to do so. The temporal expectations will be longer for more severe injuries and shorter for strong than for mild analgesics, e.g., ibuprofen versus aspirin. A key proposition of the Common Sense Model is that representations of both health dangers and procedures are abstract (e.g., labels such as diabetes, coronary disease) and concrete and/or experiential (symptoms of diabetes, effects of insulin, etc.).

Fear of a disease threat, i.e., the emotional response, can stimulate avoidance responses (minimization of the threat, avoidance of information), though these interfering effects are usually short lived and visible among individuals lacking a sense of self-efficacy. Evidence from multiple studies suggests that fear focuses attention on the danger (Lieberman and Chaiken, 1992) and encourages protective action among message recipients with high self-efficacy (Leventhal, 1970; Witte and Allen, 2000). Even individuals inclined to avoid exposure to threat information return to learn about and confront threats once their fear subsides (Wiebe, in press). Unlike planned behavior where social influences are conceptualized as norms (Ajzen and Fishbein, 1980), social influence takes multiple forms in the Common Sense Model. Observation of others, including observation of strangers, can provide information on cause, proximity and symptoms of health threats, efficacy and side effects of treatment, modeling of skills, assistance and barriers for both changing and maintaining health behaviors, and amplify or reduce fear associated with health threats and treatment procedures (Leventhal, Robitaille and Hudson, 1997).

Most of the studies guided by the "self-regulation" framework have focused on actions for primary, secondary, and/or tertiary prevention that occur repeatedly over relatively long time frames for chronic illnesses such as diabetes, cardiovascular disease and cancer (the majority of the 1,800 plus items using the keyword "self-regulation" that were entered in the PsychINFO data base since 1990 are focused on health issues (see Leventhal, Brissette, and Leventhal, in press; Petrie and Weinman, 1997). The focus on chronic illness is consistent with hypothesis and data showing that representations of health threats and the procedures for control evolve over time as a function of changes in the individual's concrete experience with illness and its symptoms and information from other persons and various media messages. Data supporting the Common Sense Model indicate that the great majority of behaviors initiated for health reasons are motivated by symptoms or functional deficits in the self or by observations of such changes in other persons. Symptoms and functional change are indicators of the state of the system, whether one is ill, stressed, or simply feeling the effects of aging, and changes in these perceptions over experienced (rather than clock) time are typically used as criteria for evaluating the efficacy of self selected and medically recommended interventions for avoiding and controlling illness threats. Although the Common Sense Model and the Social Learning Models (e.g., Bandura, 1977) were developed in parallel, they hold common assumptions about the determinants of health action.

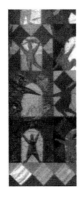

3

Health
Communication
Campaigns Exemplar

INTRODUCTION

This chapter focuses on diversity issues associated with large-scale public health communication campaigns. These campaigns include federal government-supported programs such as the National High Blood Pressure Education Program and the National Youth Anti-Drug Media Campaign; the state-sponsored antitobacco campaigns such as Florida's Truth Campaign and California's Anti-Tobacco Campaign; and privately sponsored programs such as the Campaign to Prevent Teen Pregnancy and the Avon Breast Cancer Crusade. This chapter describes how those campaigns have addressed diverse audiences and presents available evidence for their success in reaching and affecting those audiences. This analysis is based largely on the review by our Committee of approximately 18 U.S. health communication campaigns, the majority of which are national in scope and currently ongoing (see Table 3-1).

Nearly all of these campaigns indicate in their public documents that they have given special consideration to diverse audiences. A campaign may have targeted an African-American audience for enhanced levels of exposure to messages by purchasing time on stations with wide African-American listenership; a campaign may have shaped a message strategy for girls, meant to appeal to the particular beliefs that underpin their decisions about smoking; a campaign may have used actors well known to older audiences in advertisements to stimulate mammogram demand by those audiences. Often these special efforts are justified on the grounds that particular audiences are at greater risk, based on the sort of epidemiological evidence reviewed in other chapters in this volume, or more simply because different segments of the population are assumed to be responsive to different communication approaches. Nonetheless, addressing diversity is not accomplished in just one way. Although nearly all programs claim such efforts, the particular approaches they have used vary, and the level of resources applied to such special efforts varies as well. An important task for this chapter is describing the range of approaches that typically have been employed. This will be especially useful for new programs considering how to address the needs of diverse audiences. But descriptions of how programs have tried to "solve" the issue of diversity are not sufficient.

Descriptions provide little grounds for choosing among approaches or for deciding to undertake a special effort altogether. The extra resources required for special efforts to adjust programs to serve diverse audiences can be substantial, including additional research, increased production of materials, and additional purchases of media time, among other incremental costs. The justification for more resources is strongest if it relies on evidence that a particular approach to address diversity works better than programs with no diversity-based targeting approach or better than programs with alternative diversity approaches. This chapter summarizes such evidence where it exists. However, there is relatively little evidence about differential effects of campaigns on diverse audiences overall, and the evidence is even more scarce about the relative utility of the range of diversity approaches that have been used. One of the main recommendations of this volume will be to

TABLE 3-1 Campaigns—Intended Populations

National Campaign	Racial/Ethnicity
National Safe Kids Campaign	All ethnicities targeted[b]
Buckle Up America	All ethnicities targeted[b]
Child Safety Seat Distribution Program (USNHTSA)	Asian American, Hispanic/Latino, Native American/Alaskan Native
Folic Acid (March of Dimes)	High-risk populations—e.g., Asian American, Hispanic/ Latino, Asian American/Pacific Islander, Native American[b] (including Spanish); now targeting Hispanic/Latino populations
Depression Awareness, Recognition, and Treatment Program	Asian American, Hispanic, (some Asian American/Pacific Islander)
National Air Bag and Seat Belt Safety	Asian American, Hispanic/Latino; (Spanish materials)
National 5 A Day (fruits and vegetables versus cancer, sponsored by the National Cancer Institute)	Asian American, Hispanic/Latino at national level; Asian American, Hispanic/Latino, Native American/AI, Asian American/Pacific Islander at state/local level
Back to Sleep	Focus on Asian American, starting focus on Native American; generic materials for major ethnic populations also include Asian American/Pacific Islander[b]
Milk Matters Calcium Education	Native American, Asian American, Hispanic/Latino (populations with lactose intolerance)
National Campaign to Prevent Teen Pregnancy (private nonprofit)	Hispanic/Latino, Asian American
Best Start (Loving Support)	Asian American, Hispanic/Latino, (Asian American/Pacific Islander, Native American[b])

Gender	Age	SES/Social Class	Launch Date
Male, Female	≤14 years	Low income	1988
Male, Female (same)	≤14 years, parents, grandparents	General and low-income	1997
Male, Female (same)	(parents)	Low-income	2000[a]
Female	Child-bearing age	General, low SES, low education	1998
Male, Female (some different)	Older age; teenagers	—	1985
Male, Female (same)	New (and younger) parents	Low-income, low-education	1996
Male, Female (some different)	adults (25 to 55 years)	Low-income, low-literacy	1991
Male, Female (same)	Older (and general caretakers)	—	1994
Male, Female (female different)	Children, teenagers, parents	Low-income (outreach mailing—WIC)	1997
Male, Female (different)	Teenagers, parents	Low-income	1996
Female	Special materials for teenagers	Low-income, low-literacy	1997

continued on next page

TABLE 3-1 Continued

National Campaign	Racial/Ethnicity
National High Blood Pressure Education Program	Asian American, Hispanic/Latino, Asian American/Pacific Islander, Native American/Alaskan Native
Youth Anti-Drug Media Campaign	Asian American, Hispanic/Latino, Native American, Asian American/ Pacific Islander, Alaskan Native, Aleuts; (11 languages)
Florida Pilot Project on Tobacco Control ("truth" campaign)	Asian American, Hispanic/Latino, Asian American/Pacific Islander
National Truth Campaign (tobacco)	Asian American, Hispanic/Latino, Asian American/Pacific Islander
National Cancer Institute Breast Cancer Education Program Mammography (not just once)	Asian American, Hispanic/Latino, Asian American/Pacific Islander
National Breast Cancer Awareness Month	Asian American, Hispanic/Latino, Asian American/Pacific Islander; Spanish materials
National Diabetes Education Program (diabetes)	Asian American, Hispanic/Latino, Asian American/Pacific Islander, Native American
Centers for Disease Control and Prevention Flu	Asian American, Hispanic/Latino; Spanish materials
National Eye Health Education Program	Hispanic/Latino, Asian American
Feet Can Last a Lifetime (diabetes)	Asian American, Hispanic/Latino, Asian American/Pacific Islander[b]; Spanish materials.

[a]Efforts by state and local governments began as early as 1998.
[b]"Like" (i.e., racial/ethnic) models/photos used.

Gender	Age	SES/Social Class	Launch Date
Male, Female (some different)	Elderly, teenagers, youth	Low income/ education	1972
Male, Female (female different)	Youth (9 to 18 years); parents	— (rural/urban)	1998
Male, Female (same and different	Middle school students, high school students	—	1998
Male, Female (same)	Youth, teenagers, young adults	—	2000
Female	>40 years	Low SES, low education	1997
Female, Male/general public (female different)	All ages; (elderly targeted)	Low-income, (rural), low-access, low-literacy	1985
Male, Female (same)	Seniors	Low SES	1998
Male, Female (same)	25 to 54 years	—	1998
Male, Female (same)	>60 years (mostly)	Low-literacy/ low-education	1991
Male, Female (same)	—	Low-literacy	1995

gather systematic evidence about campaigns' diversity efforts and effects.

In the following sections, we discuss the definition of a campaign, the various approaches campaigns have used to address diversity, and specific evidence about diversity effects. The concluding section offers recommendations.

WHAT ARE CAMPAIGNS?

A communication campaign has been defined as an intervention that "intends to generate specific outcomes or effects, in a relatively large number of individuals, usually within a specified period of time, and through an organized set of communication activities" (Rogers and Storey, 1987). Communication campaigns can be differentiated from focused educational interventions that work entirely through clinical or other in-place institutions as well as those that are delivered individually to people (e.g., in their homes). Our focus is on a subset of campaigns that have large target audiences (for example, the entire population of a state or country). Yet even programs that fit into this category are quite different from one another. Some characteristics that are typical, although not always present, are the following:

• Communication campaigns intend to provide direct education for those people who are expected to adopt or change to a healthier behavior.

• Campaigns seek to affect large audiences and bring substantial resources to the task (sometimes monetary, sometimes voluntary, sometimes through collaboration with other institutions).

• Campaigns often use multiple channels, and may complement mediated (television, radio) channels with personal channels (health professionals, outreach workers).

• Campaigns attempt to influence adoption of recommended behaviors by influencing what consumers know and believe about the behavior, and/or by influencing actual and/or perceived social norms, and/or by changing actual skills and confidence in skills (self-efficacy), all of which are assumed to influence behavior.

• Campaigns often are sponsored by the government, sometimes in collaboration with private advocacy or professional organizations, or by national advocacy or professional organizations alone.

• Campaigns are often a component of broader social marketing programs. *Social marketing* is the application of commercial marketing ideas to help solve social and health problems (Andreasen, 1995). Social marketing programs complement communication efforts with other intervention components. For example, a social marketing campaign to encourage childhood vaccination might complement a public communication effort to promote vaccination uptake with a subsidy in the price of vaccines and an easier system for obtaining vaccines, or even a change in the rules about what vaccines can be given together.

• Even more broadly, many campaigns complement efforts to directly influence populations with efforts to affect public policy (taxes, regulation) as well as to change other aspects of the environment and the marketplace, including changes in the ways that other social institutions act. These complementary efforts would be expected to influence populations indirectly. These multilevel social change programs might include grassroots organizing, political and media advocacy, partnerships with private institutions, and the design and offering of new products. They recognize the importance of system and environmental constraints that support or impede the desired behavior changes.

Throughout the 20th century, communication campaigns were developed to address most major public health issues, including a broad array of behavioral outcomes ranging from the initiation and maintenance of preventive health behaviors to the cessation of behaviors that increase the risk of negative health outcomes. For example, health communication campaigns were developed to reduce smoking; promote compliance with high blood pressure treatment and childhood and adult vaccination schedules; promote safer sex practices to prevent HIV/AIDS; reduce illegal drug use; promote use of seatbelts, car seats, and bike helmets; reduce the practice of driving while alcohol impaired; encourage mammography and other disease-screening behavior; and promote healthy dietary choices for the prevention of cancer, cardiovascular diseases, diabetes, and other chronic diseases. Specifically, Congress authorized nearly $1 billion for the National Youth Anti-Drug Media Campaign between 1998 and 2002. California alone spent more than $634 million in its campaign against tobacco use between 1989 and 1999 (*San Francisco Examiner*, 1999), with 15 to 20 percent of those expenditures going to a continuing mass media campaign (Pierce, Emery, and Gilpin, 2002). Box 3-1 presents the outline of one campaign, the National Cancer Institute's Once A Year for A Life Time program to encourage mammograms. It incorporates many elements typical of long-lived campaigns.

Various texts provide overviews of the public communication campaign experience (Rice and Atkin, 1989, 2001; Salmon, 1989; Guttman, 2000; Hornik, 2002). We will not try to present or even summarize that literature, except to indicate that there is substantial evidence that some campaigns have affected important health behaviors, although not in every instance. For the purposes of this chapter, the essential point to understand about such projects is that they involve carrying out a series of operational tasks, and each of those tasks is an opportunity to pay more or less attention to the issue of diversity.

The major tasks to be undertaken by a campaign include (1) choosing target audience(s) and particular behavioral objectives; (2) choosing a message strategy and executions; (3) choosing the mix of dissemination channels and settings; and (4) undertaking formative, monitoring, and evaluation research to support the program. Decisions about each of these tasks will vary with the evolution of the campaign and its audience. A campaign is not defined by a specific and static mix of messages, audiences, and channels. Rather, it is defined as a program that makes decisions about these operational details, decisions that will vary over time.

Authors have broken down these tasks in many ways. Sutton, Balch, and Lefebvre (1995) acknowledge Novelli's six-step "marketing wheel" for planning a social marketing process (Novelli, 1984) that has been used in many national health education campaigns. They also point to the health communication process practiced at the Centers for Disease Control and Prevention that included a 10-step "wheel" of action (Roper, 1993). Their own system focuses on six steps: (1) defining and understanding the target audience; (2) determining the behavioral objective—that is, what action the audience should take (and not take, if there is a competitive behavior); (3) deciding what reward should be promised in the message for taking the action; (4) establishing what needs to be included to make the promised reward credible; (5) determining what "openings and vehicles" should be used—that is, how to reach audience members when they are receptive; and (6) deciding what "look and feel" or what image of the action should be portrayed in the message.

A full description of the art and science of message development is beyond the scope of this chapter. Details of these steps are not the central issue here. The issue for this chapter is how the fact of diversity has been or might be taken into account as part of the decision process in developing a campaign. We focus on the four broad tasks because they serve to illustrate the argument, while recognizing that a finer differentiation of steps may be required to implement a campaign successfully. Each of these tasks can take special account of concerns about diversity.

THE LOGIC OF SEGMENTATION AND
ITS RELATION TO DIVERSITY

Public health campaigns are designed to influence a population to maintain or improve its health status. To accomplish this, campaign developers must understand the link between behavior and health status for the population of interest. Although current reporting systems provide information on the distribution of illness and disease across broad demographic groups and are useful for identifying disproportionate risks and outcomes, this broad level of epidemiological analysis rarely proves useful in identifying the relevant characteristics that best define the audiences for a health campaign. This is because any single group characterized by these broad demographic variables is actually composed of multiple diverse segments with different needs, experiences, attitudes, and behaviors.

To address the heterogeneous nature of populations, health communication programs have applied the marketing concept of segmentation. Segmentation is the process of partitioning a heterogeneous population into subgroups or segments of people with similar needs, experiences, and/or other characteristics. A number of approaches have been developed to help determine optimum audience segmentation. Segmentation assumes that audiences that perceive a message as relevant to their interests, concerns, and problems are more likely to pay attention to the message, to process it deeply, and to remember and act on it, than are audiences that do not perceive the message as personally relevant. An elaboration of these concepts is provided in the following paragraphs.

A sensible communication campaign recognizes heterogeneity in its population. First, all members of the population do not have the same status with regard to a behavior. For a youth tobacco prevention campaign, some youth are already heavy smokers, some smoke irregularly, some have smoked in the past but have quit, and some have never smoked but are intrigued and at higher risk of beginning to smoke, while others have never smoked and, regardless of a campaign, are very unlikely to become smokers. Each of these segments of the youth population may require different interventions. The behavioral objective for the heavy smokers may be enrollment in a cessation intervention; for the casual smokers, it may be stopping all smoking; for the prior quitters, it may be developing skills to resist cigarettes in situations that signal smoking temptation; for the intrigued nonsmokers, it may be resisting offers of cigarettes from peers; and for the committed nonsmokers, it may be reinforcing their existing preference. One campaign might choose only one of these audience segments as its target, or at least begin with one of these audiences. For example, the National Youth Anti-Drug Media Campaign (1998) chose to focus on prevention of trial use of drugs among prior nonusers, and prevention of regular use of drugs among prior occasional users. It did not address current regular users, suspecting that this audience might not be responsive to its efforts.

Thus, the audience can be broken down by current behavior and the behavioral objective that campaign planners might seek for each group. However, within each of these behavioral subgroups, there is still more heterogeneity. Assume the antitobacco campaign chose to focus efforts on the intrigued nonsmokers. Some of those intrigued nonsmokers are young teenagers and some are older teenagers; some are girls and some are boys; some are surrounded by peers who smoke and others may have few friends who smoke. Some report frequent contact with prosmoking promotion by the tobacco industry that puts them at risk (Pierce and Giplin, 1995), while others do not have such frequent contact. Some may view smoking as a desirable personal symbol of rebellion against authority, while others may be more influenced by knowledge of the negative effects of smoking on athletic endurance. A single message (e.g., smoking harms your health) might affect all of these portions of the audience similarly, but much experience in undertaking these campaigns suggests otherwise. Rather, many campaigns assume that if there is heterogeneity in the causes of audience behaviors and in what influences behavior change, then there is a need for heterogeneity in message strategies as well.

Populations are heterogeneous in their behavior, and in the correlates and causes of their behavior, but they are also heterogeneous in the ways they can be reached. Some youth are devotees of MTV or hip-hop music radio stations, while others watch widely popular sitcoms or dramas, and some can be found in the audience of the teen-focused WB network. Others are regular viewers of religious television broadcasts, while still others are religiously watching rebroadcasts of the Simpsons after school. Some can be reached in school settings, while others have dropped out; some are frequent visitors to malls, while others attend rock concerts. There are many settings and channels through which intrigued nonsmokers may be reached, and different subgroups are likely to be accessible through each setting and channel. Based on an understanding of the target audience, campaign planners must seek to find the best times, places, and opportunities where the audience will be exposed and open to receiving the message.

Finally, just as heterogeneous subgroups can differ in their behaviors, in the causes of behavior, and channels and settings through which they can be reached, they can also vary in the executions of the messages that will appeal to them. The values they hold, the social groups with whom they identify, and the social activities in which they participate also will influence what messages appeal to them, and thus these factors influence campaign design. One group of youth may be accustomed to quick cuts and intense music and will pay little attention to talking heads in an advertisement. Another group will attend to slower paced ads, but pay close attention to the quality of the argument. Others are persuaded by the source: Some may be enamored of celebrities, and others by those with evident expertise.

Marketers, in recognizing this heterogeneity in the audience, attempt to define addressable segments of the audience, people who share behavioral status and a common cause of the behavior, along with other associated experiences, cultural identity, or other characteristics. Those will help define segment-specific message strategy, channel choices, and message execution choices. Health communication campaigns have selected and defined their intended audiences in very different ways. Although some campaigns divide the prospective audience into groups according to characteristics of social diversity such as age, race, income, gender, or education, this is often because only limited information is available about the potential target audiences.

The key to the effectiveness of audience segmentation for health campaigns is how well the segmentation approach identifies and separates homogeneous audience segments for which a particular message is personally relevant and motivating from those for whom it is not. The goal is to target segments of people who will respond in a similar way so that a health message can be designed to maximize its relevancy. Segmentation is now considered a necessary step in the process of design and development of communication campaigns (Atkin and Freimuth, 1989; Grunig, 1989; Rogers and Storey, 1987; Slater et al., 1996). Health campaign planners require quantitative evidence to define or identify potential audience segments and both quantitative and qualitative evidence to understand those segments well.

The idea of a heterogeneous audience is a core assumption of most current health communication programs. However, only some of that heterogeneity for a particular health behavior will correspond to the diversity categories that are the focus of this volume: race, ethnicity, gender, age, economic status and social class, education, and sexual orientation. For example, regarding marijuana use, although age matters a great deal, the genders are similar. Sexual orientation clearly is related to risk of sexually transmitted disease, but may not be a core issue for planning a campaign to encourage diabetes screening. For some behaviors and for some audiences, other factors may be much more useful for segmenting audiences than any of the focus diversity categories. For example, developers of antidrug campaigns for youth know that risk of drug use initiation is predicted by prior smoking and alcohol use and by a personality variable—sensation seeking—none of which are closely related to the traditional demographic categories used for monitoring attention to diversity (except for age). However, even in these circumstances, when the traditional diversity variables may not predict behavioral status or even the causes of behavior, these diversity categories may be relevant to the channel choices and the message executions. Thus antidrug messages may address the same behavioral target and assume the same motivations for drug use for all current nonusing youth, but use different celebrities ('N Sync for young white teens and Mary J. Blige for young African-American teens) as sources for antidrug messages or buy media time on different channels (an afternoon soap opera for girls and a football game for boys).

These strategies will be helpful insofar as the selected diversity characteristics enhance the persuasiveness of executions and access to channels and thus improve total exposure to and credibility of the antidrug messages.

Good health communication segmentation may match the diversity categories that are the focus of this volume, but there is no assurance that this will be the case. There may be a strong and legitimate political impulse to focus on groups defined by demographic or racial/ethnic categories, particularly if those groups are unequal with regard to epidemiological risk of bad health outcomes. However, the implicit assumption of targeting is that such groups are homogeneous with regard to their likely responsiveness to campaign strategies. This assumption simply may be wrong or may be a poor predictor of differences in responsiveness, which can lead to inefficiencies in campaign execution.

This discussion presents the logic and a few examples of how programs use segmentation to organize their audiences. In that context, we can review a broader set of examples, and how they have brought the focus diversity categories to bear on their choices of audiences, behaviors, assumed motivations for behavior, channels, and message executions.

Choosing Among Potential Audience Segments

The argument that audiences are heterogeneous is strong, and thus the logic of choosing to consider segmentation is strong. However, which segments deserve priority is not resolved on the basis of the division into segments. Programs use a variety of criteria for choosing among potential audience segments, including:

• *Audience need.* Higher epidemiological risk of a targeted segment based on disease morbidity and mortality, and/or prevalence of behaviors related to these health outcomes, can suggest a campaign focus.
  • *Segment size.* With limited resources, communication cam-

paigns often seek to reach the largest possible number of people who could benefit from the message.

• *Impact.* Audience segments often vary according to their potential to benefit from health messages. This may be related to their readiness to accept the message or to their likelihood of being influenced by a communication intervention. Campaign planners may give a higher priority to audiences who will take less work to change so they get the highest return on their investment. Alternately, some campaign planners will see their mission as getting the hard cases to adopt healthier behaviors, and focus their attention on the least ready. The COMMIT Program, sponsored by the Canadian Ministry of Health and carried out in Brant County, Ontario, focused on getting heavy smokers to quit but was not able to show any success. However, when the project developers refocused their analysis on moderate smokers, a secondary audience, they discovered that their intervention had a worthwhile success.

• *Accessibility.* Whether an audience segment can be reached effectively also can influence the selection of audience segments. Although a segment may be at risk for a negative health outcome, the inability to develop dissemination strategies that reach it at a reasonable cost may preclude it from the selection as an audience segment.

• *Political considerations.* The realities of the system under which many health communication campaigns are developed mean that political and legislative (or regulatory) mandates can determine the characteristics of audience segments. Representatives and advocates from particular population groups can exert considerable influence on the process of selection of topics and audiences for communication campaigns.

These are competing criteria for choosing among segments. Once they are understood, the choice among segments is not only a technical decision, but also a political/social/ethical decision. The decision thus may not belong solely in the hands of the project planners, but is appropriately negotiated among the constituencies who have an interest in the outcome. Two factors are of particular importance for these decisions: (1) the desires of the intended populations and community leaders, and (2) the projected costs and benefits associated with intervening or not intervening for a particular group.

Consideration of the desires of intended populations requires the involvement of potential audiences in the design of health communication efforts. Campaign planners and implementers must have some measure of understanding, dialogue, and mutually accepted and shared practices with intended audiences (Gbadegesin, 1998) to ensure that the communication campaign addresses shared values and goals (rather than those imposed by implementers). Challenges in identifying relevant and representative group members and social authorities, as well as in determining the degree of consent required from a group prior to the initiation of health communication interventions, are explored in our discussion about the ethics of health communication in Chapter 7.

Audience Selection: Findings from Review

The majority of health communication campaigns reviewed by this committee selected intended target populations based on need. Need was generally identified through available epidemiological and public health data sources, which characterize audiences by demographic variables (e.g., ethnicity, gender, age, educational attainment, socioeconomic status). In some cases, campaigns relied on other quantitative data for the selection of audience segments, such as survey research assessing knowledge or attitudinal, psychological, psychosocial, or behavioral characteristics of audiences, in addition to the demographic and epidemiological data available from public health sources (see, e.g., Grelen, 2001).

For example, the National Air Bag and Seatbelt Safety Campaign used available data to identify its primary audiences based on populations at highest risk for morbidity and mortality associated with traffic accidents (i.e., first-time parents, young parents, new drivers, new vehicle buyers, and ethnic minorities). Similarly, the Depression Awareness, Recognition, and Treatment (D/ART) campaign commissioned scholarly papers and literature reviews, conducted focus groups with physicians and diverse members of the public, and used available demographic data (e.g., National Institute for Mental Health Epidemiologic Catchment Area study) to determine focus areas and populations of need (see, e.g., Murray and Lopez, 1996; Davidoff, 1998; Leo et al., 1999).

In other cases, intended audiences and specific health behaviors and health outcomes were chosen because of their priority status on the nation's health agenda, as defined by Healthy People 2010 (U.S. Department of Health and Human Services, 2000) and the Initiative to Eliminate Health Disparities (Geronimus et al., 1996). Such was the case for the National Diabetes Education Program, for example, which targets ethnically diverse audiences, who are disproportionately affected by diabetes and its complications (see Chapter 5 of this volume).

Some campaigns address needs of smaller population segments, then broaden their efforts. For example, the Folic Acid Campaign first focused on women of childbearing age who were contemplating pregnancy, then broadened its audience segments in phases. Eventually, the campaign conducted communication efforts for all women of childbearing age, with a particular focus on high-risk populations (Centers for Disease Control and Prevention, 1999). On the other hand, the National 5 A Day Campaign began broadly, with all adults not meeting the guidelines for fruit and vegetable consumption. As more was learned by developers about the population, the campaign became more targeted, focusing primarily on audiences who were already trying to eat more fruits and vegetables daily and felt guilty about their poor eating habits, but believed they could not change. The campaign became even more targeted when communication strategies began to target specific socially and ethnically diverse populations, in recognition of the need to address cultural and income differences in dietary habits. This targeting generally was done on a regional rather than a national basis (Van Duyn, 2000).

Such campaigns chose to make the tradeoff between size of audience and need, starting with broadly targeted campaigns, then later focusing more on targeted groups in greater need only after more resources became available to develop and disseminate subgroup-specific materials. The Back to Sleep Campaign, which at first targeted the full population, only later developed a targeted communication campaign for Native American/Alaskan Native populations, although this subgroup has had the highest rate of sudden infant death syndrome (SIDS) (National Center for Cultural Competence, 2000). Similarly, the Campaign to Prevent Teen Pregnancy began to complement its general audience campaign with a special campaign for Hispanic populations, who have the highest rates of teen pregnancy (Brown and Nightingale, 2000; DeJong and Winsten, 1998). Another example is the Milk Matters Campaign, which began with a general audience focus, and later focused on Hispanic audiences and those who are lactose intolerant, once it had the resources and capacity to do so (Adler, 1999).

Political advocacy groups and federal health goals (and funding allocations) also guided the selection of campaign topics and audiences. For example, the Best Start Loving Support Campaign began as a cooperative agreement between Best Start Social Marketing and various federal agencies such as Women, Infants and Children (WIC), a program conducted by the U.S. Department of Agriculture, and the Maternal and Child Health Program, sponsored by an association of state and local health officials. These agencies were supported by congressionally allocated funds to promote breastfeeding among participants in the Women, Infants and Child Health programs (see, e.g., Maryland Community and Public Health Administration, 2000). The National Anti-Drug Media Campaign was launched by the Office of National Drug Control Policy in response to the Treasury-Postal Appropriations Act of 1998, in which Congress approved funding for a national media campaign to reduce and prevent drug use among young Americans. The funding included a strong expectation that specific work would be done with ethnically diverse audiences, and that has been a hallmark of the campaign (Office of National Drug Control Policy, 2000; Johnston, O'Malley, and Bachman, 2001).

Antitobacco campaigns have had a strong mandate from their funders to focus on youth. The Florida Tobacco Pilot Program originated from the $200 million initially allocated from Florida's $11.3 billion settlement with the tobacco industry. These funds supported design and implementation of a state-run program to prevent and reduce youth tobacco use (Florida "truth" campaign). Similarly, the National Truth Campaign was launched as a result of the Master Settlement Agreement among 46 states, 5 U.S. territories, and the tobacco industry, which established the Legacy Foundation and a Public Education Fund to support the campaign. Although intended audiences were predetermined by the sponsor or funding source, most of the campaigns mentioned conducted their own public relations and marketing research to identify communication strategies to most effectively reach subgroups within the diverse audience segments selected (Massari, 2000).

Campaigns often include plans to shift or expand intended audiences over time as part of their communication objectives. For example, the Folic Acid Campaign uses a stage-market segmentation plan, whereby it broadens its audience segments in progressive phases, gradually including all women of childbearing age and focusing on those who are at highest risk.

Communication campaigns often redefine their intended audiences over time, as they learn more about their audiences. In several cases, campaign implementers identified audiences who were not responding to the general campaign communication strategies, and created separate or specialized campaigns for those audiences. This was made possible by good quantitative research before and during intervention implementation, which allowed for the diagnosis of disparities in effects. Two such campaigns include the Back to Sleep Campaign and the National High Blood Pressure Education Program, both of which used continuous tracking and evaluation to identify gaps in audience knowledge and behavior and to readjust campaign strategies. Throughout the course of implementation, the National High Blood Pressure Education Program gradually targeted new and expanded audiences, such as African-Americans, women, and specific age and income groups, among others (Roccella, 2002).

Selecting particular audiences for emphasis or recognizing that the audience for a campaign is heterogeneous is a first step. However, having recognized that heterogeneity, there are many ways that a campaign can adapt to the presence of differing groups in the audience. The process of adaptation is the focus of the next section.

ADAPTATION OF HEALTH COMMUNICATION CAMPAIGNS FOR DIVERSE AUDIENCES

A campaign is made up of many components. Each opens separate avenues for adaptation to segments of an audience. There are generally three broad approaches to adaptation.

1. Create a single campaign intended to affect most audiences by focusing on what is held in common across audiences. The common approach assumes that apparently heterogeneous audiences differ in some ways, but may share enough characteristics with regard to what influences their behavior, what media they can access, and what message executions will appeal to them so that a single campaign (with its lower costs) will be effective. (An example for an antitobacco campaign, much like the Truth campaign: Focus on not smoking so as to resist tobacco industry promotion of smoking; provide messages that suggest a multiethnic, united youth movement fighting against industry manipulation; use mainstream television channels and programs watched to some extent by most youth; use multiethnic actors and language broadly used by youth in all advertising.)

2. Create a common campaign with regard to behavioral targets and essential messages, but adapt it for different audiences by varying the primary diffusion channels and specific executions of messages. (For the antitobacco campaign, purchase extra exposures in media more heavily used by African-American or Hispanic

youth; develop ad executions that feature actors of those backgrounds, and use language particularly recognized in those communities.)

3. Create largely distinct campaigns for different subgroups, varying the behavioral focus, the essential message strategies, the channel choices, and the message executions. These campaigns make the opposite assumption from the first type—that groups are so heterogeneous that if they are to be affected by a campaign, it has to be adapted closely to their unique characteristics. (For the antitobacco campaign: If it were true that resistance to authority appeals to 14- to 16-year-old teens, and reluctance to violate parental expectations appeals to those of age 11 to 13, create distinct campaigns for the two groups with different message strategies focusing on resisting manipulation and avoiding parental disappointment, purchase media time on programs particularly appealing to each group, and use different actors and settings for the advertisements.)

Specific campaigns may not fit precisely within one of these categories. If they do fit in one of them early on, they may move from one category to another as they evolve. There is no a priori assumption that following one of these approaches is better than another. It is logical to assume that per person reached, campaigns in the first category are the least expensive, campaigns in the last category have the potential to be most effective. If there is a common theme that is influential for a wide spectrum of audiences and if funds are limited, it will be quite attractive to work on a common campaign. If audiences are much more distinct and resources are plentiful, discrete campaigns make sense. The decision on how to adapt should be made in the context of available resources, behavioral focus, and the degree of actual heterogeneity with regard to influences on behavior, access to channels, and projected responsiveness to different message executions.

All three of these models contrast with tailored communication programs that are adapted to reach *individuals* rather than groups. To tailor a message, a sample of the members of the intended audience completes an assessment. Based on their answers, individuals then receive a particular form of the message (Kreuter et al., 2000b). In principle, tailoring should produce messages that are superior to group messages, because variations in behaviors and beliefs within each diverse group would be reflected in the tailored messages, as would other individual differences. However, in the context of large-scale communication campaigns, particularly those that can achieve broad reach only with the use of mass media channels, tailoring is unlikely; in that circumstance, tailoring might be used as one aspect of a targeted communication campaign, such as for a small, very high-risk segment. Thus, a mass media campaign could be used to motivate people to call a toll-free number for help in quitting smoking. At that point, they would be sent individually tailored materials to deal with their smoking patterns and quitting experiences (Kreuter et al., 1999).

There is a strong logic to attending to segmentation and, as much as possible, developing a campaign that is responsive to such heterogeneity using any of the approaches just described. However, before we look at examples, a different perspective is worth considering. Much ongoing campaign theory argues for attention to segments. In the abstract, it is easy to see the advantage, but in practice, segmentation assumes it will be possible to sort through, in fairly precise ways, which approaches will work with what audiences, and to devise channel and message strategies that will fulfill those preferred approaches. In fact, turning segmentation arguments into practice may result in any of the following three problems.

1. Resources may not stretch to cover multiple targeted subcampaigns, even if using them is the best approach. The only viable heterogeneity strategy for some campaigns may be the common-denominator version.

2. Even if resources are sufficient to pay for some targeting, it is difficult to estimate how much of an advantage there is to a particular targeting approach, for message strategy, for channels purchase, or for message execution. Often, in practice, the re-

search base for making such decisions is limited. Adaptations may focus on channel strategies (given widely available media access information) or more superficial elements of message execution targeting (e.g., employing actors of the same race in advertising). Diversity-based differentiation of message strategies is rare because these strategies are more difficult to develop and justify (due to a lack of strong evidence).

3. The logic of making micro decisions about message strategies, channels, and message executions assumes that the major path to a campaign's effect runs through individual exposure to campaign messages. However, as outlined in Chapter 2 on theory, the paths to effect of some campaigns may reflect a different path of influence as well. To achieve sustained population behavior change, successful campaigns may require supportive environments and social norms. Their effects may reflect not just individual persuasion, but shifts in social norms. An ad that may be less personally persuasive to an individual may be more likely to generate public discussion about an issue. If people across diverse subgroups share reception of messages, there may be effects that are not merely the sum of the individual effects of personal exposure. Also, communication campaigns can target secondary and tertiary audiences in an attempt to create social, institutional, and policy changes that support health behavior.

Most communication campaigns address multifaceted health problems resulting from individual, social, environmental, economic, and political factors. Increasingly, campaigns are recognizing the need to intervene across multiple levels of influence in order to have a significant impact on the relevant health behavior and to sustain it at a national level. Multilevel campaigns implement strategies to address the multiple facets of the same health problem by targeting primary audiences (for individual behavior change), secondary audiences (such as health professionals who may, in turn, reach or influence primary audiences), and tertiary audiences (to modify broader sociopolitical systems that ultimately influence individual behaviors). Such campaigns might include communication efforts that focus on social influences (peers, families), public policy and environmental influences (policy makers, legislators, enforcement agencies), organizations (employers, labor unions), institutions (schools, religious affiliations, popular media), community elements (social, cultural, and community leaders), and the health care system (health professionals). The majority of campaigns reviewed for this volume focused on health professionals, not only as sources through which to disseminate health messages to the public and diverse subgroups, but also as targets for behavioral change to support modifications in the health care environment and health care delivery system.

Furthermore, many communication campaigns advocate changes and improvements to public policies by developing communication strategies intended for policy makers at the federal, state, or local levels. Various campaigns have collaborated with corporate leaders and employers to improve worksite environments. Efforts also have been implemented to promote campaign goals by targeting faith and community leaders as a strategy to indirectly affect culturally diverse populations.

Other campaigns have employed initiatives to change the popular media or to influence news coverage in attempts to influence social norms. Campaigns have sought to achieve these goals by promoting the dissemination of campaign messages (content placement) in popular media programming, ensuring accurate and factual depictions of the targeted health issue in the media through the provision of information and technical assistance, and using popular celebrities as campaign spokespersons. Additionally, some campaigns use media advocacy activities to change how the popular and news media address particular health issues in order to influence public policy.

These approaches can be consistent with a diversity-focused approach to campaign development; many campaigns focus on reaching out to policy communities with central concerns about diversity. However, the model of effect for these campaigns reflects a complex interaction of individual persuasion, social norm changes, and institutional shifts. The tradeoff for obtaining substantial attention from external institutions may mean some loss of control of messages. If Oprah Winfrey and Peter Jennings are to address an important health issue, they will not permit campaign planners to write their scripts. Great sensitivity to diversity in campaign planning may be feasible with regard to messages diffused directly by a campaign. In contrast, when social mobilization around an issue is the goal, and it requires working indirectly through other institutions, the goals and working routines of those other institutions may determine the outcome. Scarce campaign resources may be best spent on efforts to encourage institutional actors, including mass media, to focus on an issue. Resources spent on meticulous calibration of messages may prove less relevant to such social and institutional mobilization.

One example of the tradeoffs between diversity-focused versus generalized campaigns comes from the history of HIV/AIDS campaigns. It was an epidemiological fact that some behaviors put people at greatest risk of HIV infection. These behaviors were more common in some identifiable subgroups of the population, particularly men who have sex with men. There could have been an argument that the majority of campaign efforts should have focused on communities where many individuals' personal behavior put them at risk. Indeed, many efforts focused on gay men. However, in most countries, this was only one component of a more broadly focused HIV campaign, one that declared all members of society as at risk. This strategy may have reduced infection incidence, but whether it would have done so more effectively than a campaign that focused on those at highest risk is still a question. Nonetheless, it seems clear that framing risk as broadly present in society, rather than only belonging to certain marginalized subgroups, was associated with a broadened policy concern: more health research dollars, more legislation outlawing discrimination based on HIV status, and perhaps lessened stigmatization of people living with HIV. Indeed, absent the broad policy concern, resources for an alternative focused campaign might have been missing entirely.

We continue our discussion of diversity and addressing hetero-geneous audiences by presenting examples of how various cam-paigns have worked to reach the audiences. In doing so, we leave behind this alternative perspective on how campaigns have effects, and its somewhat chastening view about limits on how far one can and should go in implementing segmentation, or at least how help-ful a research base will be in informing the right choices.

Heterogeneity in Behaviors Addressed

Health campaigns can be refined for diverse audiences by adapting behavior change goals so that they are relevant, appro-priate, and appealing to diverse audiences. A variety of campaigns reviewed for this volume capitalized on communication efforts by promoting different behavioral goals among audience segments that differed with respect to their relation to the targeted behavior or health condition.

Recognizing that an individual's relationship and exposure to a specific health risk behavior is likely to change with lifecycle stage, many communication campaigns promote different behav-ioral goals based on the various age groups in the intended audi-ence. For example, the Florida Tobacco Pilot Program promotes different antismoking-related messages to youth, depending on their age and smoking status. The focus of messages ranges from the prevention of smoking initiation among younger teens and currently nonsmoking older youth to the discussion of smoking cessation techniques and strategies to maintain cessation among current smokers and older teens.

Furthermore, because individual, familial, and societal roles change with age, some campaigns promote different behaviors to adults and youth. In effect, the campaigns develop unique inter-ventions that focus on different aspects of the same health prob-lem. For the prevention of drug use, the National Youth Anti-Drug Media Campaign promotes messages about the rejection of drug use to youth and also promotes messages to adult role models, such as parents and teachers, about the need to monitor youth behavior. Similarly, the National Campaign to Prevent Teen Pregnancy communicates messages about sexual responsibility and advocates use of safer sexual behaviors to teens. In contrast, messages intended for parents stress the importance of having open discussions with their children about issues related to sex, including prevention of pregnancy and sexually transmitted diseases.

Heterogeneity in Causes and Correlates of Behavior (and Thus in Message Strategies)

Because perceived benefits and barriers to behavior change may differ across audience segments, effective communication campaigns for diverse audiences should be adapted to appropriately frame messages to address the audience's perceived risks, costs, benefits, and social pressures related to the desired behavior change. Several examples of campaigns from this review promote the same behavioral goal through different strategies for diverse populations, including the Folic Acid Campaign. This campaign has developed different communication materials for women, focusing on the more immediate benefits to infants among women contemplating pregnancy, and the longer term benefits for those not contemplating pregnancy. Similarly, the Campaign to Prevent Teen Pregnancy has different communication strategies and materials for teenage boys and girls, emphasizing gender-specific rewards and barriers.

The National Diabetes Education Program is adapted to address the major ethnic groups in the United States. Messages promote identified cultural values that encourage diabetes self-care (cultural incentives) and challenge cultural traditions that inhibit diabetes care-related behaviors (cultural barriers). For example, messages for Hispanics to control diabetes were developed to counter the fatalistic belief that diabetes complications are inevitable, and messages for Native American/Alaskan Native populations emphasize the importance of growing older to "be around" for younger generations and to pass on traditions (Centers for Disease Control and Prevention, 1999).

On the other hand, some campaigns use information about identified audience rewards and barriers to develop general communication strategies that will be effective across all intended populations, based on similarities across diverse groups. The Best Start Loving Support Campaign developed strategies to overcome common barriers to breastfeeding identified by the mothers in their audience (regardless of age and ethnicity), including embarrassment at breastfeeding in public; competing demands of work, school, and/or social life; and lack of social support. Furthermore, campaign messages promoted identified facilitators to breastfeeding behavior change, such as the close bond between mother and baby, relaxation, empowerment, and pride.

Heterogeneity in Channels and Settings for Diffusion of Messages

Channels include all the means for communicating with the audience, such as media, interpersonal sources, and settings and promotional events. The times, places, and states of mind in which different audience segments will be receptive to messages can vary dramatically. For example, churches and other religious organizations may be appropriate openings for target audiences who attend church regularly, but they would have no influence on those segments uninvolved in organized religion.

Because the most influential channels of communication may vary with the content of the health issue and characteristics of the intended audience, formative research typically is conducted to identify the most effective communication channels. Campaigns often choose to reach particular diverse groups through different channels. For electronic media, it is possible to change the timing and placement of messages to coincide with preferred programs, listening times, or Web-surfing activities. Campaigns attempting to reach Spanish-speaking audiences commonly translate materials for communication and dissemination through Spanish-language media. Similarly, campaigns targeted at Chinese, Japanese, and Korean Americans often use ethnic radio and newspapers, which appear to be available in many geographic areas of the country where high concentrations of these populations reside (National Heart, Lung, and Blood Institute, 2000).

Different age, gender, and income groups also tend to favor different media, so it is prudent when targeting by these characteristics to investigate which media are best for each group. For example, a smoking campaign in Vermont selectively placed television spots on one or another program based on formative research the developers conducted separately with each target group (e.g., young girls and young boys) (Worden et al., 1996). Similarly, a communication campaign may use billboards and store displays to reach low-income, inner-city dwellers, and newspapers to reach suburban households. Efforts to reach gay, lesbian, and bisexual populations often supplement mainstream media with publications geared to those groups.

The Internet now offers an additional channel of communication to promote campaign messages and goals in settings that are accessible to some consumers (home, library, cafes) during times that are convenient for them. Whereas national programs traditionally have used toll-free telephone lines to offer resources and publications, support or advice, information, program and policy updates, and, in some cases, referrals, communication campaigns now can offer these information services 24 hours a day, 7 days a week through the Internet. All ongoing campaigns in the current review have developed their own Web sites, most of which offer not only campaign information and resources, but provide links to other sources of information and related sites. Some campaigns offer sites in multiple languages. Issues of access, knowledge, skills, and use related to Internet health communications across diverse income, education, age, and ethnic groups are further explored in Chapter 6 of this volume.

The Internet has also afforded campaigns the opportunity to tailor communications[1] to individuals through regular e-mail up-

---

[1]Tailored messages are used most often in print channels, but also can be applied to CD-ROMs, the Internet, telephone counseling, and video kiosks (Kreuter et al., 2000b).

dates to Web site visitors (e.g., Folic Acid Campaign), tailored e-mails to campaign members or volunteers through electronic mailing lists (e.g., National Truth Campaign), and personalized reminders to promote the desired health behavior (e.g., annual mammogram reminders by the National Alliance of Breast Cancer Organizations). Some campaigns have developed Web sites that are responsive to the unique needs of diverse audience segments, such as the National Youth Anti-Drug Media Campaign, which offers content-based Web sites for parents (http://www.theantidrug.com), teens and "tweens" (http://www.freevibe.com), teachers (http://www.teachersguide.org), student journalists (http://www.StraightScoop.org), and other audience segments.

Heterogeneity in Message Executions

Message executions involve many specific decisions. Two important ones include the basis offered for the credibility of a promised reward and the image projected by a campaign. One important basis of credibility is the source or person(s) communicating the message. Different audience subgroups may find different sources of information to be persuasive. For example, scientific findings from an expert source may be the most important and credible evidence to one audience segment, while information on social norms from a peer may increase perceived self-efficacy and offer better support to another audience segment.

The source and support for messages may reflect the health issue or topic of communication as it is seen by a particular audience. Some issues may be naturally "medicalized" for a particular audience and thus there is a reliance on sources that offer immedi-

---

Most applications of tailored messages to date appear to use criteria other than diversity—broad demographic categories (Kreuter et al., 2000b). The types of criteria used most often are based on behaviors and beliefs derived from psychological theories of behavior change and may therefore meet criteria for attending to relevant aspects of cultural process.

ate expertise. Examples for some people might include having regular mammograms, increasing folic acid intake, improving diabetes self-care behaviors, and encouraging parents to place babies on their backs when sleeping. In contrast, the promotion of health behaviors that are for some people largely mediated by social influences and norms, such as teen pregnancy, tobacco and substance use, and breastfeeding, may be more credibly communicated through peer groups, family or community members, celebrity role models, or religious leaders. Finally, messages that attempt to achieve change in environmental issues or politically mediated public health problems, such as traffic safety or the sale of alcohol and cigarettes to minors, may be communicated most effectively through authority figures and representatives of law enforcement agencies.

Most of the health communication campaigns included in this review used multiple sources of support to most effectively reach the diverse segments of their intended audiences. As an example, the National Safe Kids "Get Into the Game" Campaign relies on relevant celebrities and spokespersons to enhance the impact of messages. Different sources are chosen to reach different age and gender groups. For example, to reach adult audiences, the Surgeon General, injury experts, and Al and Tipper Gore (when he was Vice President) were used as sources of support for campaign messages, while injured children and famous athletes were used to convey messages about safety to children (Cruz and Mickalide, 2000; National Safe Kids, 2000). Similarly, the National Campaign to Prevent Teen Pregnancy reaches a wide range of audiences through credible religious leaders, political leaders, health and research experts, popular and news media, and celebrities selected to be appropriate for populations of different ethnic, gender, and age groups.

The image projected by a health communication campaign is another important element that can be modified for diverse audiences. A health campaign's image often is referred to as its tone or personality. It can be developed through the type of format, style, music, characters, and so on that are used in the creative execution of messages. The tone of a message should "speak the language" of intended audiences. For example, a serious message using spokespersons in their late sixties more likely would be perceived as talking to an older target segment than would a trendy or hip message using today's rap stars. Even when the underlying message is the same, the way it is communicated may differ among audience segments.

Executions can vary their slogans, visuals, actors, language, and music, among other things. Perhaps the most common means of altering the image of a communication campaign to appeal to diverse audiences is to alter the language, terminology, or slang used in communications. This is easiest to accomplish with print materials (such as newspapers, magazines, and flyers) and televised public service announcements using a voice-over. For example, materials can be produced in Spanish, standard English, and inner-city slang.

Another option is to use the actors or models who look like members of the intended audience. Print materials for different ethnic groups, genders, and age groups frequently convey the intended audience by use of pictures. For example, the Best Start Social Marketing Service (a nonprofit organization working under a contract with the Centers for Disease Control and Prevention, or CDC) and the Loving Support Campaign (a CDC effort to promote breastfeeding) created billboards, posters, pamphlets, and mail inserts that featured photographs of people of different ethnic groups. The National Cancer Institute's Once A Year for A Life Time mammography campaigns combined graphics featuring women similar in appearance to the ethnic and age groups of intended audiences. Although the creation of television public service announcements is costly, a few campaigns have produced parallel executions for television aimed at different groups, such as the National Truth Campaign and the National Youth Anti-Drug Media Campaign, which produced separate advertising for African-American and Hispanic audiences.

Certainly, a wide range of creative efforts has been employed by communication campaigns to project appropriate images that are credible, attractive, and appropriate for intended audiences. Some campaigns have conducted extensive research to develop a consistent, carefully designed "signature" image or symbol (known as "product branding" in social marketing), which speaks the language and conveys the culture of the audiences of interest. Although these campaigns are in the minority, they have made exemplary efforts to portray trendy images that "speak the language" of their intended audiences, using creative products, interactive technologies, celebrity role models, high technology, and sometimes controversial advertisements to attract their attention. Examples include the National Truth Campaign, and its predecessor, the Florida Tobacco Pilot Program. The campaigns represent images of hip, empowered youth making healthy decisions for themselves. The cool, controversial, and rebellious images of the Florida and National Truth campaigns are further promoted through products (e.g., "Truth gear"), innovative events (e.g., "Rip It Out," teen truth tours, the "reel truth" advocacy campaign), and the Tobacco Memorial erected in Washington, D.C.

EVIDENCE THAT DIFFERENT APPROACHES TO DIVERSITY IN CAMPAIGNS HAVE DIFFERENTIAL SUCCESS

In the previous sections, we described the logic of addressing audience heterogeneity and provided a range of examples of how this has been done in practice. The logic of segmentation often makes sense. Now we ask: Have the particular ways that programs have addressed segmentation in practice proved productive? Is there evidence that paying attention to heterogeneity matters empirically, particularly with regard to the diversity categories featured in this volume?

This section begins with a discussion of what types of evidence would be telling in this regard. Next, it presents the evidence that is available. There will be a large gap between the type of evidence that would be telling and the published evidence base. As a result, we conclude the section by presenting an agenda for such diversity-related research, rather than a summary of what is known.

Good evidence exists that the periods of operation of some national campaigns have been associated with periods of improving overall levels of problematic health behaviors and health outcomes. The operation of the National High Blood Pressure Education Program (Roccella, 2002), National Cholesterol Education Program (2001), Back to Sleep Campaign (Willinger et al., 2000), the CDC AIDS campaign, several European AIDS campaigns (Wellings, 2002; Dubois-Arber et al., 1997), the urban vaccination campaign in the Philippines (Zimicki et al., 1994), and the California (Pierce, Emery, and Gilpin, 2002), Florida (Sly et al., 2001), and Massachusetts (Siegel and Biener, 2000) antitobacco campaigns all are associated with periods of sharp change in their target behaviors. Although simple association of trends over time with campaign initiation is not sufficient grounds for claiming a causal effect, many of the evaluations have additional reasons for attributing the observed change to their efforts. These include reports of high exposure to their messages, evidence for change in intermediate process variables that were the direct targets of the campaigns, and evidence that those reporting more exposure to the campaigns were particularly likely to change (Hornik, 2002).

However, evidence that some campaigns are associated with good outcomes is not evidence that their particular strategies for dealing with diversity were effective, particularly when compared with alternative approaches. What sort of evidence would be relevant to the diversity issue? We outline a variety of levels of evidence that might bear on this issue.

Evidence About Effects on Outcomes

Evidence That a Campaign Had Differential Outcomes for Subgroups of Its Target Audience

This evidence would require examination of the trajectories of the subgroups over the period of campaign operation. Presumably, this examination would focus on comparison between groups known for disparities at the start. The analysis would evaluate whether target groups differed in their rates of change, and if so which group was favored. This sort of analysis would provide useful information for an operating campaign because it would indicate whether what it was doing was affecting a known gap between groups. However, it would not indicate whether an alternative diversity strategy would be better or worse for this purpose.

Evidence That Different Diversity Strategies Produce Differences in Effect

Four strategies can be used to compare evidence, as described in the following paragraphs:

1. *Comparison across periods of the same campaign, when, for example, the campaign moved from a unified campaign strategy to one of multiple diversity-based substrategies.* The focus comparison would be whether the relative trajectories on outcomes were more favorable to the disadvantaged subgroup during one period than in the other. Such comparisons over time would be compelling if there were no other changes across the time periods. A particular concern would be that those who were slower to change are those who were the leftover targets for later time periods. This would happen if those individuals who were ready to change were shown to have been positively affected in the first campaign periods.

2. *Comparison across distinct campaigns with the same behavioral objective and broad target audience, but with different diversity strategies.* For example, if one state youth antitobacco campaign followed one diversity strategy and another followed a different one, how would the relative trajectories of the target subgroups vary? Again, this comparison would be telling if the comparison units (e.g., states) could be assumed to be otherwise similar.

3. *Comparison of distinct campaigns with the same behavioral objectives, but different diversity strategies, to examine*

whether they produce differential rates of change for the disadvantaged population. For example, a focused campaign to reach Native American populations to stimulate active care seeking for diabetes might begin operating soon after a national campaign with the same objective. Is there evidence that the focused campaign produces higher rates of care seeking among Native Americans than the national campaign, particularly in the context of relative costs per person reached?

4. *Comparison across campaigns that differ in diversity strategy, but also differ in other important aspects, such as in their behavioral foci (tobacco versus drugs; blood pressure versus cholesterol).* This evidence would be useful, but would depend on offering a credible argument that the other differences between the comparison campaigns were not so large as to confound the diversity differences. The credibility of claims based on this evidence would be greater if it was based on multiple comparisons rather than on just one comparison.

Evidence About Differential Effects on Process Variables

Evidence That Diverse Subgroups Respond Differentially to Message Strategies

The discussion about theory (Chapter 2) describes the basis for justifying the use of different message strategies for different subgroups. It argues that different strategies were justified when there was evidence that for specified groups, different sets of beliefs were predictive of their behavior. For example, for the youth antitobacco campaign, one subgroup's discussion about beginning to smoke might be related to its belief that a person's athletic endurance would be damaged by smoking. Another group might exhibit a stronger association of concerns about parental disapproval of their child starting to smoke. A campaign might develop messages that embodied each of those ideas, then they might be tested with members of both subgroups. The test could be done in a constrained way: asking subgroup members to evaluate the ads and their arguments, with an expectation that subgroups will identify the arguments in *their* ad to be more important and more likely to be persuasive. The test also could be done in a more elaborate way, relying on a pilot study with three arms: one of which used both ads, one of which used the preferred ad for each subgroup, and one of which used the not-preferred ad for each subgroup. The outcomes would be belief change with regard to the argument made and movement on intention to initiate smoking. The expectation would be that the "correctly targeted" strategy would be the best, and the "incorrectly targeted" strategy the worst, for all groups. However, any advantage of the "correctly targeted" strategy would have to be evaluated in the context of the possible additional costs associated with double production of materials and extra delivery resources required (e.g., broadcast time).

Evidence That Diversity-Based Targeting Produces Improved Campaign Exposure

Is there evidence that target groups reported more frequent exposure to messages when the channel strategy was targeted to maximize their exposure than when it was not? At some level this is not a controversial issue. In general, if campaigns use conventional channels, publicly available data (such as Nielsen ratings for television programs) can provide reasonable projections of exposure by important subgroups. Evaluations of alternative diversity strategies for channel selection are more interesting when:

• The issue has to do with the cost-efficiency of purchases— that is, whether the additional reach associated with targeted purchases justifies the additional expense of such purchases.

• The diversity strategy involves subgroups whose access to media is not available from publicly available data sources, such as groups who differ in sexual orientation.

• The channels being considered are not conventional ones, for example, if there were to be consideration of the tradeoff between relying on conventional media channels and institutional channels (churches, community groups) to reach out to the African-American community.

Examination of this evidence might begin with simple cross-group comparisons with regard to achieved reach overall and for each of the specific channels used. Comparison would begin with evidence about differential access to channels, but would include evidence of recall of messages transmitted over each channel, and perhaps reports that the exposure to the message produced subsequent conversation. As the first test described under the approaches to evaluating outcome effects of programs, this approach would provide useful information about what exposure was being achieved across diversity subgroups for a particular campaign. However, in isolation it would not indicate whether a different diversity channel strategy would improve relative exposure among groups.

Comparisons of diversity strategies might rely on the more elaborate comparison tests parallel to those described for the outcome analyses. They would be used with a focus on recalled exposure rather than effects on outcomes.

Evidence About Diversity Effects for Message Executions

There is an easy argument that subgroups will respond differently to messages with varying sources or with varying styles or images, even if the message strategy does not vary. On the other hand, every new execution adds to the cost of the campaign, and if it is meant to complement a differential channel purchase strategy, those additional costs can be substantial. The issue is not whether such varied executions would be helpful, but rather how much of such executional variation should be done, and the extent to which the advantage counterweighs the cost. What evidence might be useful to support targeting execution strategies rather than using a common-denominator execution strategy (e.g., having ads that feature boys and ads that feature girls versus ads that feature both)? Logically, the same sort of evidence that will be persuasive for message strategy variation also will be persuasive for message execution variation. At the simplest level, assessment of alternative executions across target subgroups will provide some picture of whether something can be gained. At the next level, systematic testing of alternative executions, on the model of the three-armed strategy test described earlier with belief change as the outcome, would provide a more credible and more expensive exploration of adapting to diversity in message executions.

These are the forms of evidence that would support decisions about how much and how to adapt communication campaigns to maximize effectiveness across diverse subgroups. For each of these types of evidence, what is the extent of the evidence base? Our review of the available documents suggests that the evidence base is quite limited. Most of the evidence that was found that bears directly on the diversity issue is evidence about differential effectiveness of existing campaigns across subgroups, responding to the question just asked. In addition, there is little evidence about differential reach of projects across important subgroups. We uncovered no evidence that systematically compared effectiveness across diversity strategies.

Evidence About Differential Effectiveness

Florida Tobacco Pilot Program

The ongoing Florida Tobacco Pilot Program (currently known as the National Truth Campaign) aims to reduce teen smoking through a wide variety of activities, including media promotion, in-school education, contests, and enforcement. Initial results are positive for both middle and high school youth. Rigorous tracking and ongoing outcome evaluations of the program have revealed that knowledge of tobacco possession laws increased for all grades and ethnic groups and both genders, while the number of middle and high school students who bought cigarettes decreased in the first 2 years of implementation. Importantly, current cigarette use declined significantly in both the first and second years of the campaign among middle and high school students, boys and girls, and non-Hispanic white, non-Hispanic Black, and Hispanic students (other ethnic groups not reported) (Florida Department of Health, 2000a). The overall rates of decline in Florida's teen smoking occurred at a significantly faster pace than that of the national average. Between 1998 and 2000, current cigarette use in Florida declined 54 percent among middle school students and 24 percent among high school students, though rates of decline varied by age, stage of smoking, ethnicity, gender, and geographic region. For example, there were greater reductions in cigarette use among high school girls (6.2 percent) than among high school boys (3.3 percent) (Florida Department of Health, 2000b). Why the campaign had less impact on high school boys than girls is unknown.

Variances in smoking rates among different ethnic groups also were found on several measures. In the first year of the campaign, cigarette smoking declined among non-Hispanic whites and non-Hispanic Blacks, but not among Hispanics and Native American/ Alaskan Native youth (Florida Department of Health, 2000a). By the second year, there was a decline among whites, Blacks, and Hispanics, with no figures reported for Native Americans (Florida Department of Health, 2000b).

National High Blood Pressure Education Program

The National High Blood Pressure Education Program was implemented with the goal of reducing the incidence of death and disability related to high blood pressure, including heart disease and stroke. The campaign assessed progress and program impact by conducting its own surveys and studies, evaluating the results of other major studies, and tracking national surveys such as the National Health Interview Survey and the National Ambulatory Index, among others. At the time of program initiation in 1972, less than one-fourth of the American population was aware of the relationship between hypertension and stroke or heart disease, and misperceptions about high blood pressure were widespread, despite the fact that one in six Americans suffered from the condition. Only 51 percent of people with hypertension were told by physicians that they had elevated blood pressure and only 16 percent of them were taking medication to control it.

After the first 5 years of campaign implementation, reports of the National High Blood Pressure Education Program indicated that 69 percent of survey respondents had learned something about high blood pressure and 30 percent of the general population believed they could define normal blood pressure, though this was true of more whites (33 percent) than African-Americans (18 percent). Subsequent communication efforts focused on African-American audiences and their physicians. By the end of the 1970s, hypertension awareness had increased among African-American men (from 41 to 66 percent) and African-American women (from 53 to 87 percent). Actual treatment rates for hypertension among African-Americans increased from 24 to 35 percent for men and from 40 to 63 percent for women. However, African-Americans were still less aware and less likely to be treated for high blood pressure when compared to their white counterparts.

By 1994, three-quarters of the American public reported having their blood pressure measured every 6 months. Significant improvements were observed in awareness and treatment of hypertension among those with hypertension (Cooper et al., 1997), and age-adjusted mortality rates had declined by 53 percent for coronary heart disease and 60 percent for stroke since the 1970s. Mortality declines were observed for both genders and for African-Americans and whites (National Heart, Lung, and Blood Institute, 2000). Although mortality rates for coronary heart disease have declined substantially for all groups, the greatest decline by 1994 was documented for white males and the smallest decline was evident for African-American males (National Heart, Lung, and Blood Institute, 2000).

By 1999, reports of the Behavioral Risk Factor Surveillance System (BRFSS) indicated that as little as 0.3 percent (median) of the general population had never had their blood pressure taken by a health professional, while the median prevalence of blood pressure screening in the past 6 months was nearly 75 percent (Behavioral Risk Factor Surveillance System, 1999b). Past 6-month prevalence of reported blood pressure screening was higher among women (78 percent) than men (70 percent) and increased with age, though there did not seem to be any significant differences by levels of income or educational attainment. Interestingly, African-Americans (79 percent) were most likely to have been screened for high blood pressure within the past 6 months, followed by whites (75 percent), Hispanics (69 percent), and all other ethnic groups (69 percent). Importantly, between 1986 and 1996, overall death rates from cardiovascular diseases decreased an additional 21 percent (American Heart Association, 1998); differences by ethnic group and gender are discussed in Chapter 1.

These impressive declines in high blood pressure and stroke rates closely match the timing of the National High Blood Pressure Education Program. In addition, evidence that some of the specific targets for the program (e.g., awareness and care seeking) were affected along with morbidity and mortality supports an argument that they are related to program efforts. However, the communication-specific program elements were only one component of the broad program, and the program itself operated as a complement to other changes in the environment. It is not possible to make any precise claims as to how much of the effects might have been lost absent the communication-specific elements of the program.

Back to Sleep Campaign

The Back to Sleep Campaign was launched in June 1994 to disseminate the recommendations of the American Academy of Pediatrics, advocating the back (supine) infant sleeping position to help reduce the risk of SIDS. Continuous evaluations to monitor changes in knowledge and behaviors regarding infant sleeping practices are available to the campaign through various surveys. These include the National Infant Sleep Position Study (NISP), an annual telephone survey of nighttime caregivers of infants under 8 months of age, and national surveys of the National Institute for Child Health and Development (NICHD), such as the National

Study of SIDS, which has evaluated sleep position practices since 1992 (Willinger et al., 1998). These ongoing assessments have allowed for the identification of high-risk populations and existing barriers to behavior change (National Institute for Child Health and Human Development, 1998; 2000).

Intermediate outcomes indicated that between 1994 and 1998, twice as many child caregivers (38 versus 79 percent) reported receiving the Back to Sleep recommendation from at least 1 of 4 sources (physician, nurse, reading materials, or radio and television) (NISP, 1998). Outcome measures have revealed a drop in prone sleep positioning among the general population, from 70 percent in 1992 to only 21 percent in 1997, with a corresponding drop in the incidence of SIDS rates of nearly 40 percent since 1992.

Between 1994 and 1998, stomach placement decreased 27 percentage points among whites but only 21 percentage points among African-Americans (Centers for Disease Control and Prevention, 1999). Overall, prone infant sleeping placement was 32 percent for African-Americans compared with 17 percent of whites in 1998 (Nagourney, 2000). Indeed, the gap between whites and African-Americans increased from a 9-percent difference in 1994 to a 17-percent difference in 1998. Lower rates of reduction in the incidence of SIDS have been noted among southern states and population groups of lower socioeconomic status, those living in either rural or inner-city environments, African-Americans, and Native Americans/Alaskan Natives. However, rates of change in sleep positioning behaviors have differed between Native Americans/Alaskan Natives and whites, suggesting that the continued high incidence of SIDS among the former group may be because of a higher prevalence of environmental risk factors (e.g., household smoke) in this population (Centers for Disease Control and Prevention, 1999).

Once A Year for A Lifetime

Mammography is among the few areas of health behavior where there is impressive evidence for a clear narrowing of the gap

TABLE 3-2 Mammography Use—Women 40 Years of Age and
Older (Health United States, 2001)

	Percent of Women Having a Mammogram in the Past 2 Years					
	1987	1990	1991	1993	1994	1998
White, Non-Hispanic	30.3	52.7	56.0	60.6	61.3	68.0
Black, Non-Hispanic	23.8	46.0	47.7	59.2	64.4	66.0
Hispanic	18.3	45.2	49.2	50.9	51.9	60.2

Health United States, 2001. Department of Health and Human Services. Centers for Disease Control and Prevention, National Center for Health Statistics.

between major ethnic and racial groups. Table 3-2 presents the proportion of women over age 40 who had mammograms in the previous 2 years between 1987 and 1998. A large gap in 1987 between African-Americans and whites had nearly disappeared by 1998, while the Hispanic to non-Hispanic gap had narrowed markedly, but remained. There were many changes in the environment, as well as a wide variety of other interventions operating during this period. Thus, the narrowing of the gaps may have many causes. Still, "Once A Year for A Lifetime," described in the Annex, is among those interventions that operated during this period. It is not possible to suggest how much of the closing of the gap, if any, can be attributed to the campaign. Still, it is a first step to be able to report an association between the period of the campaign and the period of the closing of the gap. Specific claims of attribution will need more elaborate evidence.

CONCLUSIONS

This review of the communication campaign literature has produced a variety of findings, some of which are assertions about what the committee found to be true, others of which are statements about what was not learned and needs to be better understood.

1. Nearly all campaigns recognize heterogeneity in the populations whose behavior is of concern. The populations are heterogeneous with regard to the current level of their behavior, the likely causes of their behavior and of behavior change, and the channels and message executions that will be effective in reaching them. Most campaign strategists, recognizing that this heterogeneity will likely make different groups differentially open to campaign influence, choose only some segments of the population for their focus. Sometimes the aspects of heterogeneity that differentiate segments will match the diversity categories of this volume, but often they will not.

2. Three broad approaches can be used in campaign message development to address heterogeneity. The first is to look for a common-denominator message that will be relevant across most populations. The second is to vary message executions to make them appeal to different segments, while retaining the same fundamental message strategy. The third is to develop distinct message strategies and/or interventions for each target segment. We assume that the first is the least costly and that the third is the most likely to be effective, although the third is often beyond the reach of many campaigns.

3. Although our survey of campaigns was limited, we believe that nearly all major campaigns plan, and most create, implementations recognizing segment differences. Many of those implementations involve differences in message executions and channels for racial and ethnic groups, for age groups, or for men and women. Perhaps fewer of those campaigns choose different behavioral targets and basic message strategies.

4. Little evidence has been published about the differential effectiveness of particular diversity strategies across groups. There is limited available evidence about the less subtle questions concerning the extent to which effectiveness of campaigns varied

across diverse groups. As often as not, this evidence shows equal responsiveness across target subgroups, although there are exceptions. However, given that these comparisons do not allow simultaneous comparison to diversity strategies and may not focus on the segments that were the targets of the campaigns, they are of only limited helpfulness. We do not know whether and to what extent the special considerations given by campaigns to diversity subgroups pay off.

RECOMMENDATIONS

These findings led the committee to make some essential recommendations both about the construction of communication campaigns and about what needs to be better understood.

1. There is an urgent need for evidence about differential effectiveness of campaigns in the context of particular diversity strategies. All campaigns, and most experts in health communication, act as if diversity matters. However, they do so with a remarkably thin evidence base about which ways of addressing diversity matter, and how much they matter given their cost.

2. It makes sense to segment a population under many circumstances, reflecting the recognition that populations vary in their behaviors and causes of behavior, as well as in the message executions that will appeal to them and the channels through which they can be reached. However, in choosing which segments are appropriate for a campaign focus, campaigns should clearly identify the rationale for the selection of the populations to be addressed, including ethical considerations. These rationales sometimes will lead to segment choices matching one or more of the diversity groups that are the focus of this volume; however, this will not always be true. Sometimes racial or ethnic groups, gender groups, and others will be quite heterogeneous with regard to a behavior and to their susceptibility to a message strategy. If other segmentation schemes better locate homogeneous groups for effective behavior change, they should be preferred.

3. There are alternative strategies for addressing multiple audiences, as already described; a particular program will need to choose its approach depending on what resources it has available for creating multiple campaigns and on the observed variation across populations with regard to behaviors and promising message strategies.

4. Research with consumers is an essential aspect of all health communication interventions. Campaigns need to be committed to systematic formative and statistically projectable monitoring research among different potential segments of the population. Such research is needed to understand the target audiences within their cultural context as a basis for designing effective communication strategies. The research should prove more productive if it is driven by theory, as described in Chapter 2. For example, behavior change theory will suggest what the potential causes of behavior are, and drive the search for appropriate message strategies.

ANNEX:
CHANGING HEALTH BEHAVIORS:
THE MAMMOGRAPHY CASE STUDY

In the late 1980s, most women in the United States were not getting regular mammograms. Over the past two decades, mammography screening rates have increased significantly for women age 40 and over across all races. Although it is difficult to ascribe causal relationships, one can make the case for associating increases in screening rates with national campaigns initiated at this time. The synergy of these often opportunistic national activities as well as a multitude of local interventions track with increases over time. Government agencies, nonprofits, activists, and corporations have played a role. Although there was considerable focus on communications to women, broad, multilevel strategies addressed research, screening guidelines, access to mammography services, insurance coverage, and changes in regulation, legislation, and judicial actions (e.g., malpractice suits). The multilevel efforts targeting individual, system, and environmental changes demonstrate the magnitude, scale, and duration of initiatives needed to achieve behavior change.

As the lead federal agency, the National Cancer Institute (NCI) had a central role in increasing mammography rates. In support of its screening guidelines, NCI launched a mammography campaign called Once A Year for A Life Time. The initial message strategy for the campaign encouraged all women age 50 and over to get annual mammograms, not only those who had found a lump or had a family history of breast cancer.

The NCI campaign used multiple materials and distribution channels. There were also distinct campaign executions to increase the relevance of the message to African-American and Hispanic audiences. Once a Year produced print background, media, and public education materials on breast cancer and mammography in English and Spanish. These were widely distributed to national community-based organizations and print media and made available through NCI's 1-800-4-CANCER telephone line. In partnership with the Susan G. Komen Foundation, NCI distributed television public service announcements featuring singer Nancy Wilson, placed the spots on two home video releases of movies with particular appeal to African-Americans (*Glory* and *Strapless*), and began a television publicity effort on Nancy Wilson's involvement.

NCI also began several major public-private partnerships to leverage additional resources. The campaign placed emphasis on reaching diverse audiences through celebrity involvement. One example was two half-hour television specials produced by Revlon/ University of California-Los Angeles' Women's Cancer Research Program. The programs differed not only in language, but also in the use of culturally specific settings and celebrities. Jane Pauley and actress Phylicia Rashad hosted the initial English version. The program was aired during prime time by NBC and its affiliates. The Spanish program, hosted by Edward James Olmos and Cristina Saralegui, a Spanish talk show host, was aired by Univision in more than 600 cities.

Additional strategies designed for African-American and Hispanic audiences included annual efforts for Minority Cancer Awareness Weeks and NCI's early detection campaigns—Spike Lee's Do the Right Thing and Una communidad saludable. Para toda una vida. NCI also worked with the YWCA and the Auxiliary of the National Medical Association to conduct community outreach with free and low-cost mammograms in poor urban areas.

At the same time, the Centers for Disease Control and Prevention (CDC) became active in improving access to mammography. In 1990, CDC block grants created the country's first national screening program for cervical and breast cancers. Nearly half of all screening tests provided have been for women of racial and ethnic minorities.

Activists played a key role in lobbying for regulatory changes and pressuring government agencies to put breast cancer high on their agendas. As noted, the Komen Foundation played a key role in NCI's early efforts, initiating White House Breast Cancer Summits and the successful Race for the Cure, the largest series of 5-kilometer runs/fitness walks in the world, raising more than $300 million.

In response to concerns that many providers were using mammography procedures of insufficient quality, Congress enacted the Mammography Quality Standards Act in 1992, requiring all mammography facilities to meet quality criteria in order to operate. The Food and Drug Administration now certifies all mammography facilities in accordance with the act. Important gains also have been made in insurance coverage. In 1985, only two states, Illinois and Virginia, required health insurers to cover the cost of screening mammograms. As of March 15, 2000, all but five states required some insurance coverage. Legislation also has been proposed for Medicaid coverage of annual mammograms and enhanced reimbursement under the Medicare program.

National Breast Cancer Awareness Month—originating as an effort by pharmaceutical companies—is another annual breast cancer awareness promotion, occurring every October. The most obvious activity is the pink ribbon signifying support for the fight against breast cancer. Breast Cancer Awareness Month is now sponsored by a variety of partners, including the American Cancer Society, American Society of Clinical Oncology, American Academy of Family Physicians, CDC, and NCI.

During the past decade, breast cancer became an appealing cause for many corporations to adopt as "good citizens." Avon has been one of the most notable. In 1991, it launched its pink ribbon campaign, selling pink ribbons through its catalog and sales representatives to raise funds for local community efforts such as mobile mammography vans and local education. In its first year, Avon raised $6 million. Avon continues to sell pink ribbon products today and supports a variety of breast cancer-related activities through its an annual 3-day walking event. General Electric, a manufacturer of mammography equipment, and Kellogg's were also among the early participants, running breast cancer awareness advertising in the early 1990s in support of their corporate positioning. Today, countless corporations involve themselves in breast cancer promotions and cause-related marketing. American Airlines, American Express, and Yoplait are only a few of the corporate partners helping the Komen Foundation to support its annual run.

The issue of mammography also has been kept alive by scientific disagreement over the benefits associated with screening. In 1993, debate occurred over the recommendations of when women should start getting mammography. For example, the American Cancer Society recommended baseline mammograms at age 35 in contrast to NCI recommendations. Scientific debates continue to play out in the media today, as researchers debate mammography and its ability to reduce mortality given new screening procedures and advanced forms of treatment (e.g., high-dose chemotherapy procedures).

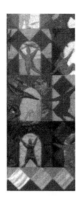

4

The Mammography Exemplar

WHY MAMMOGRAPHY IS A USEFUL EXEMPLAR

Strong evidence shows that health communication programs have played an important role in reducing disparities in mammography use among diverse groups. The committee chose mammography as an exemplar for this reason and several others. First, the risk of death from breast cancer, the most frequently diagnosed nonskin cancer among women in the United States, can be reduced significantly for women age 40 and older who get regular mammograms (see, e.g., National Institutes of Health Consensus Development Panel, 1997; American Cancer Society, 2001; Wingo, Calle, and McTiernan, 2000). Second, in 1987, when major promotions of mammography began, there were significant differences in use of mammography by age and ethnicity, including large disparities between African-American and white women. Over the past decade, these differences have been reduced so dramatically that national differences in screening rates for African-American, white, and Hispanic women no longer exist. Moreover, overall mortality from breast cancer has decreased, partially because of increases in screening (Wingo, Calle, and McTiernan, 2000).

A third reason mammography was chosen as an exemplar is because variations still exist in incidence and mortality rates by age and ethnicity that require further attention. For example, although incidence rates are higher for white women with higher incomes, African-American women and women who have low incomes and lower levels of education have the highest mortality rates from breast cancer—a finding that is attributed partially to delayed diagnosis. Figures 4-1 and 4-2 show breast cancer incidence and mortality rates by race and ethnicity (National Cancer Institute, 2002; Edwards et al., 2002). Recent data (Caplan, May,

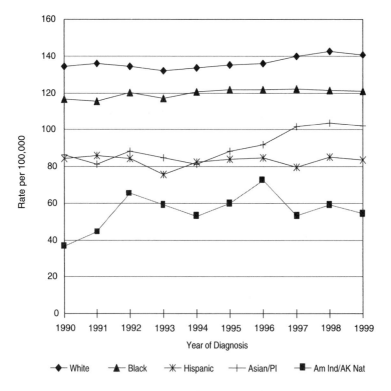

FIGURE 4-1 Breast cancer incidence rates by race/ethnicity, all ages. SOURCE: National Cancer Institute, 2002.

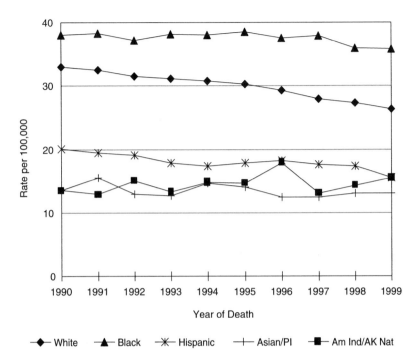

FIGURE 4-2 Breast cancer mortality rates by race/ethnicity, all ages. SOURCE: National Cancer Institute, 2002.

and Richardson, 2000) indicate that African-American and Hispanic women had the longest intervals between abnormal mammogram and diagnosis of breast cancer, while Asian women and women in the "other/unknown" category had the longest treatment intervals.

A fourth reason for choosing this exemplar is that important lessons from mammography may be applied successfully to other health behaviors. These include the effectiveness of simple interventions, such as tailored and untailored reminders and brief counseling, that are effective for all populations. The addition of access-enhancing interventions improves mammography outcomes for diverse populations.

Most important, there is an extensive literature on interventions and their effectiveness for increasing the use of mammography (e.g., Rimer, 1994; Snell and Buck, 1996; Wagner, 1998; Yabroff and Mandelblatt, 1999; Legler et al., 2002). This literature has three areas of strength: (1) studies have assessed a wide range of interventions both individually and in combination; (2) many of these interventions were grounded in behavioral and social science theory; and (3) many well-designed experiments have been conducted that provide solid outcome data. Moreover, many of the studies were directed toward or included diverse populations. When taken together, a strong case can be made for the effectiveness of several approaches to generally increase mammography use.

Although few studies were designed with enough statistical power to evaluate interventions in white versus diverse groups, a recent review of mammography-enhancing interventions for diverse women found that the same interventions that were effective for mainstream groups of women were effective for diverse groups, with the powerful exception of the addition of access-enhancing interventions for the latter group (Legler et al., 2002). Hundreds of useful mammography studies have been conducted. In this summary, we focus primarily on data from meta-analyses and other reviews of the intervention literature.

Before reviewing and assessing research on the design and evaluation of the interventions, we present a brief overview of (1) breast cancer incidence and mortality, with a focus on diverse populations, (2) the role of mammography in early detection and data on screening use, and (3) the common and culturally specific behavioral, geographic, and economic barriers to mammography use identified in the literature.

THE EFFECT OF BREAST CANCER
ON DIVERSE POPULATIONS

In 2001, there were 203,500 new cases of invasive breast cancer and 40,000 deaths from breast cancer among women (American Cancer Society, 2001). These cases are disproportionately distributed by age and ethnicity, as can be seen from the National Cancer Institute's Surveillance, Epidemiology, and End Results (SEER) data and mortality data from the National Center for Health Statistics (National Cancer Institute, 2002) (see Figures 4-1 and 4-2). For example, more than three-fourths of all breast cancers are diagnosed in women age 50 and older (American Cancer Society, 2002). White women have the highest incidence rate for every age group, while Native American, Aleutian Islander, and Alaskan Native women are least likely to develop breast cancer (see Figure 4-1).

Although the racial/ethnic patterns for mortality differ only slightly from incidence patterns, the highest mortality rates are found among African-Americans, followed by white and Hispanic women (see Figure 4-2). SEER data from the National Cancer Institute (http://www.seer.cancer.gov/) suggest that the higher mortality rate for African-American women is partially because their cancer tends to be diagnosed later, when cancer is less amenable to cure (National Cancer Institute, 2002).

Progress is being made in the fight against breast cancer. In the last period for which comparisons were made, 1987–1999, there was a 0.5 annual percentage change (APC) in breast cancer incidence; the incidence increased, partially because of continued increases in mammography use. The incidence increase was 0.4 APC for whites and 0.9 APC for African-Americans (Edwards et al., 2002). In part, this probably reflects the somewhat later adoption of mammography by African-American women. From 1990 to 1998, breast cancer-related death rates decreased for white women (2.5 percent per year) and Hispanic women (1.2 percent per year), and did not change for African-American, Native American/Alaskan Native, and Asian/Pacific Islander women (Garguilly et al., 2002). In the latest statistics, from 1995 to 1999, breast cancer mortality decreased 3.2 percent per year for all ages, 3.5 percent per year for whites, and 1.2 percent per year for African-Americans (1993 to 1999). This reflects important improvement in reducing deaths from breast cancer.

THE ROLE OF SCREENING MAMMOGRAPHY
IN THE EARLY DETECTION OF BREAST CANCER

Screening mammography is the most effective method for early detection of breast cancer (National Institutes of Health Consensus Development Panel, 1997). Strong evidence from randomized, controlled trials conducted around the world shows that regular screening mammograms can reduce breast cancer mortality by about 30 percent for women in their 50s and by 17 percent for women in their 40s (Hendrick et al., 1997; Berry, 1998). Thus, regular screening mammography is now recommended by most medical organizations for women age 40 and older (see, e.g., American Cancer Society, 2001; Eastman, 1997). Controversy remains, however, fueled most recently by a *Lancet* meta-analysis (Olsen and Gatzsche, 2001) that found no benefit from mammography for women of any age. However, reviews of this report have been conducted by the National Cancer Institute, the American Cancer Society, and other organizations. Despite the announcement that the U.S. Preventive Services Task Force will recommend regularly scheduled mammography for women age 40 and over, there is not widespread agreement among medical organizations that regular mammography should be recommended for women in that age group. Major efforts to promote screening mammography have been underway since 1987, with lead roles played by the American Cancer Society, National Cancer Institute, Centers for Disease Control and Prevention, associations of health professionals, and consumer advocacy groups, such as the Susan G. Komen Foundation and the National Alliance of Breast Cancer Organizations.

Since 1987, the proportion of women age 40 and over who report receiving regular mammograms has increased dramatically. The proportion of women age 40 and older who had a mammogram in the previous 2 years increased from 29 percent in 1987 to 68 percent in 1998. For women ages 50 to 64, the proportion increased from 34 percent to slightly over 75 percent during the same time interval (Breen et al., 2001). Data for 1998 show that mammography use is now similar nationally for all ethnic groups— 68 percent for white women; 66 percent for African-American women; and 60 percent for Hispanic women. Increased use of mammography from 1987 to 1998 is also evident for different age groups, with the most striking changes noted among women over 60, whose rates have nearly tripled. However, some important disparities remain. For example, Wu, Black, and Markides (2001) recently reported that older Hispanic women were less likely than other women to have had recent mammograms and Pap tests.

However, there are still cultural groups for whom mammography use is lower. For example, in some areas of the United States, Hispanic women are less likely to have mammograms than women of other racial/ethnic groups (Breen et al., 2001). Recent immigrants also have lower use. In some areas of the country, such as eastern North Carolina, African-American women have lower rates of screening (e.g., O'Malley et al., 2001). A recent analysis of Behavioral Risk Factor Surveillance System (BRFSS) data with a focus on Appalachian women found that rates of mammography use were slightly below the U.S. population. Women over age 60, those with less than a high school education, and women who had not seen a doctor in the past year were also less likely to have had mammograms (Hall et al., 2002). Coughlin and Uhler (2002) reported BRFSS data from the United States and Puerto Rico for Hispanic women. The findings were similar in terms both of proportion screened and the variables that predicted underutilization. These data highlight the importance of educational and economic characteristics as determinants of screening. As Coughlin and Uhler stressed, more efforts are needed to provide access to services for the medically underserved.

The lowest mammography rates currently are found among women who have low incomes (rates are between 43 and 54 percent, depending on age) and who do not have high school diplomas (between 47 and 58 percent, depending on age). For example, women age 50 and older who live below the poverty line are 21 percent less likely than women living above the poverty line to have had a mammogram in the previous 2 years. Also, women in this age group who do not have a high school education are 20 percent less likely to have had a mammogram in the previous 2 years compared to women with a high school education or higher (Breen et al., 2001). Screening rates are also lower among women who lack health insurance. There are other predictors of screening rates, but these are among the most important. However, in spite of the remarkable increase in the proportion of women who report ever having had mammograms, as well as having had recent mammograms, most women still are not getting regular mammograms (Breen et al., 2001).

PREDICTORS OF MAMMOGRAPHY USE IN MAINSTREAM AND DIVERSE POPULATIONS

This volume presents an integrative model that summarizes key concepts from various behavioral theories (see Chapter 2). We use this theoretical model to highlight the factors that have been important in predicting use of mammography. We examined the factors that seem to be shared across diverse populations as well as those that appear to be unique to one or more groups. Understanding these issues is important to determine whether audience segmentation is needed for diverse populations. We focus our discussion on three elements of the integrative model that have the most relevance for mammography use: (1) attitudes and beliefs toward mammography screening; (2) perceived norms; and (3) environmental influences. The literature on predictors of mammography has less to say about the role of self-efficacy (personal agency), intention, and skills in women's compliance with recommendations on screening mammography. This is partly because, unlike changing diet, mammography, while volitional, is primarily under the control of health professionals. Some studies (e.g., Ryan et al., 2001) have asked women if they feel confident they could get a mammogram if they wanted to do so and have provided tailored advice in this area.

Our review and analysis of the literature on factors that influence the use of screening mammography are organized in accordance with this integrative model. We covered a large number of peer-reviewed articles published between 1985 and 2000, with a focus on identifying variations among diverse groups. As noted earlier, although we reviewed articles that reported the results of individual studies, as well as meta-analyses, this chapter relies primarily on meta-analyses and reviews. There are a series of well-executed reviews that cover the literature. As the sections to follow show, many similarities exist between the general population and diverse groups in terms of their response to communication interventions. In fact, there are many more similarities than differences. In general, there are probably as many variations among women in any ethnic, income, or other group as between groups. Where differences were identified, they will be highlighted.

Attitudes and Beliefs

Knowledge, attitudes, beliefs, and behaviors are important factors that motivate people to take appropriate health actions. Most theories agree that getting a mammogram is partly a function of one's beliefs that performing the behavior will lead to certain outcomes. It is assumed that a person will not perform a behavior (or form an intention) if the costs of performing the behavior outweigh the benefits. Thus, the most commonly used models in some way assess women's perceived pros and cons or their perceptions of the benefits of and barriers to getting mammograms. Knowledge is a part of some behavioral theories, such as the Health Belief Model (Strecher and Rosenstock, 1996), and has been a consistent predictor of mammography use.

In 1987, when mammography use was significantly lower than it is today for all groups of women, the National Health Interview Survey reported that the most common reasons women gave for not having mammograms were (1) they had not thought about it; (2) it was not necessary because there were no problems/no symptoms; and (3) it had not been recommended by a physician (Rimer, 1994). Overall nationally, these are the most important attitudes and beliefs about mammography, regardless of age, ethnicity, income, or education, although some regional differences exist. Mammography use is higher among women who understand the purpose of mammography, especially its value in the absence of symptoms, and the recommended age-based intervals (McDonald et al., 1999; Lee et al., 1999; Maxwell, Bastani, and Warda, 1997, 1998a, 1998b; Wismer et al., 1998; Fernandez, Tortolero-Luna, and Gold, 1998; Rimer, 1994). This is true across populations, including African-American and Hispanic women (e.g., Valdez et al., 2001). Older women who recognize that age is the most important risk factor for breast cancer and that older women are more likely to get breast cancer are more likely to report having had mammograms (Fox, Murata, and Stein, 1991; Fox, Roetzheim, and Kington, 1997). Similarly, physician knowledge of screening recommendations is an important predictor of physician practices, although this factor has received less attention in the literature (Fox, Roetzheim, and Kington, 1997).

A recent report indicated that Hispanic women were more likely than non-Hispanic women to agree with the statement that *once you get cancer you will always die from it* (Puschel et al., 2001). Health providers reported that Hispanic women were more likely than non-Hispanic women to resist breast exams, which providers ascribed to women's fears of anything that might threaten their integrity as women (Puschel et al., 2001). Other studies have shown that older Hispanic women know less about breast cancer screening than other women (Puschel et al., 2001; Calle et al., 1993; Lantz et al., 1994; Stein and Fox, 1990; Fox et al., 1998). Most recently, Valdez et al. (2001) showed that Hispanic women who were more fearful were less likely to have had recent mammograms. In general, the low levels of knowledge about cancer screening among Hispanic women are more likely to be accounted for by socioeconomic factors, such as low education and low income, than by acculturation, language, or ethnicity (Zambrana et al., 1999; Schur, Leigh, and Berk, 1995; Fox and Roetzheim, 1994). Indeed, language is not a major barrier to screening if health care is accessible (Zambrana et al., 1999).

Further evidence of the role of cultural beliefs in women's decisions to have a mammogram has been observed across cultural groups, including a reluctance to use Western health care among Chinese-American women (Facione, Giancarlo, and Chan, 2000); cultural beliefs about fate among Filipino Americans (Maxwell, Bastani, and Warda, 1997) or karma among Cambodian-American women (Taylor et al., 1999b); concerns about modesty (Schulmeister and Lifsey, 1999; Dibble, Vanoni, and Miaskowski, 1997; Kelly et al., 1996); and beliefs that breast cancer is tied to guilt and punishment among Arabian women (Brushin, Gonzalez, and Payne, 1997).

Perceived Norms

The factors discussed in this section include perceived norms about mammography—influences from providers of health care services, family, and community groups. Norms include the overall perception about what most "important" others are saying and doing about the behavior. According to a number of reviews (Snell and Buck, 1996; Wagner, 1998; Rimer, 1994; Rimer et al., 2000a), the strongest predictor of mammography use is a recommendation or referral from a physician, arguably the most "important other" in relation to recommended medical practices such as mammography. This finding is consistent across all ethnic and age groups (Burack and Liang, 1989; McDonald et al., 1999; Maxwell, Bastani, and Warda, 1997; Risendal et al., 1999; O'Malley et al., 1999). Moreover, this finding has been robust over time. Valdez et al. (2001) reported the importance of a doctor recommendation for low-income Hispanic women. Some studies indicate that women in lower socioeconomic areas who receive their health care from emergency rooms and clinics are less likely to be advised to have mammography recommended by their health care providers (Snell and Buck, 1996). O'Malley et al. (2001) noted that only about half the women in their study of low-income women in North Carolina reported that their physicians had advised them to have mammograms. White women were more likely to report such recommendations than African-American women (55 percent versus 45 percent, odds ratio = 1.49). When education and income were controlled, the race difference disappeared. However, socioeconomic characteristics were related strongly to use of mammography.

A number of studies conducted in community health centers indicate that women in these settings are being screened at higher rates than the general population (e.g., Rimer et al., 1996; Zapka et al., 1993). Lower screening rates are found for Asians/Pacific Islanders who are treated by physicians of similar origin. Perhaps their providers reinforce the cultural belief that screening is needed only when changes in the breast are found through clinical examination (McPhee, 1997a, 1997b; Wismer et al., 1998). Thus, there is variation in the proportion of diverse women who report being advised by their providers to get mammograms. Women who have regular providers, including those at community health centers, are more likely to report having had mammograms when their providers advised them to do so. Also, women who report more physician visits are more likely to report having had mammograms (Wu, Black, and Markides, 2001). This is understandable because more visits may represent more opportunities to make a recommendation about and referral for mammography.

The patients' ability to communicate effectively with their providers about cancer screening also influences screening practices. Patient age, for example, influences communication with physicians. Physicians are less likely to recommend screening mammography to older patients than to younger patients (Fox, Roetzheim, and Kington, 1997).

Another important factor in encouraging the use of breast cancer screening by women is the behavior of people around them— that is, the norms for performing the behavior within women's social networks. Women who perceive that more of their friends and relatives had mammograms are more likely to have mammograms themselves (e.g., Rimer, 1994; Kang and Bloom, 1993; King et al., 1993). This finding is consistent across age, ethnic, and other diverse characteristics. One study found that Asians were more likely to have screening mammograms if they perceived that family and friends were also having them and were supportive (Maxwell, Bastani, and Warda, 1997). Another study suggested that African-American women with large social networks were more likely to have mammograms than those without large networks (Kang, Bloom, and Romano, 1994). The way in which larger networks may operate to increase mammography use is not well understood.

Environmental Influences

A range of environmental influences may either pose barriers to or facilitate women's use of mammography screening. Lack of access is the most important environmental influence for women with a lower socioeconomic status, especially those who live in rural areas (Breen et al., 2001). These findings are confirmed across all ethnic groups (Mickey et al., 1995; Pinhey, Iverson, and Workman, 1994; Serxner and Chung, 1992; Morgan, Park, and Cortes, 1995). One study (Kreher et al., 1995) reported that urban and rural women did not differ in their expressed intent to have mammograms in the next 2 years, but nearly twice as many urban women as rural women reported having had mammograms. Similar concerns have been observed for other groups as well; Kelly and colleagues (1996) reported that barriers for Cambodian women who should be getting mammograms included lack of transportation and fear of a large, technical medical center.

Indeed, access also may involve issues of comfort with health care systems. Women who do not speak English may have difficulty navigating the health care system, as shown by Morgan, Park, and Cortes (1995) in a study conducted on disadvantaged Hispanic women living in Bronx, New York. Foreign-born Hispanic women who are recent immigrants to the United States (and who have low levels of acculturation) are less likely to use mammography than Hispanics who have lived here for some time (O'Malley et al., 1999). Access factors may account for these differences, however. Indeed, access to screening appears to be a stronger predictor of screening than language and ethnic factors—indicators of acculturation. Like all women, Hispanic women with access to health care are more likely to be screened than are women without access to health care. A disproportionate percentage of Hispanic women, however, are low income; Hispanics are also more likely to report health insurance inadequacies and poorer quality of life, factors that are likely to interfere with maintenance of screening behaviors (Fox and Roetzheim, 1994; Zambrana et al., 1999). Nonetheless, whereas financial costs and inadequate reimbursement are barriers to screening, interventions directed only at screening costs have not been particularly effective in the absence of patient education. Indeed, even when the poor have adequate health insurance, they encounter more barriers to screening than upper income groups (Fox, Roetzheim, and Kington, 1997).

It is important to consider the assets and resources on which women of diverse groups may draw. As noted in the following sections, interventions can be designed to build environmental supports for screening. System-directed, access-enhancing, and policy-directed interventions provide important means of building these supports; indeed, access-enhancing strategies, including the provision of transportation or free mammograms, play a particularly crucial role in increasing screening rates.

THE IMPACT OF MAMMOGRAPHY-ENHANCING INTERVENTIONS ON DIVERSE POPULATIONS

This section provides a brief overview of the major findings on interventions designed to facilitate use of mammography screening. In 1994, Rimer reviewed the trends in interventions in the United States in the following areas: mass media campaigns (e.g., A Sa Salud project), individual directed (e.g., letters from physicians, mailed reminders, telephone counseling, posters), system directed (e.g., systemwide prompts, computer-generated reminders), access enhancing (e.g., mobile vans, special programs with cost subsidies), social networks (e.g., community-based programs such as Save Our Sisters), policy directed (e.g., changes in regulations), and various combinations of the strategies listed. Selected interventions in each of these areas have made a positive impact on mammography use. This review places health communication interventions, such as mass media campaigns and individual-directed communication, in the broader context of public health interventions, including those aimed at contextual influences and environmental constraints.

As discussed throughout this volume, broad groupings—such as by race, ethnicity, or age—provide little information on which to base intervention development. Rather, women's life experiences and social contexts, regardless of their age or ethnicity, play important roles in their attitudes and beliefs toward mammograms, in the social norms and environmental constraints they experience, and in the potential impacts of health communications. It is important to incorporate this information into the development of interventions for diverse groups of women. For example, understanding and addressing women's barriers to and concerns about screening have contributed to effective interventions delivered to shoppers at Asian grocery stores (Sadler et al., 2000) and among Cambodian women (Kelly et al., 1996).

Meta-Analysis Methods

We relied on meta-analyses conducted by Meissner et al. (1998) and Legler et al. (2002) for this review; other reviews and meta-analyses provided confirmatory information (Yabroff and Mandelblatt, 1999; Yabroff et al., 2001; Bonfill et al., 2001).

Meissner et al. (1998) used Rimer's (Rimer et al., 2000a) categories to examine the critical elements included in the published literature on breast and cervical cancer interventions. Of 528 studies identified, 58 screening mammography articles met the inclusion criteria: (1) the study measured the impact of an intervention to increase use of mammography and/or Pap smears in asymptomatic populations, and (2) the study focused on mammography; those focusing exclusively on breast exams (self or clinical) or an abnormal finding were eliminated. For each study, Meissner and colleagues assessed the presence and quality of the reported needs assessment, intervention, study design, analysis methods, and study outcomes, specifically:

- From 1960 to 1997, most studies were system/physician directed, individual directed, and access enhancing. There was one social network intervention, and no policy interventions.
- Of the 58 studies, 21 were based on a behavioral theory. The largest number used the Health Behavior Model, followed by Social Learning Theory and the Stages of Change Model.
- Studies were conducted in 20 of the 52 states and territories.

Legler et al. (2002) conducted a meta-analysis to determine which types of mammography-enhancing interventions are most effective for groups of women with historically lower use of mammography. The groups include the following categories under the label "diverse": high school education or less; low income (defined by study authors); ethnic or racial group; age 60 or older; and/or living in a rural or inner-city area. Studies in any of these categories potentially were eligible for inclusion if they met other inclusion criteria as well. Ideally, one would want to compare the same interventions for diverse and mainstream populations, but the studies were not constructed to facilitate such analyses. Based on principles of targeting and tailoring, the interventions developed for diverse women often have had elements or nuances specific to those populations. Similarly, interventions developed for mainstream populations may have had insufficient numbers of diverse women for subgroup analyses. Here we first present the results of a meta-analysis to answer the following question: *What is the effectiveness of different mammography-enhancing interventions for specific populations of diverse women?* Then, we compare these results to the more general mammography meta-analysis literature in order to extract some lessons about how intervention effectiveness varies when the general literature is compared to that for diverse populations.

The methods for the meta-analysis are described more fully elsewhere (see Meissner et al., 1998, and Legler et al., 2002). Briefly, using accepted meta-analytic methods, the authors conducted extensive searches of the literature, then constructed a database of the 51 studies that focused on breast cancer screening. Articles that were retained in the analysis were those that met the following criteria:

- Objectives were to increase use of mammography among asymptomatic women in diverse populations;
- Reports of intervention outcomes were based on actual receipt of mammograms, either by self-report or verified report in a clinical database or medical record; and
- Studies used experimental or quasi-experimental designs.

Ultimately, 38 controlled, experimental, and quasi-experimental interventions that specifically focused on or reported separate mammography outcomes for diverse populations were included in the meta-analyses.

Interventions were categorized according to Rimer's (Rimer, 1994; Meissner et al., 1998; Rimer et al., 2000a) typology: access enhancing (e.g., transportation to appointments, mobile vans, vouchers, and reduced-cost mammograms), system directed (e.g., provider prompts), individual directed (e.g., one-on-one counseling, tailored and untailored letters and reminders, telephone counseling), community education, social network (e.g., peer leaders, lay health advisors), mass media, and multistrategy interventions (see Table 4-1).

The outcomes were study-specific adherence rates. The definition of adherence was provided by each study author. This allowed for the inclusion of a wider range of studies both with respect to followup time and study type. Because the field has been evolving, definitions have changed over time. Generally, study outcomes typically were described as obtaining a mammogram within a specified number of months; the time period varied from study to study.

TABLE 4-1 Estimated Intervention Effects

| Intervention Type | Number of Studies | Combined Estimate Difference | | Combined Estimate Odds Ratio (95-percent confidence interval[a]) |
		Unadjusted (95-percent confidence interval[a])	Adjusted for Months[b]	
Access enhancing[c]	14	18.9 (10.4, 27.4)	16.5	2.3 (1.7, 3.1)
Individual directed associated with a health care setting	15	17.6 (11.6, 24.0)	14.1	2.5 (1.9, 3.4)
Individual directed associated with a community setting	13	6.8 (1.8, 11.8)	7.0	1.3 (1.0, 1.6)
Community education[a]	14	9.7 (3.9, 15.6)	10.4	1.5 (1.2, 1.9)
Media Campaigns[a]	6	5.9 (0.3, 11.5)	11.4	1.3 (1.0, 1.8)
Social Network[a]	7	5.8 (-0.2, 11.9)	13.0	1.4 (1.0, 2.0)

Estimated combined effect sizes with confidence limits for each intervention type. Random effects models. Studies may be classified as implementing more than one type of intervention. Entire group comparisons for primary outcomes.

[a]Confidence intervals only approximate because cluster randomization is not taken into account.
[b]Model includes outcome months.
[c]Control groups do not include strategies of the same intervention type.

Results of Meta-Analysis for Diverse Populations

As the preceding sections of this chapter demonstrate, many effective interventions have been developed over the past decade. A substantial body of research has focused on identifying and overcoming women's, physicians', and system barriers to mammography (e.g., Rimer et al., 2000a; Meissner et al., 1998; Calle et al., 1993; Clemow et al., 2000; Fox, Roetzheim, and Kington, 1997; Hiatt and Pasick, 1996; Lane et al., 2000; Rimer, 1994; Vernon, Laville, and Jackson, 1990; Yabroff and Mandelblatt, 1999; Mandelblatt and Yabroff, 1999; Bonfill et al., 2001; Yabroff et al., 2001; Sin and Leger, 1999). In addition, there have been striking gains in U.S. mammography use by age-eligible women (Martin et al., 1996; Breen and Kessler, 1994).

A reasonable question is whether the interventions that have been developed to date for mainstream populations are effective for diverse populations of women. Often an assumption is made that special interventions are needed for diverse populations—that is, that health communications to segmented audiences will be more effective than generic communications. It is important to examine the data because the development of special interventions requires resources that many communities lack. Several recent meta-analyses of mammography interventions have shown that relatively simple interventions, such as reminder letters, telephone calls, and counseling, increase mammography use across population groups (Yabroff and Mandelblatt, 1999; Mandelblatt and Yabroff, 1999; Snell and Buck, 1996; Wagner, 1998). This is an important finding. However, the meta-analyses conducted to date have not focused on strategies most effective for diverse groups of women. Several authors of the meta-analyses mentioned this and called for a greater focus on diverse populations (Yabroff and Mandelblatt, 1999; Snell and Buck, 1996; Wagner, 1998; Bonfill et al., 2001). However, until recently, there were not enough studies to permit analyses by various subgroups.

Table 4-1 shows mammography effects by intervention type. Access-enhancing interventions had the greatest impact on mammography use, with an estimated intervention effect of 18.9 percent (95-percent confidence interval [CI]: 10.4-27.4; 14 studies). These studies all used multiple types of interventions; the majority involved some form of person-to-person contact in addition to access-enhancing strategies, such as mobile vans, transportation to appointments, facilitated appointments, and vouchers for low-cost or free mammograms. A recent report by Segura et al. (2001) supports this conclusion. The authors found that for low-income women in Spain, the combination of a personal letter of invitation and direct contact with women in their homes by a trained woman of similar age was most effective in motivating women to get mammograms.

The magnitude of the impact of individual-directed interventions in health care settings was nearly identical to that of access-enhancing strategies, with an estimated effect of 17.6 percent (95-percent CI: 11.6-24.0; 15 studies) (see Table 4-1). Individual-directed efforts in community settings yielded effects of 6.8 percent (95 percent CI: 1.8-11.8; 13 studies), whereas effect sizes for community education, media campaigns, and social network were 9.7 percent, 5.9 percent, and 5.8 percent based on 14, 6, and 7 studies, respectively.

The use of multiple intervention types was effective, with intervention effects averaging 13.3 percent overall (95-percent CI: 8.6-18.0; 26 studies). With the exception of social network interventions, the estimated intervention effects were significantly greater than zero for all of the groupings. However, each grouping exhibited significant heterogeneity. The most effective combination of intervention types appears to be access-enhancing interventions combined with individual-directed interventions. These studies had an estimated combined intervention effect of 26.9 (95-percent CI: 9.9-43.9; 9 studies). The next largest effect was for the 5 studies combining access-enhancing and system-directed interventions; their effects were 19.4 (95-percent CI: 8.2-30.6). Caution should be used in interpreting these results because the number of studies available to examine pairs of combinations was quite small.

Additional analyses were conducted to examine the combined intervention effects for specific diverse populations (see Figures 4-3 and 4-4). The estimated intervention effect was greatest for older women—7.9 percent (95-percent CI: 10.5-25.4; 11 studies)—followed by an estimated effect of 12.7 percent (95-percent CI: 7.3-18.1; 26 studies) for comparisons consisting of more than 40 percent low-income women. When comparisons were made for intervention groups with more than 40 percent nonwhite women, the estimated effects were 12 percent (95-percent CI: 6.7-17.4; 24 studies) and 11.6 percent (95-percent CI: 6.4-16.7; 16 studies) if comparisons are limited to 40 percent or more African-American women. Again, significant heterogeneity between the studies was evident for each of these groupings.

As other Institute of Medicine reports (e.g., 2000, 2001) have recommended recently, the strongest interventions were those that increased access and addressed structural, economic, and geographic barriers to mammography use, along with intrapersonal and interpersonal factors (Skinner, Arfken, and Waterman, 2000; Skaer et al., 1996; Taylor et al., 1999; Rimer et al., 1992; Kiefe et al., 1994). That is, they combined communication interventions with others that were designed to enhance access. After all, mammography use does not occur in a vacuum. But individual-directed interventions in health care settings also showed impressive effects. Overall, the outcomes of combinations of certain kinds of interventions had the greatest impact on diverse women.

These results cannot be compared directly to studies conducted only among mainstream populations. However, the results can be compared to other mammography meta-analyses. Several meta-analyses of mammography-enhancing interventions previously have been reported. Although they all used different categories and inclusion/exclusion criteria, making direct comparisons impossible, the conclusions for general populations are consistent with, but not identical to, findings for diverse populations.

Wagner's (1998) review focused on mammography reminders for general populations, and concluded that women who received reminders were more likely to be screened than those who did not

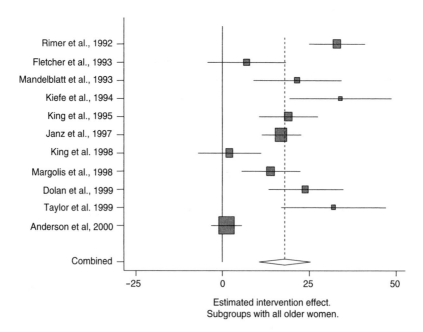

FIGURE 4-3 Individual and combined intervention effects for specific subgroups. Estimated intervention effects for individual studies and combined intervention effect estimates for studies with all older women and more than 40 percent with low incomes.

(OR = 1.48, p < .001 for n = 11 studies). Tailored reminders were more effective than generic ones, and effects of reminders were strongest in non-U.S. studies. Other reviews (e.g., Balas et al., 1997) have found that telephone calls to women increased mammography use.

Yabroff and Mandelblatt's (1999) review employed a different categorization scheme. However, it had some important similarities to the analysis by Legler and colleagues (2002). Their access-enhancing category (effect size 18.9 percent, 95-percent CI: 10.4-27.4; 14 studies) was similar in content to Yabroff and Mandelblatt's (1999) patient-targeted sociological interventions (effect size 12.6 percent; 95-percent CI: 7.4-17.9; 8 studies). Yabroff and Mandelblatt's (1999) categories of behavioral (effect size 13.2 percent; 95-percent CI: 4.7-21.2; 5 studies) and cognitive

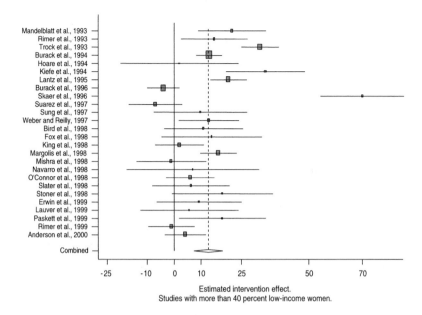

FIGURE 4-4 Individual and combined intervention effects for specific subgroups. Estimated intervention effects for individual studies and combined intervention effect estimates for studies with all older women and more than 40 percent with low incomes.

interventions (effect size 23.6 percent, 95-percent CI: 16.4-30.1; 2 studies) paralleled Legler's individual-directed interventions (effect size 17.6 percent, 95-percent CI: 11.6-24.0; 15 studies). Legler and colleagues used different intervention categories and limited the focus to studies involving diverse populations, while Yabroff and Mandelblatt's earlier analysis addressed general populations with fewer studies. Nevertheless, the results for diverse populations are similar to the findings for the general literature.

Yabroff and colleagues (2001) published an updated review that is particularly germane to the current volume. They examined the respective contributions of inreach and outreach interventions. What they found is noteworthy; the approaches had only modest differences. In every case, interactive strategies, delivered in person or by telephone, were much more effective than static interventions. Theory-based educational strategies delivered interactively increased mammography use by 10.7 percent in inreach settings and 19.9 percent in outreach settings. Communications of theory-based educational strategies combined with behavioral interventions had even greater impact—14 percent for inreach and 27.3 percent for outreach. Of special note for this volume, effects were similar across populations. The authors concluded that "the interventions should be similarly effective in minority or medically underserved populations" (p. 170). As Legler et al. (2002) and others have reported, sociologic interventions, such as lay health advisors, had a very modest impact, with effect sizes in the range of 10 percent. In a systematic review, using similar categories to those used by Legler et al., Sin and Legler (1999) concluded that "simple, brief, and effective interventions exist to boost breast cancer screening uptake. More complicated approaches are not necessarily any more effective" (p. 170). They went on to suggest that the most effective interventions are likely to be multistrategy, consistent with Legler et al.'s conclusions. They emphasized that such interventions should be suited to local needs.

In another meta-analysis, Bonfill et al. (2001) concluded that the most effective interventions were, in order of effect, mailed educational materials (2.81), letters of invitation plus phone calls (2.53), training and direct reminders to women (2.46), letters of invitation (1.92), and home visits (1.6). Their review included few, if any, of the studies Legler categorized as access enhancing. The strongest interventions fell into a category comparable to the individual-directed group. Similarly, Bonfill and colleagues concluded that combinations of effective interventions could have an important effect. The authors specifically recommended studies to explore the effect of interventions on diverse subgroups. Thus, previous reviews generally are consistent with Legler's conclusions about the efficacy of individual-directed interventions, although effect sizes vary. Focusing on studies of diverse populations revealed the importance of access-enhancing approaches, along with individual-directed interventions in health care settings.

The results of the meta-analysis of mammography interventions for diverse populations show that the past decade's investment in such interventions has translated into effective interventions for these groups. In general, the interventions for general populations are not so different from those that are effective with diverse populations, with the exception of the importance of access-enhancing interventions. This makes sense because access barriers may exert considerable negative impact for the women characterized here as diverse. But similarly, the interventions that have been effective in general, such as tailored and untailored letters and reminders and various forms of counseling, also are effective for diverse populations. Also encouraging is the fact that interventions aimed at diverse populations had strong effects. However, the results suggest that some interventions—such as social network and media interventions alone—that are widely used for diverse populations may not be sufficiently powerful to justify their use for these groups without additional interventions.

All interventions are not equal. In some cases, combinations of interventions will be needed. For example, mass media interventions can be used to increase awareness, while access-enhancing and individual-directed interventions can be used to overcome individual women's barriers to getting mammograms. The forthcoming *Guide to Community Preventive Services* (http://www.thecommunityguide.org/), led by the Centers for Disease Control and Prevention (CDC), will provide more detailed information on which interventions are most effective.

CONCLUSIONS

• Further research is necessary to characterize the relationships between the race, ethnicity, and language of women and their health care providers in order to identify factors that contribute to differential patterns of communication and behavior change relevant to screening mammography. Examples of such factors might include social norms of the patient-provider relationship, training of practitioners, and communication norms around issues of breast health and cancer screening. One frequently ignored aspect of the mammography experience is communication between women and radiologic technologists (Moyer et al., 2001). As noted by Moyer and colleagues, some racial and ethnic minority women (e.g., African-Americans) are less likely to understand the benefits of mammography, more likely to view cancer as fatal, and more likely to be more anxious about getting mammograms. Thus, communication and the opportunity to improve communication and increase the probability of subsequent adherence may be especially important for diverse populations.

• The process of intervention development needs to take into account women's life experiences and social contexts, which may not be reflected in their race/ethnicity, age, or other broad categorization.

• Health behavior change is influenced at multiple levels, including at the individual, interpersonal, institutional, community, and policy levels. Health communications targeting individual or interpersonal factors alone are likely to be insufficient in the absence of environmental interventions, such as those that enhance coverage or increase access. Interventions to reduce access barriers to mammography are important if remaining disparities in screening use are to be reduced.

• The mammography literature shows that, overall, women are more similar than different. However, although the predictors of mammography may be the same for diverse populations, their levels and intensity may vary. It is critical that interventions be built on a strong theoretical foundation using data accumulated from well-designed qualitative and quantitative studies to provide understanding of the variables that affect mammography for diverse populations. Health communications will be most effective when they are relevant, appropriate, and appealing to the specific audience targeted by the communication. Evaluations should include and report measures of fidelity and quality of intervention delivery.

RECOMMENDATIONS

• Theory-based interventions need to be developed, tested, and disseminated to increase screening utilization among women who have never been screened and to facilitate regular screening among all women. Qualitative and quantitative research is needed to identify specific barriers and to develop interventions appropriate for this population. Research on mammography and related areas suggests that combinations of inreach and outreach strategies may be especially effective.

• Authors should report sufficient detail about their interventions to enable readers to understand what was actually done. Where journal limitations preclude this, we encourage authors to put descriptive materials, including intervention descriptions, materials, and/or instruments, onto accessible Web sites.

• We advocate the use of standardized, validated measures for breast cancer screening behaviors that will permit meaningful comparisons of outcomes across studies. This would include use of standardized mammography utilization questions from the National Health Interview Survey and the Behavioral Risk Factor Surveillance Survey.

• Effective interventions should be widely disseminated. Practitioners are strongly encouraged to use previously validated, evidence-based interventions. The cancer screening chapter in the CDC-led *Guide to Community Preventive Services* should be a great advance in this regard (http://www.thecommunityguide.org).

• Future research must be directed toward studies that are adequately powered to permit subgroup analyses of potential differential impact of intervention activities.

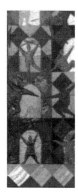

5

The Diabetes Exemplar

INTRODUCTION

Although a number of useful studies have been conducted on clinical interventions for Type 2 diabetes (e.g., Diabetes Prevention Program, 1997-2002; United Kingdom Perspective Diabetes Study, 1987-2001), the literature is disappointingly sparse on communication interventions to change behavior related to the prevention and treatment of diabetes in diverse populations. Unlike our experience with mammography and large campaigns, we found few published examples of systematically evaluated communication interventions for diabetes. Thus, we present diabetes as a challenging opportunity for developers of health communication programs.

Diabetes is a widespread disease that is differentially distributed among diverse populations, and it requires complex and continuing behaviors for prevention and management. In this chapter we review data that illustrate the effects of diabetes on diverse populations; discuss behavioral factors important for the prevention and control of diabetes; review the few studies on communication interventions for the control of diabetes and its various sequelae in the general population and in ethnic minority populations; and present factors to be considered in developing effective and testable communication interventions for the prevention and control of diabetes in the future.

WHY DIABETES?

Five sets of factors make diabetes an ideal exemplar of communication programs that encourage decisions for and the adoption of health-promoting behaviors by members of ethnic minority populations. The first factor is the systemic nature of the disease. Diabetes can affect every organ system of the body and has severe consequences. Second, it is among the most prevalent of all disorders (Diabetes Prevention Program Research Group, 2001) and it has been more prevalent and more virulent among minority ethnic groups. Third, its impact covers the human lifespan. Diabetes affects the very young, adolescents in increasing numbers, adults, and the elderly. Its effects on the body and on physical and mental functioning change with advancing age. Fourth, diabetes is responsive to behavioral interventions. Unlike many other chronic conditions, both preventive and treatment behaviors are of proven effectiveness for avoiding and/or controlling the various insults of diabetes at all times in life (Diabetes Prevention Program Research Group, 2001; Saaddine et al., 2002).

The fifth and final factor concerns the way in which diabetes is experienced by individuals, their family, and their friends. Diabetes means different things to different people, and different things to the same people at different times. The somatic effects of diabetes and its treatment create an ever-changing array of experiences and feared consequences; different behaviors are required to control these unwanted events. Most important, the patient's perspective on the disease and treatment—his or her representation as to how the disease and the treatment are affecting his or her body—will differ in a number of ways from the perspective held by those not affected. Thus, beliefs about the symptoms and causes of diabetes, the time frames for its consequences, and the procedures and

time frame for its prevention and the control of its adverse consequences differ for medical practitioners who embrace a biomedical
perspective on diabetes, patients who hold to cultural and experience-based common-sense beliefs of the disease, and family members and friends whose perspective on diabetes and its control is
shaped by cultural knowledge and observation of diabetic persons.

Understanding the various perspectives on diabetes and how
they may affect one another is essential to creating communication
programs that are effective in changing patterns of behavior to
improve diabetes control. The life-span nature of the disorder and
the long developmental history for the most common variety of
diabetes, Type 2, require that messages address different behaviors
at different times. Although some behaviors, such as dietary practices, may be valuable throughout the natural history of the disease, others play a more central role in avoiding the occurrence of
diabetes (primary prevention). Still others are important for early
detection and treatment (secondary prevention), and still others
are needed for the avoidance or control of the dangerous sequelae
of the diabetic process (tertiary prevention). Different actions will
coincide, therefore, with the different time points in the individual's
life history as well as with different time points in the life span of
the disease.

Communication strategies are complicated by the time course
of the disease. For example, successfully changing beliefs for better control of blood sugar at an early stage of disease may create
belief systems that interfere with the acceptance of messages recommending the adoption of behaviors for controlling risks at later
stages of the disease, such as foot care to manage diabetic neuropathy. The common-sense belief systems affecting the performance
and self-appraisal of preventive action differ among individuals,
change at different stages of the disease, and differ among members of an individual's social network. As a consequence, programs designed for diabetes control may succeed at some times
and in some places, but fail at other times and in other places.

DIABETES AND DIVERSE POPULATIONS

Three sets of concepts and data comprise the "bedrock" for the development of messages and programs for diabetes control from the framework of the biomedical model: (1) physiological concepts and data describing the underlying disease process, (2) data on the consequences of failure to achieve diabetes control, and (3) epidemiological data on disease prevalence, age-related incidence, and environmental causes. Differences among populations can be found in each of these areas, and these differences affect how diabetes is experienced and understood by each group's members. The translation of disease biology and epidemiology into cultural and individual beliefs may result in common-sense models of diabetes, its sequelae, and prescriptions for prevention that bear only partial resemblance to the models of biomedicine (Garro, 1990, 1995, 1996; Bruyère and Garro, 2000).

Biology and Prevalence in Diversity and Primary Risk

Diabetes is a systemic disorder that can affect many parts of the body. This complex metabolic disorder involves abnormalities in carbohydrate, lipid, and protein metabolism. The absence of insulin, insufficient quantities of insulin, or insensitivity of cellular receptors to insulin results in deficits in the transport of sugars across cell membranes. The result is elevation of blood sugar (hyperglycemia) and the appearance of symptoms such as polyuria or sweetened urine. These symptoms were identified more than 3,000 years ago; Susruta, the "father of medicine in India," labeled the disorder diabetes mellitus.

Type 1 diabetes, the less common form, affects 5 to 10 percent of diabetics. It is caused by the absence of insulin because of viral destruction of the insulin-producing cells of the pancreas in genetically susceptible individuals (LaPorte, Matushima, and Chang, 1995). In Type 2 diabetes, the form afflicting 90 to 95 percent of diabetics, the pancreas produces insufficient amounts of insulin and/or the cells of critical storage tissue are less responsive to insulin, resulting in the failure of transport of sugars across cell membranes; the net result is elevated blood sugar levels (American Diabetes Association, 2000; Centers for Disease Control and Prevention, 2000a). In addition to being far more common, Type 2 diabetes is slower to develop, usually diagnosed in adults over age 40, and most commonly diagnosed in adults over age 60. The consequences of diabetes, such as blindness, kidney failure, neuropathy, ulceration, and foot amputation, develop over lengthy periods of time and appear later in life. The difference in rate of onset led to using this variable in the statistical formula once used to distinguish Type 1 from Type 2 diabetes (American Diabetes Association, 2000; HeliosHealth.com, 2000; Songer and Zimmet, 1995). This formula is no longer useful because Type 2 diabetes now appears in adolescents, especially in minority populations. As the age of onset differs dramatically across ethnic groups, we can expect that diabetes will be seen as a disease of aging only in those communities where it is late in onset. When Type 2 onset is early in life, individuals may fail to distinguish Type 2 from Type 1 and develop beliefs about the disease incompatible both with its biology and with recommendations for behavioral change.

Prevalence

Diverse groups show substantial differences in the prevalence of Type 2 diabetes and the frequency of various complications, including heart problems and end-stage renal disease (Karter et al., 2002). Higher diabetes rates have been documented in African-American communities across all social categories (Hendricks and Haas, 1991), though prevalence is highest among women (especially those who have been previously diagnosed with gestational diabetes), the elderly, and individuals who have a positive family history for diabetes, who have fewer years of formal education, who have lower incomes, and who live alone (Brancati et al., 1996; Gaillard et al., 1997; Hendricks and Haas, 1991; Lipton et al., 1993; McNabb, Quinn, and Tobian, 1997). Statistical comparisons show non-Hispanic African-Americans to be 1.4 to 2.2 times more likely to develop diabetes than age-matched non-Hispanic whites (Bonham and Brock, 1985; Carter, Pugh, and Monterrosa, 1996; Harris, 1991; O'Brien et al., 1989; Wetterhall et al., 1992). The rate among African-American women over age 55 (25 percent) is double the rate of white women of similar age (Hendricks and Haas, 1991).

Although the overall picture for Hispanics is similar to that for African-Americans, the epidemiological data clearly indicate the importance of distinguishing among Hispanic populations. Thus, the rates of diabetes are two to five times higher among Hispanics than non-Hispanic whites, controlling for age (Carter, Pugh, and Monterrosa, 1996; Flegal et al., 1991; Gardner et al., 1984; Hamman et al., 1989; Hanis et al., 1983; Samet et al., 1988; Stern et al., 1983), but differ among Hispanics by national origin. Type 2 rates are lowest for Cuban Americans, approximately 16 percent of those ages 45 to 74 (Carter, Pugh, and Montenosa, 1996), and higher for Mexican Americans (24 percent) and Puerto Ricans living in the United States (26 percent). Major predictors of diabetes among Hispanics, namely female gender, lower levels of physical activity, and greater waist circumference (Tucker, Bermudez, and Castaneda, 2000), are similar to those for African-Americans.

Type 2 diabetes is also more prevalent among Asian Americans/Pacific Islanders. For example, rates are three to four times greater among Asian migrants to Hawaii, such as Japanese, Koreans, and Chinese, relative to those not of Asian origin (Carter, Pugh, and Monterrosa, 1996; Hendricks and Haas, 1991; Huang et al., 1996), with the highest prevalence for Filipinos. A similar trend has been noted among Asian-American communities in west coast cities of the United States, where prevalence rates are two to three times the national rate (Fujimoto et al., 1994; Hendricks and Haas, 1991).

The highest rates of Type 2 diabetes have been observed among Native Americans and Alaskan Natives. Prevalence among these groups is often 2.5 and more times greater than among non-Hispanic, age-matched samples (Acton et al., 1993; Carter et al., 1989; Carter, Pugh, and Monterrosa, 1996; Farrell et al., 1993; Freeman et al., 1989; Stahn, Gohdes, and Valway, 1993; Hendricks and Haas, 1991; Johnson and Strauss, 1993; Martinez and Strauss, 1993; Muneta et al., 1993; Murphy et al., 1992; Rith-Najarian, Valway, and Gohdes, 1993; Schraer et al., 1988; Sugarman and Percy, 1989; Valway, Linkins, and Gohdes, 1993). Native American tribes such as the Pima of Arizona suffer what may be the highest rates in the world, with prevalence rates as high as 50 percent, or 10 to 15 times higher than the overall prevalence of diabetes in the United States.

The differences in diabetes rates in age-matched, white, middle American, and ethnic populations, and the recall of past rates by members of each ethnic community, will affect both the perception of diabetes and trust in those recommending behavioral changes for prevention. If members of ethnic communities see these differences as stigmatizing and caused by intrusions from the "majority" Anglo culture, it can affect their trust and understanding of messengers and messages recommending behavior change, and undermine their sense of efficacy in achieving change for prevention. These differences will be examined later in this section.

Risk Factors

Both fixed and alterable lifestyle changes have been identified as risks for diabetes (Black, 2002), though the notion of a fixed factor is more elastic than one might suspect. For example, genetic susceptibility, age (over 45), and family history of diabetes are fixed once known, but family history changes when a family member develops diabetes, and genetic susceptibility can move from unknown to known with genetic testing and counseling. Historical factors, such as having a history of gestational diabetes and giving birth to babies weighing 9 pounds or more, fall within the set of unalterable factors for women for whom this is past history, but they also may indicate the possibility of dietary interventions for avoiding excessive fetal weight gain among women who have not yet given birth.

An estimated 97 million adults in the United States are either overweight or obese, and approximately 75 percent engage in no or only minimal physical activity on a regular basis (National Institutes of Health, 1998; U.S. Department of Health and Human Services, 1996). Smoking cessation, increased physical activity, and dietary regulation are prime targets for intervention, as these changes would reduce weight, lower low-density lipoproteins, increase high density lipoproteins, and improve glucose tolerance. Factors working against such interventions in diverse populations include the adoption of "Westernized" lifestyles, inadequate community and economic resources to access diabetes-safe diets (such as absence and/or high cost of appropriate foods in markets), and some traditional dietary practices. These factors, which are at extreme levels in many diverse communities, may be responsible for increasing rates of obesity in these communities and their disproportionate rates of Type 2 diabetes (Nakamura, 1999).

The same factors—high-fat diets and little physical activity—are likely to be the cause of the recently reported surge in Type 2 diabetes among U.S. children, many of whom are of African-American, Hispanic, or Native American/Alaskan Native descent (Libman et al., 1998; Neufeld et al., 1998; Pinhas-Hamiel et al., 1996; Rosenbloom et al., 1999; Scott et al., 1997). As many as 8 to 45 percent of children newly diagnosed with diabetes have Type 2. Libman and Arslanian (1999) reported that in 1994, 33 percent of the individuals diagnosed with diabetes were 10 to 19 years of age. Children at highest risk have a family history of diabetes, are in the middle to later years of puberty (age 10 or older), and are overweight.

Although much remains to be learned about the interacting processes responsible for the onset of Type 2 diabetes, the correlations among these risk factors and their association with Type 2 diabetes across ethnic groups reinforce the assumption that interventions effective in initiating and maintaining lifestyle changes do reduce the prevalence of this disease (Diabetes Prevention Program Research Group, 2002; Black, 2002).

Social and Cultural Disparities in
Medical Consequences of Diabetes

Not only is diabetes more prevalent among diverse populations, but its consequences are more serious. Moreover, the costs
are not evenly distributed: They are borne more heavily by ethnic
minorities. Compared with their white counterparts, African-
American diabetics are much more likely to develop hypertension
and cardiovascular disease (Harris, 1990), and twice as likely to
suffer from diabetes-related blindness, lower limb amputations,
and end-stage renal disease (American Diabetes Association; Harris et al., 1998; Kahn and Hiller, 1974; McNabb, Quinn, and
Tobian, 1997). Hispanics are also at significantly greater risk for
diabetes-associated illness at the time of initial diagnosis
(Hendricks and Haas, 1991; Hoy, Light, and Megill, 1995). Specifically, Hispanics have higher rates of diabetic disease of the
retina (retinopathy) than non-Hispanic white diabetics when they
are diagnosed (American Diabetes Association, 2000; Haffner et
al., 1989; Harris et al., 1993) and are three to seven times more
likely to develop end-stage renal disease in comparison to non-
Hispanic white diabetics (Carter, Pugh, and Monterrosa, 1996;
Hendricks and Haas, 1991; Pugh et al., 1988, 1995).

End-stage renal disease is the only complication of diabetes for
which sufficient data are available to compare Asians/Pacific Islanders with other ethnic groups (Carter, Pugh, and Monterrosa,
1996). Although the rates of end-stage renal disease are lower
among Asians/Pacific Islanders in comparison to other ethnic minorities, its overall prevalence is still higher than that for non-Hispanic white diabetics (United States Renal Data System, 1993).
Diabetic complications are especially prevalent among Native
American/Alaskan Native populations: Native Americans with
diabetes have significantly higher rates of cardiovascular disease,
stroke, end-stage renal disease, lower limb amputations, and diabetic retinopathy (American Diabetes Association, 2000; Carter,
Pugh, and Monterrosa, 1996; Hendricks and Haas, 1991; Hoy,
Light, and Megill, 1995; Hoy, Megill, and Hughson, 1987; *Mor-*

bidity and Mortality Weekly Report, 2000; Nelson and Bennett, 1989; Quiggins and Farrell, 1993; Stahn, Gohdes, and Valway, 1993). As the cohort of youngsters projected to be obese and to suffer with diabetes ages, the United States will experience an increase in elderly Type 2 diabetics suffering from cardiovascular disease, diabetic retinopathy, blindness, kidney damage and failure, neuropathy, and foot amputation (American Diabetes Association, 2000).

Diabetes Knowledge, Attitudes, and Behaviors

Four broad sets of factors affect whether and how a person takes action to prevent and control the threats associated with diabetes: (1) beliefs about the recommended action; (2) self-efficacy and related behavioral skills; (3) the social or interpersonal environment; and (4) the wider economic and physical ecology (see discussion in Chapter 2 on theory). The ecological framework provides both opportunities and barriers for action that both facilitate and constrain action-related beliefs, self-efficacy, and social influences. Low-fat and low-sugar foods will not be consumed if they are unavailable or unaffordable. Furthermore, an individual's behavioral beliefs, sense of efficacy, and social factors will not affect choice of foods if there is no way to identify which foods are inappropriate. Efforts to enhance health through changing individual beliefs and practices must not ignore such contextual factors (Lorig et al., 1999; Gohdes et al., 1996).

Ecological factors aside, can we identify social/cultural and individual beliefs and practices related to diabetes prevention and treatment, and do these beliefs and practices have a direct relationship to behaviors that put individuals at risk for diabetes and its complications? Furthermore, is there evidence to support the hypothesis that the cultural and individual beliefs responsible for prevention behaviors differ among minority ethnic groups? Theories describing the processes underlying individual decisions and actions and models of communication would assert that beliefs about the procedures for the prevention and control of diabetes are shaped by multiple sources of information (as noted in the discussion of behavioral theory in Chapter 2). We can expect differences among ethnic communities to reflect differences in such exposures. We can also anticipate that the differences most strongly related to behavior and most difficult to change will be cultural and personal beliefs about treatment based on direct experience with the disease and its consequences (Brownlee, Leventhal, and Leventhal, 2000). Personal experiences with diabetes and its prevention and treatment, observations of diabetic individuals and their family members and friends, and contacts with medical practitioners will provide both visual and auditory images to shape preventive practices.

The social environment, generally accepted beliefs expressed in culturally specific media, and beliefs expressed by family and friends will influence individuals' representations of specific preventive procedures. Individuals' common-sense models, self-efficacy expectations, and behaviors will be shaped further by observations of the preventive efforts of others; their conditions for performance, difficulty, efficacy, and other factors; and others' comments about preventive efforts (Leventhal et al., 2001; Leventhal, Hudson, and Robitaille, 1997; Leventhal, Diefenbach, and Leventhal, 1992). It can be expected that the representation of preventive actions will affect not only the performance of specific actions, but the trust in and credibility of specific sources and messages and the impact of these messages on individuals' belief systems and perceptions.

Knowledge, Beliefs, Experience, Emotions, and Action

The differences in knowledge and beliefs across ethnic communities should not obscure the commonalities—and there are many. Individuals in all communities express beliefs about the causes and consequences of diabetes, its susceptibility to control, and its symptoms, and all express beliefs about the procedures for preventing and controlling the disease and who is responsible for its control. Emotional distress and depression are also present among diabetic individuals in all communities. Differences appear, however, in the prevalence and precise meaning of the factors within each domain. For example, the nearly universal expressed belief that one has no control over diabetes seems to be directly related to the failure to take preventive actions, but lack of control appears to depend on a number of more fundamental, experiential factors, including personal and observed experience with the chronic, consistent worsening of diabetes-related dysfunction; beliefs placing causal responsibility on the larger, external culture (those who are responsible for causing it are responsible for curing it); and experienced difficulty in performing specific activities for diabetes control, such as exercise (Garro, 1995; Blanchard et al., 1999). Social barriers also play a critical role. Barriers may include pressure to eat traditional foods that are inappropriate for diabetics and lack of control over meal preparation.

Cause and Control

Diet

Foods high in fats and sugars are perceived as critical causes of obesity and diabetes, whether one is African-American (Blanchard et al., 1999; Liburd et al., 1999; Minnesota program); Hispanic (Hunt, Valenzuela, and Pugh, 1998; Zaldivar and Smolowitz, 1994); Native American, such as, Dakota Sioux (Lang, 1985, 1989) or Ojibway (Garro, 1990, 1995); or Asian American. Studies show that food-related causal beliefs differed among these communities, as did the association of such beliefs with behavior. As diabetes was absent prior to the change from traditional diets to store-bought foods, Native Americans identified it as a "whiteman's sickness" (Garro, 1995). This focus appeared to facilitate beliefs in other "external" causes, such as hormones injected into animals and insecticides sprayed on crops. "Personal causation," a second theme, linked diabetes to excessive drinking and overeating. Garro's findings suggest that the externalization of the cause to relatively uncontrollable factors will lead to low community efficacy, with adverse effects on personal efficacy.

Problems controlling diet were pronounced and common to all groups. One problem was lack of knowledge. For example, group members lacked the knowledge to accurately identify foods that were free of salt or sugar and to prepare healthy yet tasty meals (Hispanic participants in the Minnesota program). Another problem was social issues, such as the effect of diabetic dietary restrictions on family relationships (Hmong community participants in the Minnesota program) because (1) culturally valued foods were not among recommended healthy foods (Native Americans: Parker, 1994) and (2) adhering to "proper" diets interfered with social relationships that required sharing traditional foods (Lang, 1995). Avoiding traditional foods was seen as a sign of disrespect to those offering them (Pacific Islanders: Wang et al., 1999). Barriers to dietary adherence also existed in a variety of contextual factors, ranging from the difficulty of preparing two menus to the availability and greater cost of healthy foods (Hispanic communities: Hunt, Valenzuela, and Pugh, 1998). Many of the variations on the diet/food/obesity theme are not ethnically specific, and the absence of data from specific ethnic communities likely reflects the focus of the investigator or the special circumstances of the respondents.

A few studies reported data suggesting that latent cultural and individual values may play a critical role in dietary practices. Liburd and colleagues (1999) examined perceptions of preferred body size among African-American women with Type 2 diabetes. As these women "understood" the relationship of weight to diabetes, two-thirds of them expressed a desire to lose weight. However, when confronted with images of thin, mid-sized, and large bodies, they rejected "thin" bodies as unhealthy and perceived mid-sized to large bodies as signs of good health. African-American women living in less safe, low-income areas also appeared to see large body size as a safety factor; a large person appeared more formidable and less likely to be attacked. Implicit beliefs such as these can create a sense of unease and hesitation to adopt and adhere to weight reduction programs.

Another example concerns the role of symptoms and feeling states as motivators and deterrents to diabetes-healthy diets. Members of Hispanic communities reported (Hunt, Pugh, and Valenzuela, 1998) that how they felt determined when and how they used medication and complied with diabetes-healthy diets; if they felt "well," they didn't need either. Respondents also reported tradeoffs between medication and dietary behavior. They increased medication in response to dietary indiscretions, a phenomenon that has been documented previously in the anthropological literature (Garruto et al., 1999; Trostle and Sommerfield, 1996). The somatic sensations and sense of well-being generated by consuming large amounts of food also emerged as a deterrent to consuming meager, diabetes-healthy diets among Native Americans from the Dakota tribe (Lang, 1985, 1989). Thus, weight reduction can involve a tradeoff between diabetes control and good health and perceived safety for African-American women, and between diabetes control and somatic feelings of fullness and well-being for Hispanics and Native Americans. Similar findings regarding the use of symptoms to regulate medication for hypertension have been reported for low-income whites and African-Americans; respondents were more compliant with medication and had better blood pressure control if they believed their medications reduced their blood pressure symptoms (Meyer, Leventhal, and Guttman, 1985). Unfortunately for these respondents, symptoms are unrelated to blood pressure.

Exercise

Although the findings for exercise are similar in some ways to those for diet, differences emerge. Hispanic women believed exercise was important for diabetes control (Hunt, Valenzuela, and Pugh, 1998), but Pacific Islanders did not attach a high priority to this behavior (Wang et al., 1999). Comparisons between African-American and white women showed less frequent and less intense exercise by the former (Summerson, Konen, and Dignan, 1992). Barriers to exercise were reported by women from all ethnic communities, though income level affected the frequency with which specific barriers were mentioned. For example, women from low-income areas were more likely to report difficulties in finding a safe and appropriate place to exercise and an inability to afford child care. Pain and distress from exercise are commonly expressed barriers among older, female respondents, who are most susceptible to diabetes and its complications (Leventhal et al., 2001). The negative perception of exercise by Hispanic respondents—that exercise posed the danger of rapid declines in blood sugar levels and symptoms of hypoglycemia—represents another barrier that is likely based on direct observation either of other persons or personal experience. Thus, perceived features of the environment and experienced somatic effects, such as pain, appear to be the main barriers to exercise, or at least are reported to be.

Hopelessness and Personal, Medical, and Social Support for Diabetes Control

The prescription for lifestyle changes in diet and exercise for diabetes prevention and control gives the at-risk individual two complex behavioral tasks that are difficult to initiate and more difficult to sustain. The difficulties in changing behaviors that are the major targets of prevention programs are consistent with data showing a high level of fatalism and hopelessness regarding diabetes prevention. African-American respondents are reported to experience a nearly overwhelming sense of powerlessness and lack of control over the development and management of their diabetes, a feeling made more extreme for respondents experiencing one or more complications of diabetes (Blanchard et al., 1999). Powerlessness was felt by African-American and Native American participants in the Minnesota program, and by low-income Mexican Americans (Schwab, Meyer, and Merrell, 1994). Hispanic respondents expressed their sense of powerlessness in different ways. Some attributed diabetes to prior and unchangeable life traumas such as auto accidents and prior illnesses (Hunt, Valenzuela, and Pugh, 1998). Others believed diabetes was caused by fate or God (Quotromoni et al., 1994). Still others perceived diabetes as incurable (Weller et al., 1999), and others saw it as a source of frustration and blamed themselves because they could not follow a proper lifestyle (Native Americans: Parker, 1994).

Not surprisingly, hopelessness is associated with beliefs in the importance of external support from family and health care providers. A supportive family is seen as critical for adoption and maintenance of preventive behaviors, and a sympathetic and caring medical provider is essential to provide the emotional reassurances and educational input needed for understanding the disease and developing the skills needed for more complex, and potentially risky and threatening, self-regulation behaviors, such as use of insulin. These feelings were expressed by African-American, Hispanic, Chinese American, and Native American respondents. As is the case for other chronic, difficult-to-understand, and seemingly intractable conditions, respondents vacillate between traditional and "Western" biomedical systems and their respective treatments.

Intervening for Diabetes Prevention and Control

Preparing recommendations for future programmatic communication research would be much easier if one could draw on a body of studies that have identified communication factors known to facilitate effective preventive behaviors. Although studies of communications targeting diabetes-related behaviors are sparse, a substantial number of studies provide information important for the future development of communication research. These studies have three objectives: (1) demonstrating the efficacy of specific treatments for reducing complications of diabetes, (2) evaluating the efficacy of different interventions for changing behavior in the hope of achieving improved control, and (3) attempting to translate efficacy findings to community and treatment settings, such as carrying out studies of effectiveness. Communication broadly defined, both mass media and interpersonal communication of various types (e.g., doctor and investigator with participants, participants with family members and friends), is involved in all three types of studies. Studies that provide evidence for the contribution of a specific type of communication or media to behavioral change are lacking.

Treatment Efficacy

Drug Trials: Studies of treatment efficacy provide compelling evidence of the effectiveness of specific treatments for controlling adverse outcomes of diabetes, though the largest randomized clinical trials have been conducted with Type 1 diabetes. For example, the 1993 publication of findings from the Diabetes Control and Complications Trial Research Group showed that intensive therapy (use of an external insulin pump or 3 or more daily insulin injections guided by frequent blood glucose monitoring) in comparison to conventional therapy (one or two daily insulin injections) resulted in a 76-percent reduction in retinal pathology and a 60-percent reduction in neuropathy in 1,440 persons with insulin-dependent diabetes. Although the differences are of a lesser magnitude, these early dramatic effects were sustained 4 years after completion of the trial (The Diabetes Control and Complications Trial, 2000).

The UK Prospective Diabetes Study, begun in 1978, is a large clinical trial study involving more than 5,000 patients suffering from Type 2 diabetes (Kothari et al., 2001). The main focus has been on glycemic (blood sugar) control by using insulin and sulfonylurea drugs instead of on diet modifications. The intensive drug treatments were found to be effective in reducing the various negative outcomes of Type 2 diabetes such as progressive retinopathy. Treatments augmented with beta-blockers helped reduced cardiovascular complication associated with Type 2 diabetes. Metformin (an organic enzyme) alone reduced myocardial infarctions (heart attacks) in obese patients, but combinations of metformin and sulfonylurea drugs had an adverse effect. This has been carried out over a long time period with a median followup of 11 years. More than 60 research papers have published findings from this program.

Behavioral Studies: A meta-analysis reviewing the efficacy of a behavioral intervention offers encouragement regarding the efficacy of exercise as a means of reducing glycosylated hemoglobin (HbA1c). Twelve aerobic and two resistance training studies found postintervention HbA1c to be "lower in the exercise groups compared with the control groups," a difference that "should decrease the risk of diabetic complications" (Boule, Haddad, and Kenny, 2001).

The Diabetes Prevention Program (Diabetes Prevention Program Research Group, 2002) found that both lifestyle changes and drug treatments were effective in reducing the incidence of Type 2 diabetes. In this study, 2,324 nonaffected individuals who had elevated glucose concentrations but did not have diabetes were randomly assigned to one of three experimental conditions: lifestyle modification (diet and exercise), metformin administration twice daily, and placebo. The baseline characteristics of the study population included both genders; several ethnic groups (white, African-American, Hispanic, Native American/Alaskan Native, and Asian American/Pacific Islander); and variations in age, weight, family history, body-mass index, leisure physical activity, and blood glucose levels. The average followup was 2.8 years after the beginning of the trials. Although some disparities in occurrence of diabetes were found across ethnic groups, lifestyle changes provided the best outcome for all groups. Overall, lifestyle interventions reduced the incidence of diabetes by 58 percent relative to the placebo, while metformin reduced the incidence by 31 percent. Asians had the lowest incidence rate when following the lifestyle intervention, and African-Americans had the lowest incidence rate when administering metformin. Approximately half of the participants in the lifestyle treatment group met the weight loss goal of 7 percent, and three-quarters met the exercise goal of 150 minutes per week (at 6 months); at the 2.8-year followup, the percentage that had maintained these goals over time was 38 percent and 58 percent, respectively.

Behaviors such as dieting and exercise for weight loss define two of the complex, difficult-to-change behaviors important for both primary and secondary prevention: Dieting requires regulating an appetitive response, while exercise requires the introduction of a time-consuming change in lifestyle that can be physically distressing. Few studies have collected evidence on long-term adherence (Diabetes Prevention Program Research Group, 2002). Evidence is mixed for success in generating adherence to a variety of relatively easy-to-perform self-monitoring behaviors important for secondary prevention, including weighing oneself, daily examination and cleansing of feet, and simple protective behaviors such as wearing shoes both inside and outside the home when there is evidence of neuropathy. Behavioral interventions that encourage testing blood sugar and self-administering medication (oral medication and insulin, although the latter is used less often to control Type 2 diabetes) appear more effective, but the intervener confronts an additional set of factors important for behavioral change—the abilities to self-administer medications and to manage the threats that arise if the medications are administered incorrectly. For example, excessive doses of insulin can generate life-threatening attacks of hypoglycemia. Fears of such attacks are associated with less adequate control and increased threat of long-term complications.

Two points should be kept in mind when using the results of studies of behavioral interventions to draw conclusions relevant to communication campaigns for changing these same behaviors. The first, and most important, is that the individuals in these studies either have or are at risk for diabetes and, therefore, are willing and/or motivated to participate. There is an enormous gap between the disinterested or hostile nonparticipant and the willing recruit; to a substantial degree, the latter individual is on the same page as the investigator. The proportion of "eligible" elderly, those most at risk for chronic disability from conditions such as diabetes and arthritis, who are willing to participate in efficacy trials on exercise and other health behaviors is distressingly small (Leventhal et al., 2001). Second, it is worth noting that the goals for a particular behavior can differ depending on the stage of disease and the presence of other treatments. For example, variation in sugar intake will have relatively little immediate effect on those with Type 2 diabetes not using medication to control blood sugar levels, but can have important, immediate consequences for those with Type 2 diabetes who have used excessive amounts of insulin or oral medication.

Sustaining Weight Loss and Exercise Behavior

An enormous number of studies have been conducted on weight loss and regular exercise. Both of these behaviors have been difficult to influence, particularly over the long term, with the initial effects of cognitive behavioral interventions generally dissipating over a year or two (Wing et al., 1986, 1998). Although the subset of studies on samples of those with diabetes or individuals at high risk for diabetes is smaller than that for those who do not suffer from diabetes, a meta-analysis of 72 randomized trials with diabetic participants (Norris, Engelgau, and Narayan, 2001) suggests that it is possible to initiate changes in knowledge and self-management practices, such as frequency and accuracy of self-monitoring of blood glucose and self-reported dietary habits. Effects of interventions on lipids, physical activity, weight, and blood pressure were variable, and most beneficial effects were observed for 6 months or less. It may be more difficult to sustain alterations in dietary practices and exercise among those with Type 2 diabetes than among those who do not suffer from the disease. Failure to sustain dietary and exercise changes often are attributed to the complexity of these behaviors, which may be more rigorous for regimens to control diabetes than more usual everyday dietary or exercise practices. Such explanations likely fall short, however, of capturing critical factors that investigators need to recognize. Differences reflecting less favorable levels of adherence for those at risk suggest that worsening consequences, and attributions to uncontrollable causes, may undermine self-efficacy motivation, resulting in failure to sustain behavioral change.

An Education Program to Influence Behavior

The National Diabetes Education Program (2002) was developed in the mid-1990s to raise awareness about the causes and treatments for diabetes, to promote early diagnosis, and to prevent the onset of Type 2 diabetes. It is a large-scale program that includes a number of communication interventions. We describe this program because of its scale and its work with diverse populations; however, no systematic evaluation has been done on the program's impact, particularly regarding potential differential effects on diverse populations. The program is sponsored by the National Institute of Diabetes and Digestive and Kidney Diseases and the Centers for Disease Control and Prevention's Division of Diabetes Translation. It has private and public partners who are asked to provide information about their organizational structure, size, and activities. Activities of concern may include a range of communication strategies, including newsletters, personal communication, and materials on prevention and care. Partners are provided with media kits and guidelines for developing campaigns. A Web site (http://ndep.nih.gov/) offers links to information about the program and about diabetes and its prevention, procedures for conducting an awareness campaign, and applications for becoming a partner. Six organizations are working with the program's minority work groups to distribute culturally appropriate education messages. These include the Association of American Indian Physicians, Association of Asian Pacific Community Health Organizations, National Asian Women's Health Organization, National Council of La Raza, National Hispanic Council on Aging, and Urban League of Nebraska.

The program's messages promote identified cultural values that encourage diabetes self-care (cultural incentives) and challenge cultural traditions that inhibit diabetes care-related behaviors (cultural barriers). For example, messages for Hispanics to control diabetes were developed to counter the fatalistic belief that diabetes complications are inevitable, and messages for Native American/Alaskan Native populations emphasize the importance of growing older to "be around" for younger generations and to pass on traditions (Centers for Disease Control and Prevention, 1999).

A Community-Level Behavior Study

Daniel et al. (1999) used social learning principles based on cognitive behavioral theory, in comparing an experimental community to two control communities. The majority of communications were delivered to the entire community, though the subset assessed for knowledge gains and physiological changes had a more intimate relationship with the program investigators. The approach was multilevel because it included television, radio, and newspaper coverage of program activities and individuals could participate in physical activity classes, health events, cooking demonstrations, information forums on diabetes, and if diabetic, a diabetes support group. Relative to the two control communities, the intervention community showed positive gains for systolic blood pressure, but did more poorly than the controls for the glycated hemoglobin (HbA_{1c}) test. However, all differences were minimal for the relatively small sample of individuals repeatedly assessed.

RECOMMENDATIONS

Given the paucity of well-planned and well-evaluated programs for communication for behavior change related to primary and secondary prevention of diabetes, this section discusses factors that should be considered in developing such interventions in the future.

A hypothesis that is both implicit and explicit throughout this volume is that a message that takes account of the knowledge, beliefs, and cultural and ecological contexts of its audience should be more successful in achieving its goals. Until goals and audiences are specified, however, this assumption remains little more than an empty truism. The hypothesis, that behavioral theory has a critical role to play in assuring success, has a similar empty status until theory is translated into specific communication content and structure, and delivered in appropriate channels. The following recommendations and suggestions should assist investigators and program planners with these tasks.

Behavioral Goals and Disease Status

Selection of an attitudinal or behavioral goal for communication, an essential first step in comprehensive planning for a diabetes prevention program, should reflect the nature of diabetes as a chronic, lifelong disease that may require the segmentation of the population with respect to its medical status. Possible population segments include those who are at risk but not yet diabetic; diabetic but without neurologic or cardiac complications; or diabetic and with specifiable complications. Planners and developers of communication interventions should consider the following points:

1. Evidence that links behavior change to disease risk and progression should be communicated.

2. Some goals are important across disease states, such as maintaining appropriate blood sugar levels, while others, such as neuropathy and avoidance of ulceration, will vary. A different set of specifiable behaviors will come into play for different end points.

3. There is the possibility that increased awareness, screening, and other factors encouraged by the program can lead to apparent increases in prevalence that will be reported by local media and interpreted by the community as a sign of program failure.

Behavioral Goals and Disease Beliefs

Self-regulation models of behavior suggest the need to consider a number of social-psychological issues and/or constraints when selecting a target behavior.

1. Does the behavior make sense given the model of the disease held by the recipient audience? If diabetes is understood as a blood sugar problem, it makes sense to reduce sugar consumption and to use a medication to reduce blood sugar. It may make less sense, however, that exercise can affect blood sugar, or that the neuropathy and the absence of foot pain means that blood sugar is causing a serious disease threat that could lead to ulcers and foot amputation.

2. Communication to enhance effective self-regulation should consider the structure of the recommended behavior and present an appropriate plan for action (Leventhal, 1970; Gollwitzer, 1999). Areas to be explored may include whether the program can select a target behavior that is relatively easy to perform and an early step in a lengthier, more complex sequence of actions, and whether the program can generate actions that enhance self-efficacy and encourage the performance of subsequent, more difficult-to-perform actions.

3. Will the recommended behavior lead to noticeable outcomes that will be perceived as indicators of success in preventing diabetes and one of its feared outcomes? Any relief of patient anxiety or discomfort will be an experiential reinforcement for the recommended behavior.

4. Communications to regulate behaviors that produce intense and rapid feedback must include careful instructions for performing the action, criteria for interpreting behavioral feedback, and behaviors to provide control and create a sense of control over potentially threatening feedback. For example, improper dosage of insulin can create reactions that will be perceived as, and that can be, an indicator of a serious health threat. Awareness of these somatic changes and ways of controlling them should be considered.

5. Realistic criteria should be provided. Messages that encourage behaviors that have effects that appear over long time frames (such as weight loss or reduction in blood sugar) should provide reasonable and achievable intermediate outcome expectations for the behavior. It is too easy for a recipient to assume that

he or she has failed to change behavior if the criteria for evaluating success are inappropriate. For example, if expectations for weight loss are unrealistic, such as 5-pound changes in a week, appropriate changes of 1 to 2 pounds a week may be read as failures, leading to nonadherence and rejection of prior and future health messages.

6. The complexity of each behavioral goal suggests different strategies for communication. For example, mass media may be useful for defining broad goals, such as weight loss, and even for defining sensible criteria, such as weight loss of 1 to 2 pounds a week. The skills needed to achieve weight loss, such as food preparation, may be better presented through print media, television food programs, and direct instruction.

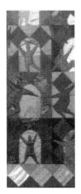

6

New Communication Applications and Technologies and Diverse Populations

THE CHANGING HEALTH COMMUNICATION LANDSCAPE[1]

Communication applications and technologies changed dramatically over the 20th century. The telephone did not become a routine means of communication in the United States until World War I (Mandl, Kohane, and Brandt, 1998). In the early years of its use, there was concern that the telephone might harm doctor-patient relationships. Now we accept the telephone as part of everyday life and as an essential part of health care. The committee recognizes that telephone coverage averages about 95 percent for the United States, but noncoverage varies from 1.8 percent in Delaware to 13.3 percent in New Mexico. Telephone coverage also is lower for some population groups, e.g., Blacks in the South, persons with low incomes, and people in rural areas (Cen-

[1]We are grateful to David Gustafson and Bernard Glassman for their contributions to this chapter. We also thank Lee Rainie, Director, Pew Internet & American Life Project, for generously sharing information.

ters for Disease Control and Prevention Comparability of Data, http://www.cdc.gov; Behavioral Risk Factor Surveillance System, 2000). The evolution of social activities and social relations brought about by the telephone pales in comparison to the communication revolution being propelled by the Internet. Health communication is at the forefront of that revolution.

The last decade of the 20th century was distinguished by massive changes in the way people get information, including health information. By the beginning of the 21st century, there were more communication channels than ever before—not only face-to-face, print, telephone, radio, TV, fax, VCR, DVD, and CD-ROM, but also the many options possible through personal and networked computers, including the Internet, with both wired and wireless options. New phrases such as "instant messaging" became part of the global vocabulary nearly overnight. The early 20th century discussions about the impact of the telephone were replaced by commentaries about the impact of e-mail on doctor-patient relationships. Perhaps no other innovation has transformed communication as quickly and with as much reach as the Internet (Lucky, 2000). As Bandura (2001:6) observed, "new ideas, values, behavior patterns and social practices now are being rapidly diffused by symbolic modeling worldwide in ways that foster a globally distributed consciousness."

The growth of new technologies parallels changes over the past half century in the patient role and the patient-physician relationship. Increasingly, patients want to play an active role in making decisions about health (see, e.g., Chen and Siu, 2001; Edwards and Elwyn, 1999). Across a number of health topics, patients say they want to receive as much information as possible (Chen and Siu, 2001; Fallowfield, 2001; Cassileth, 2001; Bluman et al., 1999). Furthermore, whether they want to play an active role or not, the evolution of the health system may force them to play that role to an ever-increasing extent. Physicians and other health professionals may have less time available to follow up aggressively with patients. Patients and their families may assume increasing responsibilities for negotiating their way through the system, obtaining prevention information, finding appropriate care, and gaining follow-up advice.

This chapter will explore the use of new health communication technologies and new uses of current technologies, with a focus on diverse audiences. We will describe the nature and potential benefits and limitations of these communications, summarize the evidence especially with regard to diverse populations, and recommend several actions to reduce the barriers to their use and to speed access to a range of new communication applications and technologies, including Internet-based applications among all population groups. Our recommendations also include potential research. A caveat is in order: Little research has been published on the experience of diverse populations with these new technologies. The research that is reported generally includes few controlled trials, and many of the samples are still small. In most cases, if there are data on diverse populations, they are in the context of studies that include both diverse and nondiverse populations. Like other good interventions, computer-based applications should be developed and measured with theory as a foundation, as described elsewhere in this volume (Chapter 2). Moreover, they should specify the linkages among cognitive/affective domains, behavioral objectives, and program content (Rhodes, Fishbein, and Reis, 1997).

INNOVATIVE USES OF CURRENT TECHNOLOGIES

New uses of current and widely accessible communication media, such as print and telephone, have been possible because of computer applications that have permitted content to be tailored to individuals, allowing people to use older tools in new ways. Tailored print communications (TPCs) and telephone-delivered interventions (TDIs) are among the most widely used innovations. The potential of these media for reaching those with and without Internet access, and people with highly diverse linguistic and cultural requirements, should not be underestimated, nor should the challenge of harnessing the new media to reach diverse audiences.

Tailored Print Communication

TPCs are printed materials created especially for an individual based on relevant information about that person, usually from the person (e.g., by telephone interview or self-administered questionnaire) with or without other data (such as medical records) (Skinner et al., 1999; de Vries and Brug, 1999; Kreuter and Skinner, 2000; Kreuter et al., 2000b). At least theoretically, computer-tailored print materials permit the reach of mass media, with content that is relevant and appropriate to recipients. This is why tailored approaches have been referred to as mass customization. Where generic materials might include a substantial amount of irrelevant content for any individual, tailored materials can provide information needed to modify specific antecedents of behavior change and enhance skills for a particular individual. For example, tailored materials can suggest dietary changes based on the recipients' eating patterns and preferences. Tailored information is different from personalized information, which may be as simple as putting a name on a brochure, and has no demonstrable impact on behavior change (Kreuter et al., 1999; Kreuter and Skinner, 2000b). Tailored information also is distinct from targeted communication, which is based on the social marketing principle of market segmentation, using group variables such as ethnicity to design special communication to meet group needs. Segmentation is discussed further in Chapters 2 and 3.

Tailored interventions range from those that are very simple and tailor only a few variables, perhaps in a letter, to more elaborate tailored booklets based on algorithms that have potentially billions of combinations of pieces of health-related information. Tailoring can range from the most precise algorithm that adjusts individual words and phrases within a sentence to methods that choose whether to include a whole topic (Bental, Cawsey, and Jones, 1999). Some systems allow specific questions to be answered (Buchanan et al., 1995). Many formats are possible, including tailored letters, booklets, calendars, newsletters, games, and church bulletins. The possibilities are nearly limitless, but should be appropriate to particular audiences. Like any good intervention, tailored interventions should reflect participation of potential users at every stage. As with other print interventions, some are designed better than others.

Bental, Cawsey, and Jones (1999), Dijkstra and de Vries (1999), Kreuter et al. (1999), Rimer and Glassman (1999), and Kreuter et al. (2000b) provide more detail about how tailored communication is created. Briefly, tailored materials require: (1) identification of relevant individual-level characteristics; (2) a message library; and (3) an algorithm that specifies the decision rules for assigning particular messages to individuals (Dijkstra and de Vries, 1999). A fundamental part of developing TPCs is the creation of a message library that contains all possible messages that could be given to an individual under different conditions (Rimer and Glassman, 1999; Kreuter et al., 1999; Kreuter et al., 2000b). For example, a woman who is thinking about getting a mammogram would get a very different message from a woman who has never considered having one.

More than 40 studies of TPCs have been reported, and several summary articles have been published (see, e.g., Strecher, 1999; Rimer and Glassman, 1999; Dijkstra and de Vries, 1999; Skinner et al., 1999). As Table 6-1 shows, reports of TPCs have covered a wide range of health-related behaviors, including diet, exercise, smoking cessation, weight reduction, mammography, prostate cancer screening, hormone replacement therapy, health risk appraisal, and multiple risk behaviors. More recent studies, as well as some that are ongoing, have extended tailoring to new formats and variables, including the use of cultural tailoring (Kreuter et al., in press; Lukwago et al., in press; Lukwago et al., 2001).

TPCs that were tested in these studies used many kinds of tailoring based on theories such as the Elaboration Likelihood Method (Petty and Cacioppo, 1979b; Kreuter et al., 2000; Kreuter and Holt, 2001), Stages of Change Model, Social Cognitive Theory, and the Health Belief Model, and using variables such as self-efficacy, perceived susceptibility and risk, as well as barriers and facilitators to behavior change (Glanz, Rimer, and Lewis, in

TABLE 6-1 Evidence for the Effectiveness of Tailored Print
Communications

Impact	Significant Outcome by Author[a]	
	Yes	No
More likely to be read, recalled, rated more highly, discussed with other people, and perceived as interesting and relevant	Brinberg and Axelson, 1990 Campbell et al., 1994,[b] 1999,[b] 2002[b] Skinner et al., 1994 Dijkstra et al., 1998a Strecher, 1999 Brug et al., 1996, 1998 Lipkus et al., 1999,[b] 2000 Kreuter et al., 1999, 2000b Rimer et al., 1999,[b] 2002 DeBourdeaudhuij and Brug, 2000 Etter and Perneger, 2001 Nansel et al., 2002[b] Blalock et al., 2002 McBride et al., 2002[b]	Curry et al., 1995 Bull et al., 1999a
Significant main effect or subgroup effect on smoking cessation	Dijkstra et al., 1999 Strecher, 1999 Lipkus et al., 1999,[b] 2000 Velicer et al., 1999 Orleans et al., 2000 Prochaska et al., 2001 Becona and Vazquez, 2001[b] Etter and Perneger, 2001 Lennox et al., 2001 McBride et al., 2002[b]	Curry et al., 1995 Dijkstra et al., 1998b Campbell et al., 2002[b]

TABLE 6-1 Continued

Impact	Significant Outcome by Author[a]	
	Yes	No
Significant decrease in dietary fat intake	Brinberg and Axelson, 1990 Bowen et al., 1992 Campbell et al., 1994,[b] 1999,[b] 2002[b] Kreuter and Strecher, 1996 Brug et al., 1996, 1998 DeBourdeaudhuij and Brug, 2000	Siero et al., 2000[b]
Significant increase in fruit and vegetable intake	Brug et al., 1998 Campbell et al., 1999,[b] 2002[b] Kristal et al., 2000 Delichatsios et al., 2001	Campbell et al., 1994[b] Brug et al., 1996 Lutz et al., 1999
Significant effect on weight reduction	Burnett et al., 1985	
Significant effect on exercise behavior or main effect on those not exercising at baseline	Kreuter and Strecher, 1996 Bull et al., 1999a Marcus et al., 2000[b] Bock et al., 2001 Campbell et al., 2002[b]	Bull et al., 1999b Blalock et al., 2002
Increased adoption of home and car safety behaviors among parents of young children	Nansel et al., 2002[b]	
Increase use of calcium supplements to prevent osteoporosis among persons thinking about but not appropriately performing the behaviors	Blalock et al., 2002	

continued on next page

TABLE 6-1 Continued

| Impact | Significant Outcome by Author[a] | |
	Yes	No
Improve decision making about HRT	McBride et al., in press[b]	
Significant main effect or subgroup effect on use of mammography	Skinner et al., 1994 Rakowski et al., 1998 Rimer et al., 2001, 2002 Valanis et al., 2002	Meldrum et al., 1994[b] Drossaert et al., 1996 Rimer et al., 1999[b]
More accurate assessment of breast cancer risk	Lipkus, Rimer, Strigo, 1996 Rimer et al., 2002 McBride et al., in press[b] Skinner et al., in press	
Improved completion of multiple tests needed by women	Harpole et al., 2000[b]	
Increased adherence to early detection for prostate cancer	Myers et al., 1999[b]	
Increased adherence to cervical cancer screening	Campbell et al., 2002	
Improved knowledge about genetic testing and related issues and increase accurate assessment of risk of being a mutation carrier	Skinner et al., in press	

[a]Note: Only first or first and second author(s) listed here in order to conserve space, co-authors can be found in reference list.
[b]Focuses on or analyzes impact on diverse populations.

press). In some cases, pictorial material was tailored, as were variables such as personal risk, self-confidence, smoking characteristics, and specific behavioral recommendations. Very different approaches to tailoring have been used. For example, some studies have created materials that are stage matched and tailored, while others have been tailored entirely for individual items or variables. No reported study has compared the effects of different tailoring systems.

Although the data are not unequivocal, most studies have shown main effects or important interactions. In some cases (e.g., Lutz et al., 1999; Lennox et al., 2001), tailored materials outperformed the control group, but were no better than nontailored materials. More research is needed to understand the mechanisms underlying both effective and ineffective TPCs and whether some tailoring algorithms and approaches are better than others. Substantial evidence shows that TPCs are more likely to be read and kept, that they are rated more highly than generic materials, and that they produce changes in knowledge, beliefs, and behaviors. Where they are effective, their success seems to be partly because of the greater level of attention paid to tailored communication (de Vries and Brug, 1999; Kreuter et al., 1999; Becona and Vazquez, 2001). Consistent with the Elaboration Likelihood Method, there is increasing evidence that tailoring causes recipients to pay more attention and to process more deeply, leading to improved comprehension and behavior change (Kreuter et al., 1999; 2000). When combined with a physician message that "primes" patients to pay attention to subsequent messages, TPCs may be especially powerful (Kreuter, Chheda, and Bull, 2000).

More work is needed in this area. Specifically, none of the reported studies was designed to answer the following question: Did a particular intervention perform differentially with a diverse population? However, several of the published studies focused on or included analyses of effects on diverse populations (e.g., Campbell et al., 1994, 1999, 2002; Skinner, Strecher, and Hospers, 1994; Rimer et al., 1999; Becona and Vazquez, 2001) (see Table 6-1). The results are encouraging. Skinner and colleagues showed that tailored letters about mammography had a significant sub-group effect on African-American women. Lipkus and colleagues (Lipkus, Lyna, and Rimer, 1999) found that tailored birthday letters and newsletters had a highly significant effect on smoking quit rates among low-income African-Americans, especially men. Campbell et al. (1994) showed that a combination of tailored church bulletins and other culturally appropriate interventions resulted in significant increases in fruit and vegetable consumption in a low-income African-American population. In a study of blue-collar women, Campbell et al. (2002) found increases in several behaviors, including fruit and vegetable consumption, flexibility exercise, and short-term change in fat intake, but no changes in smoking or cervical cancer screening in a worksite program that also included natural helpers. Kreuter, Vehige, and McGuire (1996) reported that a tailored calendar improved the rate at which parents adhered to their children's immunization schedules. Myers and colleagues (1999) demonstrated that an enhanced intervention composed of telephone and print materials tailored to African-American men with no previous history of prostate cancer resulted in increased adherence to early detection for prostate cancer. Becona and Vazquez (2001) showed that the combination of a standard self-help smoking cessation intervention and tailored letters resulted in a significant improvement over self-help alone for Hispanic smokers, with impressive abstinence rates.

Nansel et al. (2002) tested the efficacy of tailored print materials produced for parents to reduce child injury-promoting behaviors in the home and car in a primarily minority sample. McBride et al. (2002) extended previous work on genetic susceptibility and tobacco control by examining the use of feedback about a genetic biomarker of cancer susceptibility to increase smoking cessation in a low-income African-American population. At 6 months (but not at 12 months), there was a significant difference between those who received TPCs with biomarker feedback (19-percent quit rate) versus enhanced usual care (10-percent quit rate). These studies are encouraging. They show that for a wide range of topics, TPCs are efficacious for both white and ethnic minority populations. In one of the few studies that showed an ethnic group disadvantage, McBride et al. (in press) found that tailored materials about hormone replacement therapy were less effective for African-American women than for white women.

In many cases, TPCs are more effective when combined with other interventions. Among the most promising are telephone counseling and natural helpers (e.g., Lipkus, Rimer, and Strigo, 1996; Rimer et al., 2002; Blalock et al., 2002; Campbell et al., 2002; Earp et al., 2002). The addition of such components may be especially important in reaching women with lower levels of income and education and in explaining topics that are complex and require informed decision making. More research is needed that examines combinations of tailored interventions with other appropriate interventions. It is important to think about systems of interventions.

Telephone-Delivered Interventions

TDIs include a range of human-delivered counseling and reminder interventions delivered using the telephone and computer-generated voice response systems. These are often complex interventions that include components designed to motivate people, provide information, and overcome barriers to action. Substantial evidence-based literature documents the efficacy of TDIs across health behaviors, settings, and populations. McBride and Rimer (1999) reviewed the published literature to late 1997, with a special focus on diverse populations. TDIs have a number of variable components that, in combination, yield a broad continuum of applications (Soet and Basch, 1997). From the perspective of the intervener, calls can be initiated reactively—through calls to services or helplines, often with toll-free numbers—or proactively, via outbound calls initiated by trained interventionists. TDIs also vary by service provider (e.g., health professionals or lay staff) and whether they are paid staff or volunteers. They differ in the extent to which the call is scripted, the degree to which the script varies algorithmically with the characteristics and responses of the respondent, and the extent to which each subsequent call takes into account what was learned in previous calls or other encounters with an individual. The number, length, and timing of calls range from single contacts to multiple calls over a 12-month period. Most rely on brief calls, 10 minutes or less, although some services provide longer contacts. Increasingly, calls are based on motivational interviewing, a nondirective, behavioral process developed by Miller and Rollnick (1991).

TDIs also have served as the main intervention or as one adjunctive component of multicomponent interventions or services. This wide array of variable components increases the potential flexibility and cost-effectiveness of providing individualized services.

Examination of participation rates and demographic characteristics of study participants indicates that TDIs, particularly reactive helplines, do not have the broad-based reach that initially was expected. In one study, only 4 percent of eligible smokers in a five-county area took advantage of a telephone hotline for smokers (Ossip-Klein et al., 1991). There is no question that reactive services are underused by diverse populations. Nevertheless, the data show that TDIs are effective across different health behaviors and populations. Dini, Linkins, and Sigafoos (2000) conducted one of the few studies with substantial numbers of minorities; they reported effectiveness of brief tailored calls and/or printed reminders for childhood immunizations, with a comparison of ethnic groups versus the white population. Children assigned to the intervention groups had higher screening rates, regardless of race. One recent study (Fishman et al., 2000) compared brief reminder calls versus motivational calls as a means to increase mammography use. The study found that the reminder calls were the most cost-effective intervention. Thus, if other studies support this conclusion, we might conclude that the additional time and effort to conduct motivational calls may be unnecessary for most people. Although few studies have had sufficient sample size to compare subgroups with adequate power, the evidence suggests that diverse populations seem to benefit as much as or more than other groups (e.g., King et al., 1994).

Interactive voice response (IVR) systems are a newer variant of TDIs that allow users to call a computer to report their status and to receive information; in addition, they can be used to initiate proactive calls (Piette, 2000). The cost and complexity of creating IVR systems are now nearly as low as those for creating a Web page, with the introduction of the Voice Markup Language standard. Although still few in number, tests among diverse populations have shown positive results (Ramelson, Friedman, and Ockene, 1999; Schneider, Schwartz, and Fast, 1995; Greist et al., 1999; Piette, 1997, 1999, 2000; Piette et al., 1999). Particularly relevant to closing the digital divide, Alemi and colleagues (1996) found that low-income, chemically dependent, inner-city mothers using an IVR system of data collection, reminders, and appointment scheduling were more likely than the control group to enroll in drug treatment programs and to reduce use of health services while maintaining their health status.

Piette et al. (1999) showed that an ethnically diverse, low-income veterans population was responsive to use of automated calls for disease management. Automated calls were acceptable to both English- and Spanish-speaking patients with diabetes, including low-income patients (Piette, 1999; Piette et al., 1999). Moreover, the information people provided during the calls was reliable and clinically significant. Such calls may be useful for symptom reporting and prevention/disease monitoring in low-income and other populations. IVR and similar techniques may contribute to improved patient care without using scarce provider resources for routine monitoring (Piette, 1997).

Combinations of Tailored Print Communications and Telephone Delivery Interventions

Several studies have assessed the impact of combined interventions, such as TPCs and TDIs (e.g., Rimer et al., 1999; Lipkus et al., 2000; Blalock et al., 2002; Wakefield et al., 2002). For some topics, such as decision making about mammography, the combination appears to be more effective than TPCs alone. In a few surprising cases, TPCs performed worse than usual care, while the combination of TPC and TDI was highly effective (e.g., Rimer et al., 2001). Not enough is known about how tailored interventions work to explain these unintended effects. In at least a few studies, the use of TDIs appeared to increase the likelihood that TPCs would be attended to, read, and retained (e.g., Lipkus et al., 2000; Rimer et al., 2001). However, some studies (e.g., Wakefield et al., 2002) showed no effects—in this case, on home smoking bans, parents' smoking, or children's cotinine levels. More research is needed to determine whether there are topics that are inappropriate for tailoring as well as other macro-level conditions that should be considered. In addition, more understanding is needed of the mediators of outcome and the active ingredients in interventions. For example, Blalock et al. combined tailored print and telephone with or without community intervention. In addition, some tailored interventions seem to perform better for people in some behavioral stages. Generally, people who are not thinking about making changes are least influenced by tailored interventions (e.g., Blalock et al., 2002). All of these issues must be pursued for diverse populations.

A recent review (Revere and Dunbar, 2001) concluded that tailored intervention studies improved outcomes, as did targeting; however, little research compared tailored with targeted strategies. An important distinction must be made among these technologies. Some of them do not require users to actively seek information. TPC and TDI systems can incorporate user interaction, but do not need to do so. They can be used to reach largely passive audiences. In contrast, the IVR system assumes an active audience seeking information. Whenever a system requires active seeking of information, new questions loom. One question is the extent to which these interventions, once made available, are used by the population in the way they are intended. There is always a risk that a new technology will appeal only to the minority motivated to seek information about their health, but prove too demanding for the majority of consumers. Similarly, there is a concern that an early engagement with a technology will not be sustained. Once the first blush of technological appeal passes, there may be some tendency to reduce use. These concerns are particularly relevant in the context of diverse audiences that may vary sharply in their habits of actively seeking health information.

The next section deals with new communication technologies. In many cases, their use assumes active seeking of information by users. It will not be enough for research to show that these technologies are productive for those who use them, although that is an essential first step. The research also should address whether active audience-dependent technologies reach target and diverse audiences, and whether they can sustain active engagement among those audiences. What are the contexts in which large-scale active engagement occurs, and/or what specific incentives engender large-scale active use?

NEW HEALTH COMMUNICATION TECHNOLOGIES

The Rise of the Internet

The Internet has been adopted faster than any other known innovation in history (Institute for the Future, 1999). It took 20 years from its inception as ARPANET for the Internet to reach critical mass, where enough people were using it for it to be self-sustaining (Chamberlain, 1996). But in only 11 more years, the Internet was adopted by nearly half of the U.S. population (Rogers, 2000). In 2000, 44 percent of Americans (117 million people) reported using the Internet (U.S. Department of Commerce, 2000). Every day during the first quarter of 2000, 55,000 people became first-time users of the Internet, and 3.2 million pages of content were added.

By 2001, 54 percent of Americans—143 million people—were online (Lebo, 2001). A recent U.S. Department of Commerce (2002) report suggests that the digital divide is narrowing. Between September 1998 and September 2001, Internet use by the nation's poorest citizens—those earning less than $15,000 a year—increased at an annual rate of 25 percent. The most important reason people said they went online was to get information quickly (U.S. Department of Commerce, 2002). Over the past 2 years, there has been a trend toward more e-mail sharing of worries and seeking of advice (Pew Internet & American Life Project, 2002).

By 2001, 40 percent of African-Americans, 32 percent of Hispanics, 60 percent of whites, and 60 percent of Asian Americans/ Pacific Islanders had Internet access (U.S. Department of Commerce, 2002). All of these data are changing rapidly, and thus become outdated quickly. Moreover, the statistics vary from one report to another. Little data are available on Internet usage by some important populations, including Native Americans. In spite of large increases in the proportion of Americans with Internet access, large numbers of people still lack home access (especially important for health information) or any access at all. Numerous reports have documented the characteristics of this ever-changing population. As of 2001, although some ethnic differences in access still existed, the most profound determinants of those without access were low income and a high school education or less (U.S. Department of Commerce, 2002). Important disparities in Internet use that are relevant for health communication are as follows:

• Older Americans are less likely than younger Americans to use the Internet. Even though the number of older adults using the Internet is increasing, 85 percent of those age 65 and older, and 59 percent between the ages of 50 and 64 do *not* go online (Lenhart, 2000).

• Approximately 80 percent of people in households earning more than $75,000 have Internet access. In contrast, one-fourth of those living in households earning less than $15,000 annually have access (U.S. Department of Commerce, 2002).

• Adults without Internet access tend to have less education than those with access. Only 32 percent of Internet users have a high school education or less, compared with 71 percent of nonusers (Lenhart, 2000).

• Internet access from home for racial/ethnic groups is as follows: Asian Americans/ Pacific Islanders, 56 percent; whites, 44 percent; African-Americans, 24 percent; and Hispanics, 24 percent (U.S. Department of Commerce, 2001). Cost is the greatest deterrent to at-home access by African-Americans and Hispanics (Cultural Access Group, 2001).

• People with mental or physical disabilities (such as blindness, deafness, or difficulty walking, typing, or leaving home) are less likely than those without disabilities to use computers or the Internet (U.S. Department of Commerce, 2002). New government regulations that require all government Web sites to be configured to enhance access could make a significant difference.

• At least 50 million Americans (20 percent) are estimated to face one or more content-related barriers to the benefits offered by the Internet. These barriers include lack of local information, literacy barriers, language barriers, and lack of cultural suitability (The Children's Partnership, 2000).

A recent report by the Cultural Access Group (2001) highlighted some important ethnic differences in attitudes toward Internet use. For example, more than 60 percent of Hispanics and African-Americans said the Internet helped them stay connected to their cultures. Overall, more than 66 percent of African-Americans and Hispanics said they visited ethnic Web sites. However, more than half the African-American respondents said people of color have unique online needs, compared to only 16 percent of Hispanics and the general market. Furthermore, 66 percent of Hispanics said online content is adequate for them, compared to only 33 percent of African-Americans. A recent report by the Institute for the Future (Cain, Sarasohn-Kahn, and Wayne, 2000) concluded that significant opportunities exist to customize information to different segments of the population, based on factors such as age, socioeconomic status, ethnicity, health status, and medical condition.

The Internet is potentially one of the most powerful tools available for communicating with diverse audiences. It is critical that we understand the potential of the Internet and other computer applications for health communication with and among diverse populations.

Use of the Internet for Health Communication

The phenomenal increase in use of the Internet for health information can be attributed to many factors, several of which have particular implications for health communication for diverse audiences. Among the most important is the short time available for the health encounter (now averaging 15 minutes or less) and the increased attention to informed decision making. In the United States and most Western countries, concerns about health care costs have led to increased emphasis on the health of populations and on prevention (Eysenbach and Kohler, 2001). Many people seek health advice via the Internet to supplement their physicians' advice (Pew Internet & American Life Project, 2000b; Science Panel on Interactive Communication and Health, 1999), but there is little evidence that the Internet is replacing physician advice. In a diverse sample of Californians, including African-Americans, Hispanics, and Asian Americans/Pacific Islanders, physicians were the most common source of health information among both Internet users and nonusers. The Internet was the fifth most common source of health information, behind family/friends and various print media (Pennbridge, Moya, and Rodriguez, 1999).

By 2001, about 64 percent of U.S. Internet users said they had used the Internet for health information (Pew Internet & American Life Project, 2002). Over time, all population groups have shown a steady increase in the use of computers for health information, and this trend is likely to increase. A recent Pew Report (Pew Internet & American Life Project, 2000b) found that those seeking health information on the Internet were more likely to be members of minority groups and to have low incomes than those who use the Internet for other reasons. More than 40 percent said the information they found during their most recent search affected their health-related decisions. Half the people who sought health information on the Web said it helped them improve the way they take care of themselves (Pew Internet & American Life Project, 2000b). Forty-five percent of African-American users said the Internet helps them find health care information, compared with 35 percent of whites (Pew Internet & American Life Project, 2000a).

On one hand, these numbers are remarkable; all of them would have been near zero only a few years ago. On the other hand, they provide only the beginnings of evidence that the Internet, as it is now used, has a substantial role in health. We do not know whether those reporting Internet influence on decisions are making many new decisions about major aspects of their health or are only reporting on quite rare and/or trivial decisions, such as which brand of daily vitamins costs the least. Moreover, we do not know the extent to which self-reporting about these activities is accurate and reliable.

Networking for Health (Institute of Medicine, 1999b) identified four classes of Internet health applications: (1) real-time video transmission, (2) static file transfer, (3) remote control information search and retrieval, and (4) real-time collaboration. Each of these applications has potential uses for diverse populations that should be more fully developed.

One of the characteristics of the Internet that consumers and patients value most is access to vast amounts of information coupled with the opportunity to customize information to individual needs and characteristics. Furthermore, consumers are making use of information that until recently was available only to health professionals. For example, National Library of Medicine searches increased from 7 million in 1996 to 120 million in 1997, when free public access was inaugurated (Eysenbach and Jadad, 2001). The Internet has many other important attributes as well. Users can access information at their own pace, when and how they want, theoretically at least, 24 hours a day, 7 days a week. Communication can be real time or asynchronous, one-to-one or in a group. Multiple presentation modes can be used, such as video, audio, text, and/or animation. Moreover, interactive health communication systems can be entertaining (Lieberman, 2000).

For some health topics, such as HIV/AIDS, the anonymity afforded by the Internet may be perceived as a strong asset (DeGuzman and Ross, 1999). An excellent recent report by MacDonald, Case, and Metzger (2001) provides an overview of the range of possible uses for e-health.

Another advantage of the Internet is that it provides the latest information on given health topics. Users can obtain the level and kind of information they want—from simple explanations provided by support group participants to journal articles. Increasingly, users can select language to suit their needs, and people with visual or literacy deficits can use speech functions to receive information. Geographic boundaries per se are not a limitation, although they may reflect differences in access to certain technologies (e.g., broadband). Similarly, people with hearing limitations can use print, significantly expanding their communication opportunities. Furthermore, people with disabilities do not have to leave their homes to get information.

For sensitive topics, the privacy afforded on the Internet may be a paramount advantage, even when people have other worries about privacy. The very act of creating Web sites for the Internet can be used to facilitate the involvement of particular groups, such as teens, using action research methods (Skinner et al., 1997). In addition, e-health encounters can be self-documenting and relationship enhancing (MacDonald, Case, and Metzger, 2001). The possibilities for use of the Internet range from e-mail, support, and searches for information, to much more organized approaches, including e-health encounters (two-way exchanges of information) and e-disease management, which involves coordinated and proactive approaches to managing patients with chronic illnesses (LeGrow and Metzger, 2001). Online tools for health management can include health risk assessments, surveys, retail stores that sell health products, and home monitoring. Case managers can provide a strong link between the patient and his or her medical team.

At present, disease management appears to be attracting greater interest than e-health for prevention. This does not mean that prevention will not work online, but rather that it poses unique challenges, particularly in creating awareness and demand where none is inherently present. For example, a person's disease condition (or that of a friend or relative) may drive a search for online tools to address the problem. But because much prevention requires action in the absence of symptoms or in acute problems, the user demand for such programs will be less.

From a theoretical perspective, Internet and computer-based applications have other advantages as well. Didactic and experiential learning can be combined. Notably, these features can permit people to simulate experiences, provide believable models, and generate feedback to cue and reinforce people embarked on behavior change. People also find support through online communities. Hundreds of electronic support groups operate every day on the Internet (Winzelberg et al., 1998). The potential of these groups for health communication may be substantial. People experiencing social isolation, such as adolescent mothers with young children, can obtain a level of social support through Internet-based programs that otherwise might not be attainable (Dunham et al., 1998). A program developed for new adolescent mothers showed that the mothers used online services an average of two times a day. Low-income, socially isolated young mothers were most likely to participate. Moreover, mothers who participated most consistently had lower levels of parenting stress. The appeal of the social support components of Internet programs also was shown in a program for people with diabetes (McKay et al., 1998).

As Bandura (2002b) observed, electronic media can go beyond transmission of information. The media can be used to build virtual social networks for creating shared knowledge through collaborative learning and problem solving. One spinoff of the social support function of the Internet is especially striking. As a recent *Wired* magazine article described, some parents of desperately ill children have become Net-connected activists who not only search for and share information relevant to their children's health, but also fund medical research and contribute to research. Solovitch (2001:9) concluded, "Look online and you'll also find something more: a spirit of community, a level of candor rarely broached in polite conversation, and a warehouse of information, often routinely monitored by medical specialists." While acknowledging the questionable information on the Internet, she argued persuasively for the power and the permanence of these new Net-inspired citizen scientists who are changing not only the search for health information, but the practice of medicine and research (Solovitch, 2001).

Selnow (2000:59) provided an excellent description of the key features of the Internet:

> *Here is where I think the Internet stakes its claim. The most obvious features of the Net parallel the traditional media: like print, the Internet provides public information. Like the telephone, it permits interpersonal exchange. Like books and manuals, it offers tutorials, and like movies and TV, it provides entertainment. The Internet is a remarkable Swiss Army knife of information and communication and unlike the other media, it does the job simultaneously in print, audio and video. Unlike the traditional one-way flow of information where audiences remain passive receptacles, the Internet gives users an active role as it enables them to fulfill personal requests.*

For these reasons, Cassell, Jackson, and Cheuvront (1998) referred to health communication on the Internet as a hybrid channel. It is both transactional and response dependent and combines attributes of both mass and interpersonal communications.

A growing focus on informed decision making (IDM) assumes that consumers can be educated about health care choices (see Frosch and Kaplan, 1999; Volk, Cass, and Spann, 1999; Flood et al., 1996). The Internet may be especially promising in supporting individual autonomy and choice in decision making (Skinner et al., 1997).

Consumers value online interaction with their doctors, and they want more of it. Four million U.S. adults have e-mailed a doctor's office, and 34 million more would like to do so (Cyber Dialogue, 2000a), while only 10 to 21 percent of physicians e-mail their patients (*Journal of the Mississippi State Medical Association*, 2000; Cyber Dialogue, 2000b). Eighty percent of people surveyed in a recent poll online (Harris Interactive, 2001) said they would like to receive e-mail health reminders from their physicians. Physicians' associations such as the American Society of Clinical Oncologists and the American Gastroenterological Association have begun helping their members to create Web sites for which the associations provide content (e.g., news) and services (e.g., search functions).

A survey of patients conducted through medical oncology practices in Canada, with parallel surveys of the oncologists, confirmed the important role of physicians as sources of health information, but also shed light on why the Internet has become so valuable to patients. A majority of patients (86 percent) said they wanted as much information as possible about their illnesses (Chen and Siu, 2001). More than half the patients (54 percent) said the information from their physicians was insufficient. Most patients (71 percent) searched for information about their illness, with the Internet as the most popular choice (Chen and Siu, 2001). The overwhelming majority of patients (88 percent) said their physicians were willing to discuss this information with them and believed (70 percent) it did not adversely affect their relationships with their physicians. The corresponding view from oncologists was cautiously supportive. Most physicians (70 percent) said they searched the Internet, and one reason was to find information that might interest their patients. Like patients, the oncologists did not believe the Internet had adversely affected their relationships with patients. The patient population for this study was primarily white and with a high school education or less. More information is needed about how nonwhite patients and those with low income and education use the Internet for health information and how this affects their relationships with their physicians.

Kassirer (2000) predicted that consumers will expect more and more from the Internet in terms of health care. Not only will they demand better services tailored to their needs, but patients will want to use e-mail with their physicians and discuss with them the information they find on the Internet. Unfortunately, physicians have been slow to adopt e-mail for communication with patients. Thus, patients' preferences and physicians' behavior are likely to become more disconnected (Kassirer, 2000). Eysenbach and Jadad (2001) cautioned that although there is a strong international trend toward shared decision making, many consumers still visit health providers who favor authoritarian models for the patient-provider encounter. Patients who come to their visits with information obtained on the Internet sometimes may be rebuffed by their health providers, although specific data are needed to document both positive and negative outcomes of patients' Internet use.

Ultimately, changes will be needed in the health care system to accommodate the growing consumer demand for online support. For example, it is unlikely that physicians are going to be able to answer potentially hundreds of e-mails a day. Some practices are using technology to organize e-mail so it can be processed more efficiently, but such tools do not appear to be widely used. In addition, new kinds of human interfaces may be needed to expedite the process. Payment may be needed as an important incentive.

As a number of observers have noted, to be without Internet access today is much like being without a telephone was earlier in the century. More and more, lacking access to the Internet may limit one's potential economic growth as well as access to health information. As the Internet has grown, it has attracted more women, more ethnic minorities, and more people from different age groups (Cain, Sarasohn-Kahn, and Wayne, 2000). The Internet is not the only—or even the most important—health communication strategy for diverse audiences, but it is a vital force and it must be considered. The challenge is to harness its potential as part of the menu of communication options for diverse audiences.

To do that, a recent survey by the Children's Partnership (2000) shows that the Internet will have to provide more of the health information that diverse groups want and need. Serious barriers also will have to be surmounted. These barriers have been articulated by a number of authors and include variable quality of information, difficulty finding high-quality information because of the vagaries of commercial search engines, lack of access, and concerns about privacy (Eng et al., 1998). One of the most important deficiencies is the lack of content, the Children's Partnership notes. Moreover, most of the text on the Web is written at a reading level too advanced to be understood by many users (Graber et al., 1999; Oermann and Wilson, 2000). According to the survey, persons with low incomes want more information in their native languages, more sites written for beginning-level English speakers, and more information about health services. For those with low health literacy—a third or more of the U.S. population—this may represent a major information barrier (Eysenbach and Jadad, 2001). In addition, recent data show that consumers use search engines that may restrict their access to high-quality health information (Taylor and Leitman, 2001; Harris Interactive, 2001).

Many people in the United States and other societies, especially those about whom this volume is most concerned, lack any access to the Internet, limiting the effectiveness of Internet-based health communication. This may be a special problem for rural populations. Limitations also include the lack of verbal, aural, and visual clues (DeGuzman and Ross, 1999); the mass of information of unknown or poor quality; and the difficulty of navigation (Cline and Haynes, 2001). The startup costs of computer-based applications can be high, although efficiencies can be achieved in the long run. As discussed elsewhere in this volume, many people remain concerned about lack of privacy on the Internet.

The potential of the Internet is extraordinary, but this is not the same as the realization of the potential. Successful use of the Internet can require a fundamental shift among the population in how users make sense of the world. They need to be motivated to seek information; they need the skills to know how to frame a question, how to seek good information, and how to interpret information they receive. People commonly express their desire to move from a passive role to an active role, and the Internet offers that promise. However, what proportion of the need for information will be met in this way in practice is the hard question. It is likely to vary sharply by domain and by audience characteristics. If only a small proportion of the need for a particular domain for a given audience is actually met through active Internet use, this may create a worrisome tension. Although physicians report few negative experiences with patients' use of the Internet, they do report some negative sequelae (Potts and Wyatt, 2001). Moreover, we are still at an early point in studying how the Internet affects patients' health behaviors and their communication with health professionals. It is possible that institutions could reduce their outreach efforts after confusing the extraordinary availability of Internet information with the actual limited use of that information by the audience. They may believe the Internet has solved the problem when it has not.

Interactive Health Communication

Interactive Health Communication is defined as the interaction of an individual—consumer, patient, caregiver, or professional—with or through an electronic device or communication technology to access or transmit health information or to receive guidance and support on a health-related issue (Patrick et al., 1999). Many of the early applications demonstrated increases in users' knowledge and acceptability of the systems (Kumar et al., 1993). Most applications now are Internet based or will be in the future. IHC includes computer health enhancement systems, interactive computer games, and Web-based applications, including the Internet. IHC services can range from simple applications, such as a single article or a discussion group, to online support groups and programs that offer many services, including information, communication, analysis, and a personalized Web page or a computer-based game intended to promote a certain behavior change (see Bental, Cawsey, and Jones, 1999, for an excellent overview of computer-mediated patient education techniques). Telemedicine and telecomputing offer a host of new communication opportunities, including electronic house calls (Ostbye and Hurlen, 1997).

IHC applications operate through telephones, personal digital assistants, Internet appliances, personal computers, and public kiosks. As wireless computers become more available, there will be even more delivery options. The Science Panel on Interactive Communication and Health (SciPICH) (1999) concluded that IHC reduces disease risk, improves quality of life, and influences use of health services.

Much of the potential for IHC in behavior change can be attributed to five things this communication does well: (1) provides social support and guidance, (2) tailors messages, (3) analyzes data, (4) monitors performance, and (5) provides reminders. IHC may improve adherence by providing motivation, social support, and guidance during the early and maintenance periods of personal change. It can increase salience and relevance by tailoring for age, ethnicity, and disease characteristics. Guidance can be adjusted to reflect a person's efficacy level, unique impediments in their lives, and progress they are making (Bandura, 1997a, 2000). Information can be adjusted to reflect a person's past behavior. In addition, graphic information, such as portion sizes for dietary recommendations, can be person specific (Oenema, Brug, and Lechner, 2001). Because distance is not an issue, people who share problems can be brought together from all over the world. This is especially useful for rare conditions. In addition, the anonymity of the Internet may make it easier for people with stigmatizing conditions to disclose and discuss them (White and Dorman, 2001). Feedback can be provided in many ways.

The absence of individualized guidance places limits on the power of mass communication. The advances in interactive technology provide the means to increase the scope and productivity of health promotion and other health communication programs (Bandura, 2000). One can distinguish between the enhancement of health impacts through electronic technologies on the input side and on the behavioral adoption side. On the input side, health communication can be tailored personally to factors that are causally related to health behavior. Individualized interactivity, on the behavioral adoption side, further enhances the impact of health promotion programs. Social support and guidance during early periods of personal change and maintenance increase long-term success. Group-oriented systems often do not fare well because of arbitrary timing, bothersome accessibility, and inconvenience. Informal social systems do not necessarily provide good guidance.

Interactive computer-assisted feedback can provide a convenient means for informing, motivating, and guiding people in their efforts to make lifestyle changes. Tailored guidance can be adjusted to participants' efficacy levels, the unique impediments in their lives, and the progress they are making. The feedback may take a variety of forms, including TPC, telephone counseling, and linkage to supportive social networks. For example, the self-management model for health promotion developed by DeBusk and colleagues (1994) centers heavily on interactive guidance on the behavioral adoption side. Moreover, online support groups can be available to people 24 hours a day, 7 days a week (White and Dorman, 2001).

We provide brief descriptions and summaries of how some of these computer-based technologies have been used, especially with diverse populations, and a selective review of the evidence.

The Comprehensive Health Enhancement Support System (CHESS) developed at the University of Wisconsin is one of the best examples of the potential of IHC to improve health among diverse populations (see http://chess.chsra.wisc.edu/Chess/). CHESS was developed in 1989, has been tested in several research studies, and is now Internet based. Patients obtain access to CHESS through their health care providers. Many organizations that offer CHESS can loan computers to participants.

After entering a code name and password, users see a main menu from which they can choose a general topic, pick a particular keyword, or enter a service of interest. Descriptions of the services follow, using prostate cancer as an example:

• *Information Services* include several features. *Questions and Answers* provides brief answers to 400 frequently asked prostate cancer questions. *The Instant Library* includes more than 200 full-length articles drawn from the scientific and/or popular press available on other Web sites. *The Consumer Guide* provides descriptions of 150 services to help users visualize what it will be like to receive the service, learn to identify a good provider, and become an effective consumer. *Web Links* includes direct connections to other Web sites or specific pages in those sites. The *Resource Directory* describes local and/or national services and ways to contact them.

• *Communication Services* offer information and emotional support to users. Professionally moderated bulletin board *Discussion Groups* for patients, partners, prayer groups, and other groups are open to any CHESS user, but are limited to 50 participants. *Ask an Expert* allows people to receive a confidential response to questions from specialists at the National Cancer Institute's (NCI's) regional Cancer Information Service. Responses are made anonymously and available for all users within *Open Expert*. *Live Chats* are scheduled real-time discussions facilitated by content experts. *Journaling* provides a private (content saved only on the user's floppy disk) forum for users to write their deepest thoughts and feelings about prostate cancer in a controlled and timed environment. *Personal Stories* are accounts of how people cope with prostate cancer. *Video Gallery* allows users to see prostate cancer patients and their spouses talk about how they coped with the disease and its treatment.

• *CHESS Analysis Services* include: (1) *Health Tracking*—people enter data on their health status every 2 weeks and receive graphs of how their health status is changing; (2) *Decision and Conflicts*—patients and families examine important treatment decisions by watching video clips of prostate cancer patients talking about how they made their decision, or by using a structured decision analysis; and (3) *Action Plans*—a decision theory model helps users plan behavior changes by identifying goals, resources, and ways to overcome obstacles.

In a randomized CHESS trial of younger women with breast cancer, about one-third of the participants were low-income, inner-city African-American women. They used CHESS as much as affluent white women with breast cancer (Gustafson et al., 2000). However, they used it very differently. In particular, low-income women (older and younger) used the computer-mediated communication services (e.g., electronic discussion groups) less frequently and information services (e.g., frequently asked questions and library) and analysis services (e.g., decision analysis and health tracking) more often. A growing body of research suggests that using IHC for information and analysis is more important to improving quality of life than using them for emotional support (Bass et al., 1998; Shaw et al., 2000; Boberg et al., 1997; Smaglik et al., 1998). This suggestion may be especially relevant for diverse populations. CHESS also has resulted in quality-of-life improvements, shorter ambulatory care visits, and fewer and shorter hospitalizations (Gustafson et al., 1999). These are particularly noteworthy health services outcomes.

Computer games are another important IHC. *Packy and Marlon* is a Super Nintendo video game designed to teach children with diabetes self-management skills to address specific challenges facing diabetes patients. The characters are two adolescent elephant friends with diabetes who are going to a diabetes summer camp. The players (one or two) play the role of the elephant friends who must save their camp from rodents who have scattered the camp's food and diabetes supplies. Players must help their elephant character monitor blood glucose, take appropriate amounts of insulin, review a diabetes logbook, and find foods that contain the right amount of food exchanges. Through entertaining experiences, players learn about self-care and typical social situations related to diabetes. To win, players must learn how to engage in behaviors that help their character stay healthy. *Packy and Marlon* improved diabetes-related communication between parents and children with diabetes, increased parents' ratings of self-care and self-efficacy, and reduced clinic visits (Brown et al., 1997).

Psychosocial programs for health promotion will be implemented increasingly via interactive Internet-based systems in a variety of formats. For example, young women at risk for eating disorders often refuse preventive or remedial health services, but some may pursue online individualized behavioral guidance. In several studies, participants reduced their dissatisfaction with their weight and body shape, and they positively altered dysfunctional attitudes and disordered eating behavior by this means (Winzelberg et al., 2000).

Most studies have shown that computer-based education programs are accepted by people of different ages, educational levels, economic strata, and ethnicity (Balas et al., 1997; Krishna et al., 1997; Fieler and Borch, 1996; Bental, Cawsey, and Jones, 1999; Alemi et al., 1996; Prochaska et al., 2000; Jones et al., 2000). IHC using structured psychoeducational approaches has the potential to transfer knowledge and help people develop skills to change behaviors (Lewis, 1999). The BARN Research Group found that teenagers using IHC were more likely to remain free of risk-taking behaviors and improve risk-relevant behaviors such as stress reduction, smoking cessation, and contraceptive use (Bosworth, Gustafson, and Hawkins, 1994). Other examples of IHC for adolescents have been well received and have focused on topics such as conflict resolution (Bosworth et al., 1996) and safer sex negotiation (Thomas, Cahill, and Santilli, 1997). Chewning et al. (1999) reported significantly increased knowledge of oral contraceptives as well as increased rates of adopting (though not increased adherence to) oral contraceptives. Some of the benefit from using IHC may result from the greater involvement and deeper processing compared to passive methods.

A number of other outcome studies of IHC have been reported, several with diverse populations and across a range of health areas, including adolescent risk behaviors (Paperny and Hedberg, 1999; Bosworth et al., 1994), AIDS (Gustafson et al., 2000), exercise, diet, smoking cessation, asthma (Yawn et al., 2000; Homer et al., 2000), safe sex (Thomas et al., 1997), conflict resolution, eating disorders (Winzelberg, 2000), immunization, and skin cancer prevention (Hornung et al., 2000; Chewning et al., 1999). The results show improvements in outcomes such as knowledge and beliefs, quality of life, reduced hospitalizations, improved functional status, reduced pain, confidence in asking questions, body image, decisional confidence, self-efficacy, and knowledge. Krishna et al. (1997:25) concluded that "Computerized educational interventions can lead to improved health status in several major areas of care, and appear not to be a substitute for, but a valuable supplement to, face-to-face time with physicians." However, more studies are needed that report outcomes on diverse populations.

IHC has the capacity to provide real-time feedback to patients recovering from acute illnesses and patients with chronic diseases. For example, Brennan et al. (2001) reported on the development of HeartCare, an Internet-based information and support system for patients recovering at home after coronary artery bypass graft surgery. HeartCare provides information tailored to patients' recovery needs. Such tools may be especially useful as patients spend fewer days in the hospital. Nursing assessments and patient-specific data are used to tailor information to individual needs. Patients use "smart cards" and Web TVs to access HeartCare, thus reducing potential access problems. Although data are not yet available, systems like HeartCare are likely to become more common in the future. Moreover, by providing easy tools for access, they are more likely to meet the needs of diverse populations.

Balas et al. (1997) conducted a synthesis of published articles that reported on electronic communication with patients. Of 80 eligible clinical trials, 61 (76 percent) analyzed provider-initiated communication with patients and 50 (63 percent) reported positive outcome, improved performance, or significant benefits, including studies of computerized communication (7 of 7), telephone followup and counseling (20 of 37), telephone reminders (14 of 23), interactive telephone systems (5 of 6), telephone access (3 of 4), and telephone screening (1 of 3). Significantly improved outcomes were found in studies of preventive care, management of osteoarthritis, cardiac rehabilitation, and diabetes care. There were no reported outcomes for diverse populations.

Patients want more interactions with their physicians than physicians are willing to provide. Physicians consistently give several reasons for not participating in e-mail exchanges and what have been referred to as e-encounters. The reasons include not being reimbursed, concern about professional liability, and concern about volume (MacDonald, Case, and Metzger, 2001). These reasons will have to be addressed before major advances can be made in the use of the Internet for patient-physician (or other health professional) encounters. In addition, medical curricula should include interactive health communication (Cline and Haynes, 2001).

A recent conference on consumer health informatics concluded that "consumers want personalized relationships with their clinicians . . . so they get information that addresses their individual concerns and conditions" (Kaplan and Brennan, 2001:310). They also want interactive tools to manage their health and diseases. Today's children will grow up with interactive technologies. Thus, it is certain that acceptance will increase over time.

CONCLUSIONS

As Rainie (2002) envisioned, the Internet permits Net-savvy patients to individualize a virtual Net world to meet their individual needs. Such a world provides information and educational tools, and gives self-helpers supportive techniques and even opportunities for conversations with one's physician or other health experts. We view this world as potentially even larger, with messages and cues from the mass media part of the environment.

The Internet is likely to be used more for distance learning (e.g., Steckler et al., 2001) and as a way to collect information efficiently from potentially large numbers of people, such as stakeholders on a particular issue (Atkinson and Gold, 2001). This may be an important democratizing force in health care.

Interactive technologies offer great potential to strengthen diverse communities and improve their health. However, this is now more a promise than a reality (Bernhardt, 2000). In fact, even the very issue of interactivity is not a given: Stout, Villegas, and Kim (2001) recently examined health Web sites across different domains and found that few of them employed interactive tools. Ideally, the new communication technologies will expand choices for how people get health information, not constrain them. The new technologies, like the old, should represent a choice, not a requirement, for diverse populations.

Achieving the potential of new technologies for diverse populations requires attention to access, as well as to the acceptability, availability, appropriateness, and applicability of content. As Eysenbach and Jadad (2001) warned, without deliberate action, new computer technologies may exacerbate inequities in health and health care. Merely providing computers rarely will be sufficient. Rather, ongoing training and support will be required. As in other areas of health care, participation of community members in program planning will heighten the potential for success.

Although poor-quality information cannot be removed from the Internet, consumers can be taught how to search for information and separate the good from the bad (Eysenbach et al., 2000; Cooke, 1999). There is some evidence that consumers' search strategies are suboptimal, but training could help (Eysenbach and Kohler, 2002). Moreover, consumers should be taught to use search engines that direct them to high-quality health Web sites. Within the European Union, progress has been made in developing interoperative standards for rating health Web sites (Eysenbach et al., 2000). More attention is focusing on issues of access and usability (see, e.g., Eveland and Dunwoody, 2000), but more effort is needed (Cline and Haynes, 2001). This will benefit all Internet users.

We should not become so focused on the medium that we ignore the message. The content of health information is vitally important. As Cline and Haynes (2001) stressed, the Internet should be viewed as a communication process that activates social influence. This requires shifting focus from information alone to messages and meanings. At this point in time, a focus on all these areas, including content and quality, is needed.

More research is needed to fully understand the impact of IHC on diverse populations. This means that the mechanisms by which they operate should be examined. Today, most research on behavioral interventions using new communication technologies relies on "kitchen sink" approaches that do not permit an assessment of the individual and combined contributions of intervention components. Currently available reports in the literature focus disproportionately on nonbehavioral outcomes, such as knowledge. In addition, most studies follow participants for only short periods. Multifactorial designs should be used more, with measures of both mediators of behavior and behavioral and health outcomes. Research designs should incorporate the means to study the Internet as a communication process rather than merely a high-tech conveyer of information (Cline and Haynes, 2001). Of the computer-based studies, Winzelberg et al. (1998, 2000) were the only ones to assess mediators of outcomes.

More attention also should be paid to the relationship between behavioral determinants and individual characteristics that are identified as important for tailored and Internet-based interventions. As Kukafka and colleagues (2001:1477) noted, Web technology permits us to "deliver a tailored mix of educational content, directed simultaneously at motivations, beliefs, and skills." However, they stressed the importance of the selection of determinants and constructs: "Sophisticated tailoring to weak or irrelevant determinants and individual characteristics will yield poor results" (Kukafka et al., 2001:1477).

A recent review concluded that tailored communication can affect health outcomes more than generic, targeted, or personalized interventions. However, the review also highlighted a number of problems we have noted earlier. These include the lack of explicit theoretic basis, few studies that compare tailored approaches, and an inability to explain what design features affected the outcomes (Revere and Dunbar, 2001). In addition, few studies have assessed the impact of mobile devices for patients, except for data input and monitoring (Revere and Dunbar, 2001). Only 23 studies (62 percent) stated use of a theory to guide the health behavior intervention: 19 were print communication, and 4 were telephone (Revere and Dunbar, 2001). Moreover, more research is needed on wireless devices. Mobile systems have particular appeal because of their portability, privacy, and other features. In addition, they can provide discrete, immediate, and frequent feedback (Revere and Dunbar, 2001; Dirkin, 1994). Of course, cost and availability barriers first must be transcended.

In the future, large-scale health campaigns may look vastly different from those with which we are familiar. The mass media may be used to direct people to Internet sites from which they can receive tailored health communication programs, combining the reach of the mass media with the effectiveness of individualized counseling. Such approaches would use segmentation to capture the attention of diverse populations and tailoring techniques to reach individuals. By providing access points in communities, the digital divide could be transformed into digital access. Many new technology commentators have predicted devices that combine several elements and perform multiple functions. An even more important type of convergence may be the convergence of different media, such as mass and micro media, to achieve health communication goals.

As new communication technologies proliferate, there is a great risk that an additional divide will develop between the public health sector and other health settings. Urgent attention must be paid to how to increase the availability and use of new communication technologies within the public health sector, where they can meet specific needs of diverse populations. The private and public sectors both have roles in meeting the health information needs of diverse populations and in facilitating the dissemination of new technologies.

Although the new media world has many real and potential benefits, potential dangers also exist. The availability of large amounts of data on individual users of the Internet presents a major threat to individuals' privacy. It is not yet clear how new U.S. Department of Health and Human Services (HHS) regulations governing access to medical data will affect health communication applications on the Internet. Multiple surveys indicate the public is very concerned about privacy online, and health communication researchers and practitioners should pay attention to this issue. The Internet is a bit like the Wild West: It has vast amounts of unregulated territory and no one in charge. Many people believe the Internet is inherently self-regulating, but more regulation may be needed where health information is concerned.

Issues of privacy, quality, access, and appropriateness of content for diverse populations must be addressed if the potential of the new technologies to benefit all people is to be achieved. Finally, we want to emphasize our strong belief that although the Internet should be part of the menu of choices available to people who want health information, consumers should not be forced to use new technologies and they should not be denied information because they are nonusers. It would be unfortunate if the Internet became the voice mail of the future. Such a scenario would represent yet another way to meet demand without meeting need in an effort to cut costs.

COMMUNICATION: THE NEXT FRONTIER

The astronomical increase in wireless technologies providing Internet access through handheld devices brings new meaning to the term *personal computer.* Many new delivery devices are now available, including kiosks, interactive pagers such as the Blackberry, Web TV, and Internet appliances such as I-Opener and Audrey (designed for placement in the kitchen). Some of these, such as Audrey, already are being displaced by the next generation of technology. Internet-ready cellular phones have made instant messaging a worldwide phenomenon. The handheld devices offer new opportunities to put health messages literally in the palm of one's hand. New devices are proliferating, and more people are using them. Greater bandwidth and videoconferencing may provide new ways for patients and their health providers to interact (Jadad, 1999).

These devices often start as gadgets for the affluent, but then become tools for the masses. In a shorter and shorter amount of time, price goes down and access increases, making the devices more accessible and appealing to diverse populations. Promising examples include devices such as Web Pads, which are now being used in some hospitals to provide Internet access to patients and their families (Bennett, 2001). It may be years before these devices become household products, but now is the time to prepare for the future.

In the not-too-distant future, use of Internet radio will be even more important than it is today. Some churches and community groups already have their own radio stations. This trend is likely to increase. Partnerships between health- and faith-based organizations may provide new outlets for health messages. Parallel trends in the syndication of Internet content offer opportunities to customize health content to diverse populations as well as to individuals within those populations.

Complementary tools from science and biology will be delivered increasingly via the Internet. An example is the NCI's Breast Cancer Risk Assessment Tool, which allows women to calculate their probability of developing breast cancer and to receive feedback about potential preventive strategies. The Harvard Cancer Risk Index (http://www.yourcancerrisk.harvard.edu/index.htm) is another Internet-based tool that provides comprehensive cancer prevention assessment and feedback (Colditz et al., 2000). In the future, users of these and other individualized risk assessments will be able to receive private, individualized health advice; make plans; and track their progress. Such tools are likely to be accompanied by biological sensors carried by individuals to monitor bodily processes and provide feedback. In the future, patients may be able to access their own medical records online and to monitor their own test results. This kind of activity now occurs only in limited settings.

Instant translation services on the Internet are breaking down language barriers between people. Text-to-speech capabilities are improving and will offer further options to maximize access for diverse populations. The Simputer can read Web pages aloud in Native American languages and is one of a new generation of handheld devices that could make a tremendous difference in access to information by poor, illiterate people (Ward, 2001). Today's children and adolescents are growing up with fast-paced, high-tech computer games and television shows and movies that look like the games and vice versa. They will have a facility with computers that few of today's health professionals have developed. Moreover, their expectation for high production quality will raise the standards for health information. To compete, health communication professionals will have to partner with experts in areas such as marketing, computer design, and computer games.

To imagine health communications of the future, one can rely on both a theoretical basis and growing evidence. Undoubtedly, there will be more tailored health communication of every type, using a variety of media and formats. This communication will be increasingly interactive and based on theory-relevant variables as well as other variables, such as cultural factors appropriate to specific behavior. Ideally, this new health communication will complement other communication strategies, such as mass media, social network interventions, policies, and provider counseling. The convergence of mass media and new techniques could permit social-level attention to health issues, with the potential to individualize programs through tailored interventions. The combination of mass and micro media could produce synergistic effects leading to greater behavioral impact.

However, we must express appropriate caution. Funding of most health communication research relies on processes that are too slow to accommodate the speed of technology development. Some attempts have been made to correct this problem in other fields, and new approaches should be developed for health communication as well. In addition, public health efforts must compete with much more remunerative private health efforts. Programming and design talent are critical to creating programs that will compete in a sophisticated and information-rich environment, yet such personnel often demand salaries that exceed existing university structures. These concerns could be assuaged by greater collaboration with the private sector and by some creative restructuring of funding mechanisms that support such research.

The evolving information technologies increasingly will serve as a vehicle for building social networks. Online transactions transcend the barriers of time and space (Hiltz and Turoff, 1978; Wellman, 1997). Interactive electronic networking can link people in widely dispersed locales, and permit them to exchange information, share new ideas, and transact business. Virtual networking provides a flexible means for creating diffusion structures to serve given purposes, expanding their membership, extending them geographically, and disbanding them when they have outlived their usefulness.

Tailored technologies present challenges for delivery and evaluation—especially in public health settings that tend to be computer poor. Demand for health communication interventions using new technologies is likely to outstrip availability. Measurement challenges also exist—such as how to analyze data from trials in which every individual receives a different intervention. Today's tools will require substantial transformation to be adapted to the methods, messages, and media of tomorrow.

The rapidly changing world of the Internet also is changing the look and feel of other media. Magazines and television commercials look more and more like Web sites. In the near future, we may no longer think of mass media, new media, and old media, but many media with different and complementary uses, ultimately able to reach through and touch individuals while creating and enhancing real and virtual communities.

The result may be enhanced personal and collective efficacy and, ultimately, improved health. The borders between individuals and countries already have been reduced as health information travels throughout the world in mere seconds. The media boundaries may become indistinct as well. The messages will be far more than the media. But, in a new way, the media will be the message.

Another area offering significant, although yet unrealized, potential is disease management through remote monitoring and feedback (Patel, 2001). This may be especially true for asthma and other diseases for which meaningful information exchange and proactive partnerships are essential. Clearly, there are many privacy issues that must be confronted, among other challenges. Nevertheless, some early data suggest that diverse populations can participate in their own self-management through Internet-based assessment and capture of spirometric data (Patel, 2001).

Although the committee is optimistic about the future opportunities afforded by new technologies, we recognize that storm clouds are on the horizon. The potential of new technologies still is far greater than today's reality. As noted earlier in this chapter, the clouds include availability, accessibility, and affordability of the new technologies. Content relevant to and appropriate for diverse populations is a high-priority need. Technology is a means to an end, not an end in itself. We should not place excessive hope in the technology itself (Bandura, 2002b:4).

The growing social and economic divide between rich and poor nations presents more daunting challenges to make globalization more inclusive and equitable (Bandura, 2002b:6). Electronic technologies not only may be unaffordable in many parts of the United States and in poor nations, but such places also may lack the educational, communication, organizational, and service infrastructure to manage the use of new technologies.

On an individual level, the clouds involve not only threats to privacy, but the ways, still not well understood, in which the medium of new technologies may encourage or at least provide permission for socially unacceptable behaviors. Bandura (2002b) cautioned that concealment and depersonalization can bring out the worst in people.

Another problem, whose scope is still unknown, is the amount of incomplete or inaccurate information that is acquired on the Internet. Bichakjian et al. (2002) assessed the accuracy and completeness of information about melanoma on the Internet. Identified Web sites were evaluated by independent reviewers with high reliability. The authors concluded that the majority of Web sites that mentioned melanoma failed to provide complete information on risk factors, diagnosis, treatment, prevention, and prognosis. Fourteen percent of the Web sites included factual inaccuracies. None of the sites used innovative graphic techniques, including videos, to enhance understanding. What the authors failed to point out was that many of the Web pages in their sample were the personal anecdotes of melanoma survivors, and did not purport to be either comprehensive or medically rigorous. As a recent *British Medical Journal* editorial cautioned, there probably cannot be a single standard of quality on the Internet, just as there could not be for other media (Purcell, 2002). We should be cautious about adding new regulations.

Moreover, the Internet has an unexpected dark side. Although it is still a small proportion of overall sales, there is evidence that adolescent minors buy cigarettes on the Internet (Unger, Rohrbach, and Ribisl, 2001). In 2001, Ribisl, Kim, and Williams estimated that more than 88 vendors sold cigarettes online, and the number is growing. Connolly (2001:299) cautioned, "if the tobacco industry embraces this new unregulated medium, many of the major public interventions that we have developed to curb real world lung cancer could go up in a puff of cyber smoke. Taxes, ad bans, and youth access laws are easily eroded online."

In spite of the storm clouds and frank concerns about the new communication technologies, these technologies are diffusing widely throughout the world, with rapid and consistent growth among diverse populations. Our recommendations about the new technologies are made in light of both the vast potential and the possible pitfalls.

RECOMMENDATIONS

Previously, the Science Panel on Interactive Communication and Health made a series of excellent recommendations about priorities for IHCs (Science Panel on Interactive Communication and Health, 1999). Recommendations focused on several broad areas, including the development and application of models for quality and evaluation; improvement of basic knowledge and understanding of the uses and applications of IHCs; enhancement of capacity, particularly in the public health sector; and increased access to new technologies, especially for diverse populations. We support these recommendations. Most important, we support the goal of universal access as articulated by SciPICH (see Eng et al., 1998:1374):

> *Technology, if used appropriately, can help people increase their knowledge of health, enhance their ability to negotiate the health care system, understand and modify their health risk behaviors, and acquire coping skills and social support. Furthermore, by reducing the information divide now, the next century may bring us closer to health equity.*

The following recommendations are additional high-priority topics that must be addressed if the advances in health communication are to reach their potential for diverse audiences. The priorities are in the areas of research, practice, training, and policy:

• *Support continued experimental research to understand new communication technologies, including how they are used, how they work, and how they may be used effectively with other communication strategies, such as the mass media, natural helpers, and interpersonal counseling, to increase population reach and maximize health outcomes, especially for diverse populations.* This includes assessment of psychosocial, cultural, and other potential determinants of health behavior from the perspective of the public, patients, and health providers, and assessment of how their interactions are changed by new technologies. A goal should be to identify the "active ingredients" that provide informative guides for constructing effective health promotion programs (Abrams, 1999). Are some tailoring algorithms more effective than others? How can one enhance dissemination? Research should be sponsored by the National Institutes of Health (NIH), National Science Foundation, and other organizations, including foundations and the corporate sector. NCI is currently the only NIH Institute that has allocated research support to research designed to increase digital access. More Institutes should invest in this area. Moreover, partnerships, such as that developed by the NCI and the Markle Foundation to fund digital divide projects, can be productive.

• Increase access of diverse populations to health care information through new technologies. The roles of the public and private sectors should be examined and clarified. New public-private partnerships (some might include faith-based organizations) are needed to develop new technologies, increase access, and develop health information content appropriate for diverse populations. It is unlikely that a technological fix will be sufficient. Both access and content are important. Also important is an understanding of the sociostructural conditions that shape the use of new communication technologies.

• Support interdisciplinary training in the new technologies at multiple levels, including the next generation of health communication researchers and practitioners, as well as those currently in the field. Training also is needed to equip potential users with the skills to maximize the new technologies to meet their own needs.

• Encourage HHS to form a cross-departmental working group to make recommendations about how to interface with the commercial sector and should specifically address the issue of search engines. Commercial search engines increasingly are giving priority to paying commercial sites and bypassing public sector and nonprofit sites. This trend may pose a special threat for diverse audiences. User-friendly health portals will be especially important for diverse populations. This priority is consistent with the leadership that HHS has taken with SciPICH, its scientific panel on IHC.

• Encourage open source development of interventions using new health communication technologies, including those developed for research, to ensure that new tools have wide availability (see Schrage, 2000; Raymond, 1999). This will increase the likelihood that diverse populations benefit from advances in health communication and from the large tax-supported research investment.

• Develop and test new methods for studying and reporting the nature, uses, users, and impact of the new media. Recognizing that the new technologies create new environments, new kinds of use, and new communities, research methods must be adapted. Provide some fast-track funding to enable researchers to use new technology as developed and to obtain answers quickly.

• Create a high-level public-private partnership to focus on the multiple issues related to quality and ethics on the Internet, including the consideration of a rating system to brand Web sites that are rated as trustworthy and accurate. However, any quality system must go beyond Web site ratings and deal with content as well. Internet users should be trained to assess the accuracy of health information on the Internet. Important ethical issues are involved in health communication using the new technologies, particularly because of the potential for collecting, storing, and using personal data on Internet users (see Spielberg, 1998; Institute of Medicine, 1999b; Eysenbach, 2000; Eysenbach et al., 2000). Although the issues transcend particular populations, special attention should be paid to the concerns by and for diverse populations. We commend the Internet Healthcare Coalition for its e-Health Ethics Initiative (2000) and encourage wide participation in this effort.

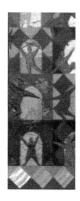

7

Toward a
New Definition of
Diversity

DIMENSIONS OF DIVERSITY

One part of the committee's charge was to review existing theory and research applications in health communication and behavior change, especially as they related to socioculturally and demographically diverse populations. Throughout this volume we have used traditional epidemiological categories to describe disparities in health risks and health outcomes for diverse populations and to characterize the research literature on communication interventions for those populations. However, there is a lack of clarity and consensus about the constructs commonly used for grouping individuals—specifically, race, ethnicity, and culture—as well as what is actually measured in studies that rely on these constructs. This makes the interpretation of the existing literature problematic.

This chapter has two purposes. The first is to comment on the broad demographic categories featured in most population-based descriptions of health status differences and most discussions of disparities. We show that even following such crude indicators, populations are more diverse—and vary more along multiple dimensions of demographic differences—than may be commonly assumed. The second purpose of this chapter is to offer an alternative concept of cultural processes that affords a more relevant base from which to understand sociocultural diversity and its implications for health communication. Our recommendations from this chapter stem from the perspective that understanding differences in health status or health behavior requires an examination of sociocultural processes and life experiences. Underlying this perspective is a radical reframing of cultural groupings because current categories are often misused in attempts to explain differences within and across groups. This new perspective suggests a fundamental reorientation in the research agenda.

In the discussion of culture and diversity in this chapter, a number of specific issues are raised, and suggestions are made to address those issues. The issues include:

• Despite a lack of *biological* evidence for racial groupings, "race" as a *social* construct continues to be a reality that is reflected in discriminatory social relationships and actions (racism, discrimination, oppression). For this reason, the construct of "race" matters in our society.

• Because these key social constructs of "race/ethnicity" (e.g. African-Americans and whites) are correlated, however imperfectly, with socioeconomic indicators, they are useful as rough indicators of health disparities. It is when we want to go beyond rough assessments of the health impacts of socially mediated macro forces that these constructs have little explanatory power, because of intragroup variation and other sociocultural and political factors that may have more important influences on behavior.

• The identification of health disparities through the use of racial and ethnic categories has also led some to equate diversity with disparity and to contribute to a view that ethnic groups are homogeneous. Neither of these is necessarily the case. In fact, the use of racial/ethnic labels reifies the groups and conveys the sense that these group labels reflect some "cultural reality" in some meaningful way. This implies that the solution lies in dealing with cultural differences even though positing a causal relationship is not warranted by the data.

• There is also a tension resulting from the focus on "groups" and the tendency to reify culture as a static experience for members of so-called "ethnic groups" versus looking at cultural and social experiences or processes as they affect people's lives and behavior. With regard to health communication efforts, the lack of a biological basis for grouping human beings means that the only avenue for the positing and creation of "groups" is in society (not in nature). Without race, experience-based constructs remain the main option for categorizing diversity. Highlighting experience does not move attention away from political-economic and structural impacts on health, but rather allows us to better grapple with disentangling and assessing the impact of the socially constructed world on the health of individuals. The sharing of socially mediated life experiences provides the basis for researchers to posit groupings that may be more meaningful for public health research in general.

• Differences in health risks and health outcomes also may reflect environmental factors ranging from socioeconomic constraints and health care access barriers to poor air quality. Behavioral factors also may be affected by social and environmental parameters and by biological factors.

• The risk of assuming that people have more power to alter their behavior or their environment than they may actually have can lead to "blaming the victim."

Problems with Traditional Categories as Used in Federal Statistics

Federal categories focus primarily on so-called "race" and "ethnicity." Diversity in the United States is culturally and socially constructed. Part of the complexity in talking about diversity is that the naming, grouping, and categorizing of perceived differences among human beings is done from a variety of perspectives, and to achieve a variety of ends.

Contradictions and inconsistencies exist in official use of terms for ethnic groups in the United States (Ahdieh and Hahn, 1996; Hahn, 1992, 1999; Hahn and Stroup, 1994). Pan-ethnic categories such as Asian American and Hispanic are largely arbitrary constructions created by demographers and social scientists for purposes of data development, analysis, and policy (Suárez-Orozco, 2000:14). For example, "Hispanic" was introduced by demographers working for the Bureau of the Census in the 1980s as a way to categorize people who are either historically or culturally connected to the Spanish language. Note that "Hispanic" has no precise meaning regarding racial or national origins, and is rejected by many individuals in favor of other terms, including Latino, Mexican American, or Puerto Rican. In addition, Latinos are white, Black, indigenous, Asian, and every possible combination thereof, and originate in more than 20 countries. They may have just arrived or been in this country for generations, speak Spanish but no English or English but no Spanish. An African-American may have been born in Nigeria, Panama, Barbados, or Britain; have lived in the rural south for generations; or be from the urban north. A Chinese Buddhist and a Filipino Catholic are both considered Asian American, though they may have little in common in terms of language, cultural identity, and sense of self (Suárez-Orozco, 2000:14).

This problem with current categories is recognized in the 1977 Office of Management and Budget (OMB, 1977a) directive, which states:

This directive provides standard classification for record keeping, collection, and preservation of data on race and ethnicity in Federal program administrative reporting and statistical activities. These classifications should not be interpreted as being scientific or anthropological in nature, nor should they be viewed as determinants of eligibility for participation in any Federal program. They have been developed in response to needs expressed by both the executive branch and the Congress to provide for the collection and use of compatible, nonduplicated, exchangeable racial and ethnic data by

Federal agencies [http://www.whitehouse.gov/omb/inforeg/stat97.
html#classdata].

These categories are even more problematic. The Hispanic
category is directly contrasted with the "race" classification that
includes whites, Blacks, American Indians/Alaska Natives, Asians,
and Pacific Islanders. Latinos are identified separately as an
ethnicity; Latinos can be of any "race." Thus, the census has racial group categories that include Latinos in the number of persons
within each racial group (e.g., whites and Blacks) and racial group
categories that exclude the portion of Latinos from the specific
racial group (e.g., non-Hispanic whites).

The more recent U.S. census categories represent an attempt to
better reflect the country's increasing diversity. The 2000 census
questionnaire is an improvement from the past in that it asks
Americans whether they belong to one or more of some 14 "races"
(though 4 are considered basic) or to some other race, and whether
they are of Spanish/Hispanic/Latino ethnicity (of which there are 3
basic varieties and an additional fill-in-the-blank option).

Race

Discussions about race can be seen as grounded in perceived
biological and physical differences. Problems with this view are
discussed in several recent Institute of Medicine reports (1999c,
2000) and in the anthropological and public health literature, as
we will describe.

The concept of biological race is inconsistent with scientific
data to the extent that "race" is not a useful shorthand for human
variation (Goodman, 2001:34). Goodman notes that:

The first leap [of illogic] is a form of geneticization, the belief that
most biology and behavior are located "in the genes". . . . Genes, of
course, are often part of the complex web of disease causality, but
almost always a minor, unstable and insufficient cause. The pres-
ence of GM allotype, for example, might correlate to increased rates

of diabetes in Native Americans, but the causal link is unknown. In other cases, the gene is not expressed without some environmental context, and it may interact with environments and other genes in nonadditive and unpredictable ways (Goodman 2000:700).

This concept has been confirmed recently by the results of the Human Genome Project, which, Collins and Mansoura noted (2001:221), "has helped to inform us about how remarkably similar all human beings are—99.9 percent at the DNA level. Those who wish to draw precise racial boundaries around certain groups will not be able to use science as a legitimate justification." Goodman (2000:701) wrote more on the subject:

The attribution of racial differences in disease to genetic differences illustrates both geneticization and scientific racialism. For example, the rise in diabetes among some Native Americans is often thought to be caused by a genetic variation that separates Native Americans from European Americans. Type II diabetes, along with obesity, gallstones, and heart disease, is part of what has been called "New World Syndrome." Contemporary variation in diabetes rates among Native North American groups is tremendous, however, and the rise in diabetes rates is a relatively recent phenomenon. Other groups experiencing shifts from complex carbohydrates to colas, from fast-moving foods to fast foods, and from exercise to underemployment have experienced very similar increases in diabetes rates. Rather than accept that diabetes is "in our blood" as articulated by the Pima [Indians], it might be more productive to locate diabetes in changeable lifestyles.

Sickle-cell anemia provides another good example of the problems inherent in racial reasoning. (Sickle cell anemia is not a "racial disease," but a characteristic of some local populations.) Livingstone's (1962) intervention four decades ago demonstrated that the frequency of this genetic trait is found among populations in tropical ecological niches in Africa as well as in certain environments in southern Europe and western Asia. He underscored the point that if sickle cell were "racial," then the so-called "race" that exhibits it "[consists] of some Greeks, Italians, Turks, Arabs, Africans, and Indians" (Livingstone, 1962:280).

"Race" may be biological and genetically meaningless, but racially defined concepts, based on presumptions of underlying biological differences, abound in the United States. The nation has the legacy of decisions like the 1896 Plessy versus Ferguson ruling, which declared a man Black on the basis of one Black ancestor among his eight grandparents (Davis, 1991). Another illustration is the debate over "blood quantum" within some Native American communities that has led to polarized positions and deep divisions over how much Native American blood is necessary for one to be considered a Native American and/or to hold tribal membership.

Racism, or the negative treatment of individuals based on perceptions of race, has been demonstrated to have negative effects on health. Krieger's (2000) recent chapter presented a comprehensive summary of "discrimination and health." James et al. (1984), Dressler (1990, 1991), and Krieger and Sidney (1996) demonstrated the relationship between self-reported experiences of discrimination and blood pressure. Many argue that epidemiological data may need to continue to be collected on the "social" categories of "race" in addition to the more logical categories of life experiences, cultural processes, and self-identity (discussed later in this chapter).

Race matters because the United States is not a colorblind society and the experience of race and racism (more than the genetics of race) has health consequences. Like other social constructs, races are often real cultural entities. For many people, membership in a racial group constitutes an important part of their social identity and self-image. "Because race and racism are sociopolitical realities, they affect individual biologies. Understanding this presents a new and radical biocultural agenda. The continuance of race and ethnic differences in health calls for an explication of the biology of inequality and racism" (Goodman, 2001:31).

Ironically, because of inequalities, groups often argue for increased political clout based on the numbers in the group—the bigger the group, the better. This is one reason Native Americans find it acceptable to be grouped together under an umbrella term, even while advocating the need for tribe-specific data. Nobles (2000:1745) notes that "racial categories on censuses do not merely capture demographic realities, but rather reflect and help to create political realities and ways of thinking and seeing." Furthermore, civil rights organizations have claimed racial categories (legal and census) have been bases of discrimination and thus bases of remedy. Racial categorization and racial data are now sometimes seen as having positive benefits, including providing a way to track the effects of racism.

A 1993 Centers for Disease Control and Prevention (CDC)/ Agency for Toxic Substances and Disease Registry (ATSDR) Workshop (Centers for Disease Control and Prevention, 1993: http:// www.rice.edu/projects/HispanicHealth/mmwr.html) on the topic generated the following statements:

• Emphasis on race and ethnicity in public health surveillance diverts attention from underlying risk factors.

• Despite the potential limitations of the categories of race and ethnicity, such information can assist in public health efforts to recognize disparities between groups for a variety of health outcomes.

• In all reports and other uses of surveillance data, the reason for analyzing race and/or ethnicity should be given, approaches to measurement of race and ethnicity should be specified, and findings should be interpreted.

This tension between the lack of scientific validity for the current ways in which Americans are categorized by OMB and other government agencies and the reality of racism and its effects was debated extensively by our committee. We agree that "race" is an inaccurate concept biologically and that direct and indirect effects of racism on health need to be acknowledged and measured. Data continue to be collected, based on the rather arbitrary OMB, census, and other classifications, which means demographic and epidemiological data exist using only those classifications. These data must be cited in order to make any statements about the distribution of populations across the country and about health disparities; however, it is important to work toward more sophisticated and accurate ways of understanding and describing the American people (Office of Management and Budget, 1997a, 1997b).

Reformulating Diversity as a Sociocultural Process

Culture

The concept of culture highlights the general potential for human beings to learn through social means, such as interaction with others and through the products of culture, such as books and television. Reliance on tools and symbolic resources, notably language, are hallmarks of culture. Language is central to social life and to acquiring cultural knowledge. Language "provides the most complex system of the classification of experience" and is "the most flexible and most powerful tool developed by humans" (Duranti, 1997:49 and 7). In addition, nonverbal-embodied ways of knowing and being take particular form in specific settings. Language also involves subtleties of meaning. For example, in one study the word "trauma" meant "injury" to a neurologist talking to the Mexican mother of a child with seizure disorders, but was often interpreted as "emotional shock" by the mother (Long, Scrimshaw, and Hernandez, 1992). Many words and phrases have no exact translation into another language because of subtleties of meaning.

It is important to note that culture is something we all have. "There is no such thing as a human nature independent of culture," noted Geertz (1973:49). Culture is the "way of life and thought that we construct, negotiate, institutionalize, and finally . . . end up calling 'reality' to comfort ourselves" (Bruner, 1996:87), and culturally grounded taken-for-granted knowledge is "often transparent to those who use it. Once learned, it becomes what one *sees with*, but seldom what one sees" (Hutchins, 1980:12). Ways of physically being in the world, such as bodily experience and the use of space, also assume cultural form without entering conscious apprehension.

Culture has many definitions, but most include the following basic concepts:

- Culture includes shared ideas, meanings, and values;
- Culture is socially learned, not genetically transmitted;
- Culture includes patterns of behavior that are guided by these shared ideas, meanings and values;
- Culture is constantly being modified through "life experiences"; and
- Culture often exists at an unconscious or implicit level.

Many people believe that specific culture can be recognized by culturally characteristic ways of being, but it is more complex than that. Although discussing culture in this way is often useful, it raises the risk of stereotyping. Intracultural variation—change and variation within a cultural group—occurs constantly. These variations occur among individuals in the same setting, across generations, between genders, across geographic and rural urban settings, and so on. As a counterpoint, much is shared across apparently diverse "cultures." For example, many U.S. television shows can be viewed in local languages in many countries. Similarly, "McDonalds" is found in most countries today.

Ethnicity

The term "ethnic group" was rarely used in anthropology before the mid-1950s. It appeared, in part, as a substitute for "race" and "tribe" and as a synonym for "cultural group" (Zenner, 1996:393). Although social science discussions of this concept proliferated and no longer assume a one-to-one relationship between ethnic identity and culture, ethnic (or "racial") groups are often talked about as bounded entities, with each one having a "culture." This view of culture assumes that people's behavior is locked in by their culture, an assumption that is incorrect and often resented as stereotyping. Imposed typologies that operationalize "ethnicity" in terms of checkboxes may, at times, be cast too broadly to relate to any meaningful discussion of cultural and social processes. As discussed earlier, examples include the conjunction of "Asian and Pacific Islander," in which many diverse groups with distinct histories are placed together, and "Hispanic," which includes people of many different origins and appearances. Ethnicity does imply some sharing of life experience and learned traditions, including meanings and values. These usually involve a shared group experience embedded in socially grounded processes, yet shared group experiences often are assumed to be a group's culture.

Cultural and Social Processes

Anthropologists have become wary of talking about culture in ways that suggest bounded entities characterized by stability, internal coherence, and homogeneity, with members of a culture recognizable by a set of stereotypical characteristics that are generationally reproduced. Much less constancy across time and much more intracultural variation exists within any social group than a discrete notion of a "culture" admits. As Sapir noted (1985:515), "The true locus of culture is in the specific interactions of individuals and, on the subjective side, in the world of meanings which each one of these individuals may unconsciously abstract for himself from his participation in these interactions."

The concept of cultural processes allows us to highlight the connections among life experiences, learning, and sharing. By learning about, belonging to, or participating in social groups, individuals become exposed to ways of thinking about the world (or specific aspects of the world) and ways of acting and responding. Culturally acquired knowledge also may reflect understandings gained through cultural products, such as books, television shows, and computer software (Garro, 2000).

Cultural processes are socially grounded ways of learning that contribute to the way an individual thinks, feels, and acts. Individual lives are embedded in a variety of cultural processes that shape the individual, although not in a deterministic fashion. For example, children who grow up in different parts of the United States, but who watch the same television programs and play similar children's games, come to share cultural understandings through their exposure to and participation in similar activities. To the extent that these life experiences differ from those of their parents, their parents will not be influenced by these same cultural processes and will differ from their children by not sharing in these same sources of experience. A strength of the concept of cultural processes is that it allows us to see individuals as unique and complex, but still exemplifying culture. It facilitates the understanding of the complexity of the multiple social and cultural influences that contribute to and shape who we are, what we do, and how we live (Garro, 2001, in press).

Paying attention to the broader community context is also important. The endorsement of the concept of cultural processes embedded in socially grounded processes that shape ways of learning and contribute to how an individual thinks, feels, and acts led the committee to adopt the concept of a "community of relevance" as fundamental to discussions on communication. Cultural processes unfold through many potential sources of shared learning, such as shared group experiences that are part of ethnic communities, training programs and professional behavior that is learned for a specific occupation, education, age, religion, language, gender, and generation. All of these sources may provide a basis for complex social groupings and contribute to intracultural variation because individuals participate in, or are exposed to, different cultural processes. Framing a message should be based on identifying the salient features for a recognized group, a subgroup, or a new composite collective based on other priorities such as region or language, which then form the community of relevance for a specific health issue, health condition, problem, or communication objective. Understanding the audience and the context it brings to the message is the first step in designing health communication interventions.

The concepts of life experiences and cultural processes need to be put into operation so that they can be used effectively in understanding and changing health behavior through communication. One way to describe these is the concept of experiential identity. Experiential identity represents the characteristics of an individual in terms of culture of origin, language, age, and gender combined with life experiences and cultural processes. Thus, someone whose parents come from different cultural and linguistic groups may have grown up in a multicultural city, lived in a rural area during college, and moved to another city with a different cultural mix from the city of origin. All of these experiences, including the learning of a profession, contribute to the individual's experiential identity. Experiential identity may be important in assessment of individual response to behavior change strategies, but most communication for behavioral change strategies examined in this volume focuses on groups. The individual is at the intersection of life experiences that are shared by others. Individuals are impacted by intersecting strands of social and cultural processes, and the strands, alone or grouped, rather than the individuals, provide the basis for health communication efforts that go beyond the individual level. Common grouping variables—age, occupation, gender—indicate greater likelihood of shared experiences among individuals, but the markers only help direct attention; they are not the focus of interest in themselves.

Good and Good (1981) discuss a meaning-centered approach to clinical practice, including some principles that could be extrapolated from application to individuals to use in the development of measures for groups. As derived from their text, these include:

- Groups vary in their style of medical complaints.
- Groups vary in the nature of their anxiety about the meaning of symptoms;
  - Groups vary in their focus on organ systems; and
  - Groups vary in their response to therapeutic strategies.

Human illness is fundamentally semantic or meaningful. (It may have a biological base, but it is a human experience.) Clinical practice is inherently interpretive. Practitioners must elicit patients' requests; elicit and decode patients' semantic networks; distinguish disease and illness and develop plans for managing problems; elicit explanatory modes from patients and families; and analyze conflict among biomedical models and negotiate alternative treatment regimens.

Adapting these principles to communication strategies for groups should help to avoid stereotyping, while analyzing characteristics that may influence the acceptability and success of the strategies (Good and Good, 1981).

Both behavior change theories (discussed in Chapter 2) and social marketing strategies (discussed in Chapter 3) contain the tools to assess individual beliefs, knowledge, and attitudes without relying on rigid categories. It is essential to use these existing tools to assess populations, rather than to make assumptions based on superficial characteristics.

Social Discrimination and Health Outcomes

In the United States, whether framed as ethnicity (e.g., Mexican American) or socially constructed as race (e.g., American Indian by the U.S. census), people of color and/or those who speak a language other than English may be treated differently and in ways that lead to poorer health outcomes. Existing evidence on poor health outcomes for particular populations supports an interpretation that links poor health with factors such as poverty, discrimination, lack of access to adequate health care, and poor nutrition.

Frequently observed differences in behavior often are attributed to "culture" without careful analysis and/or consideration of alternative hypotheses, such as the impact of the broader social/political/economic context on health behavior. For example, Young and Garro (1982, 1994) looked at treatment decision making in a rural Purépecha (Tarascan) community in Mexico, where "cultural beliefs" and "preferences" for local curanderos (curers) previously had been suggested as reasons why community members consulted infrequently with physicians. However, it was found that community members generally believed that biomedical treatment was compatible with their own understanding about illness. They did, in fact, believe biomedical treatment would result in a cure compared to their other alternatives. The relative inaccessibility of physician services, including the high costs and transportation difficulties, accounted for the observed pattern of treatment actions. This finding suggests that behavior patterns in physician consultation will be impacted not by educational efforts directed at changing cultural beliefs, but rather by reducing the financial and structural limitations that keep community members from seeking a physician's care.

Beliefs and behaviors regarding health and illness are influenced by culture and vary by "ethnicity" (Kleinman, 1980, 1986; Lindenbaum and Lock, 1993; Good and Good, 1981; Hunt et al., 1998; Rubel, O'Nell, and Collado-Ardon, 1984; Rubel and Garro, 1992; Nichter, 1981). The critique of cultural groups and the construct of "ethnicity" in this chapter applies to the terms as used in the past by anthropologists as well as demographers. Yet, as noted, people with common cultural processes and life experiences will be more likely to share health-related beliefs and behaviors. "Definitions of health are inherently subjective, influenced by the dialectic between the body and the self," noted McElroy and Jezewski (2000:191), who diagrammed the analytic domains in the experience of health and illness to include individual (e.g., age, gender, genetics, health history), microcultural (e.g., ethnicity, socioeconomic status), and macrocultural (e.g., economy, environment, health care systems) factors (2000:192). The multitude of cultural, individual experience, ethnic, biological, social, economic, environmental, and other factors complicates analyses of influences on health and illness in general and on health disparities in particular. This complexity has led to the tendency to isolate one or two factors, rather than to consider the complex whole. This is necessary, but researchers need to be aware that they are selecting factors out of context. The key is to select the relevant factors.

Also, as noted earlier, there is a tendency for the onus for health problems to be put on the individual, to "blame the victim."

Some ethnic groups or cultural groups are more likely to be impoverished, which affects their health status. The committee concluded that none of the current terms, including "race," ethnicity, and culture (interpreted as cultural group), successfully captures the complexity of people's experiences and contexts, which may explain the disparate health risks and outcomes found in American society. Thus, in order to understand and, ultimately, to contribute to the elimination of health disparities, we should think in terms of cultural processes and examine how the life experiences of people may be impacted by social forces, such as discrimination, that are based on perceptions of difference. For this reason, breaking out of ethnic and cultural boundaries to embrace the concept of experiential identity is important.

It is not within the scope of this volume to operationalize the concepts of cultural group identity proposed here. It is important for future committees or task forces to work toward ways of operationalizing "cultural group identity" that would serve as markers of increased likelihood of shared experiences among those identifying with a cultural group.

CULTURAL COMPETENCE AND HEALTH COMMUNICATION

Cultural competence has been investigated largely in the context of the delivery of health services in clinical contexts. The field of cultural competency is based on an underlying belief that disparities in health outcomes are the result of a range of social factors, including race/ethnicity, education, socioeconomic position, gender, age, and sexual orientation. A wide range of models has been offered; many of the models use cases to illustrate key points. Systematic research rarely has been applied to develop or test existing models.

Models of cultural competency and tools to assess the capacity of organizations to serve cross-cultural populations, and those designed to help practitioners provide cross-cultural services and care, point to the importance of attending to the social context of health behaviors when providing health services and when designing health communications. Models of cultural competency offer a variety of definitions that attempt to capture or expand on five elements considered essential to providing culturally competent health care across cultures. These elements are as follows:

- Valuing diversity;
- Developing the capacity for self-assessment;
- Raising awareness of dynamics inherent when cultures interact;
- Using organizational processes to institutionalize cultural knowledge; and
- Striving to develop individual and organizational adaptations to diversity.

Cultural competency models incorporate how individuals, organizations, and society at large interface with, influence, and are influenced by cultural artifacts, such as language, beliefs, and practices (Cross et al., 1989; Leininger, 1978; Tirado, 1996; Campinha-Bacote, 1994). Attitudes and beliefs and the behaviors they produce are the basis of interactions at all levels. The interpersonal dimension includes the attitudes and consciousness of individuals. Organizational contexts created by policies and procedures, leadership attitudes, and other factors also influence and reinforce individual responses that contribute to a health care organization's ability to competently serve diverse populations. In addition, cultural competency models suggest that the way society influences individuals, their communities, and health care organizations needs to be considered.

The concept of cultural competency only recently has begun to enter the health service literature. Because of its origins outside of academia and its recent appearance in the research literature, the discussion of cultural competence tends to be largely conceptual in nature.

Cultural competency implies more than beliefs, attitudes, and tolerance. It includes the ability to act appropriately in the context of daily interactions with individuals who are culturally unlike the health care providers. The providers and provider organizations need to honor and respect beliefs, interpersonal styles, and attitudes and behaviors of recipients. Cultural awareness is the deliberative and cognitive process through which an individual learns to appreciate and become sensitive to the values, lifestyles, practices, and problem-solving strategies of an individual with a different cultural background (Campinha-Bacote, 1994). Such cultural awareness includes refraining from forming stereotypes and judgments based on one's own cultural framework.

Cultural knowledge is the process of actively seeking information about different cultural and ethnic groups, such as their world views, health conditions, and practices, including their concepts of health and illness; use of home remedies and self-medication; dietary habits; pregnancy and childbearing practices; perceptions of Western medical care, health care providers, and barriers; risk-taking and health-seeking behavior; biological variations and drug metabolism tendencies; and reasons for migration and occupational hazards.

Cultural skill is the ability to discern values, beliefs, and practices in individual encounters and the ability to extract cultural or group variations in health statistics and program data. This skill is a type of cultural assessment. It is the ability to maintain an open and objective attitude about individuals and their culture and to remain open to the possibility of differences. Health providers should be nonjudgmental regarding cultural differences.

Communication is the means by which culture is transmitted and preserved (Delgado, 1983). Cultural patterns of communication affect the expression of ideas and feelings, as well as decision-making and communication strategies (Hedlund, 1988; Kretch, Crutchfield, and Ballachey, 1962). Many factors influence communication, both messages sent and those received, such as personal needs and interests; cultural, social, and philosophical values; personal tendencies; the environment in which communication takes place or the medium through which it is communicated; past experiences as they relate to message content; knowledge of the subject and basic beliefs or understandings; and how the message is understood. For example, a Vietnamese individual may smile in response to a message to avoid confrontation or to show respect for the speaker. Nodding may not be an indication that the message was understood or accepted (Rocereto, 1981).

Increased diversity and changing demographics in the United States have driven the demand for culturally sensitive public health messages. Rensnicow et al. (1999) defined cultural sensitivity as the extent to which ethnic and cultural characteristics, experiences, norms, values, behavioral patterns, and beliefs—including the relevant historical, environmental, and social forces of a target population—are incorporated into the design, delivery, and evaluation of communication messages and programs. A model for developing health promotion and disease prevention interventions should look at cultural sensitivity in terms of "surface and deep structures." Surface structures involve matching intervention materials and messages to characteristics of a target population, such as using people, places, language, music, food, locations, and clothing that are familiar to the target population. Deep structures involve incorporating the cultural, social, historical, environmental, and psychological forces of the target population in messages to influence health behavior change. The Navajo, for example, value living in harmony with nature and with other people. Illness is perceived as falling out of harmony with others and the individual's environment, and curing is believed by the Navajo to restore such harmony. Alcohol treatments and diabetes interventions designed and evaluated by scholars at the University of New Mexico suggest that the concept of harmony can be considered in ways to make these interventions more effective in health behavior change.

ETHICS OF HEALTH COMMUNICATION
INTERVENTIONS FOR DIVERSE POPULATIONS

Principles of ethics are important in developing and implementing health communication interventions. Although there are competing ways to consider ethical principles, we focus our attention on four core values that are central to effective ethical analysis for health care: respecting an individual's autonomy, providing benefit (beneficence), avoidance of harm, and treating groups and individuals justly and equitably (Beauchamp, 1994). The application of these principles to the design and implementation of health communication recognizes that the goal of improving health behavior is important, but it is not the only important goal in an individual's life. Therefore, it must be balanced against other interests, particularly in a world of divergent views, diverse cultures, and differences in understanding of health. The principles have been defined as follows:

- Respecting an individual's autonomy is based on the premise that a fundamental dignity of human beings resides in their capacity for rational choice and their right to make their own choices.
- Beneficence concerns the balance between benefits and risks; the guideline is that the benefits must outweigh or at least be equivalent to the risks the individual is being asked to take.
- Avoidance of harm involves ensuring that such actions as stereotyping, blaming the victim, and presenting conflicting messages are avoided.
- Treating groups and individuals justly and equitably suggests that all people should be treated similarly and fairly regarding the distribution of benefits and harms.

Table 7-1 provides some examples of questions guided by these principles that might be asked at different points in the design and implementation of a health communication intervention.

Implementing ethical principles can be complicated by a number of factors. First, the developers' consideration of tradeoffs

TABLE 7-1 Ethical Aspects of the Design and Conduct of
Health Promotions

Facets	Examples of guiding questions and ethical issues
The right and obligation to sponsor the intervention	• Who has the moral right to intervene on this health issue? *(respect for autonomy; utility/public good)* • Who has the obligation to intervene? *(obligation to do good)*
Framing, problem definition, and choice of strategies	• How are the causes for the problem defined? *(respect for autonomy)* • Are factors related to different levels of the health issue represented in the framing of the problem, beyond the individual level? (e.g., family relations, cultural norms, economic factors, enforcement of protective laws and regulations) *(justice)* • Are the diverse perspectives of population members or of the individual client represented in the way the problem is framed? *(respect for autonomy)* • Does the client/patient or do the intervention's populations have issues that need to be addressed that may have a higher priority than the intervention's behavior-change objectives? *(avoidance of harm)* • Does the intervention run counter to other important behaviors related to maintaining/enhancing the individual, family, or community? *(beneficence)* • Are there opportunities for the client or the population members to participate in decisions regarding problem definition and choice of strategies? *(respect for autonomy)*
Evaluation	• Are evaluation findings and conclusions made available to the population members? *(respect for autonomy)* • Are the evaluation findings and recommendations formulated in a way that they can be used for improving future activities? *(utility)*
Segmentation, targeting and tailoring	• Which segments should be targeted and on the basis of which ethical justifications (e.g., particular needs or vulnerabilities, ability to reach, relationship with sponsoring organization)? *(equity)*

TABLE 7-1 Continued

Facets	Examples of guiding questions and ethical issues
	• To what extent should messages and strategies be tailored? To whom should they be tailored? *(equity)* • Who may tailored messages offend? How would individuals who are not their intended audience respond when they are exposed to the tailored messages? *(avoidance of harm; equity)*
Persuasive and dialogical approaches	• How to attract the attention, interest, and make the health message salient without using appeals that can be considered manipulative? *(respect for autonomy)* • How to provide accurate and complete information to support the health claim without overloading the client or the intervention population with messages that may be too cumbersome or confusing? *(avoidance of harm, comprehensibility)* • Can the persuasive strategies be compatible with the culture of the population? When is it justifiable to adopt strategies that are not compatible? *(avoidance of harm, providing benefit)*
Cultural symbols and themes	• Is there a possibility that the use of cultural themes may serve to stereotype the population? *(avoidance of harm)* • Are there any individuals or groups that may be excluded and even stigmatized when certain cultural themes are made a dominant part of the intervention? *(avoidance of harm)*
Information	• Is the information presented in a way that all members of the population, regardless of language skills or cultural background, are able to relate to it and understand the messages for health behavior change? *(equity, comprehensibility)*
Deprivation	• Do certain practices that the health interventions aim to eliminate have important sociocultural or personal gratification functions? Would people, particularly members of vulnerable populations, be deprived in any way? *(avoidance of harm, equity)*

continued on next page

TABLE 7-1 Continued

Facets	Examples of guiding questions and ethical issues
	• Does the intervention proffer alternatives for practices that fulfill an important function for the population? *(avoidance of harm, equity)*
Responsibility	• How are responsibility and irresponsibility defined? *(avoidance of harm, respect for autonomy)*
	• Is culpability implied in messages related to responsibility? *(avoidance of harm)*
	• Are messages that appeal to responsibility using high emotional appeals? *(respect for autonomy, justice)*
	• What is the ethical base of appeals that relate to obligations to significant others and the community? *(respect for autonomy, justice)*

among efficiency, cost, and improving the health of the most in need versus a broader range of persons can lead to conflicting goals. Second, the design of a communication strategy guided by ethical principles for one segment of the population may not be appropriate for another segment. Third, there is always the opportunity for unintended consequences, even with the most well-intentioned and well-executed health communication interventions. Possible outcomes for diverse populations include confusion about the meaning of the message, manipulation of individuals or groups without their understanding or consent, unwarranted anxiety resulting from implying individual culpability, and the stigmatizing of certain cultural practices.

In the interest of providing benefit and supporting the individual's autonomy to choose, it is important for the message to be truthful and clear. This may require providing risk probabilities of specified health-related behaviors. The format in which probabilities of risk and benefit are presented can significantly affect the way people estimate the probability of their own risk (Singer and Endreny, 1993; Slovic, 1987; Slovic et al., 1987; Tversky and Kahneman, 1981).

Because health communication initiatives often encourage individuals to take responsibility for their own well-being (Kirkwood and Brown, 1995; Knowles, 1977; Guttman, 2000), it is important for developers to assess environmental constraints, access to health care resources and facilities, and the values and beliefs of the group. In some health communication interventions, people may be urged to make prudent and responsible choices about food consumption, leisure activities, intimate relations, and other lifestyle options. In response, those who are economically or otherwise disadvantaged might be compromised in their ability to follow the recommendations and may, as a result, be viewed as lacking motivation to change, being "difficult to reach," and deserving of negative health outcomes (Daniels, 1985). Although health messages do not usually blame individuals for being responsible for their illnesses, they may frame disease prevention as if it were primarily a matter of individual control (Wallack, 1989). In doing so, they deemphasize structural factors related to employment and housing, access to health care, access to healthy and inexpensive food stuffs, pollution, and other factors that can precipitate or exacerbate serious health risks. Such messages also may deemphasize the importance of institutional changes that may supersede changes by individuals alone (e.g., Ellison et al., 1989; Coreil and Levin, 1984; Glanz and Mullis, 1988; Glanz et al., 1995; Green and Raiburn, 1990; Milio, 1981; Wallack, 1989; Williams, 1990).

Appeals to personal responsibility also may be viewed as manipulative (Bayer, 1996; Niebuhr, 1978; Veatch, 1982). Persuasive messages using personal responsibility as an emotional appeal may warn people that failure to adopt a responsible lifestyle may lead to illness or disability, which could turn them into a burden on their family or society as a whole. Health behavior change messages may imply that people have an obligation to help promote or protect the health of significant others. For example, people may be told that they should help their spouses maintain a healthy diet, insist that their adolescent children use seatbelts, and support the efforts of siblings and friends to quit smoking. Such messages can reinforce moral commitments such as service, responsiveness to others with special needs, fidelity, compassion, kindness, and keeping promises (Baier, 1993; Pellegrino, 1993). These ethical imperatives also can be associated with the ethic of care and other principles that emphasize the importance of being connected to others (Hallstein, 1999; Nodding, 1990; Pellegrino, 1985). These kinds of messages can cause dissonance when, for example, family members become antagonistic toward one another in the name of promoting their health (Kleinman, 1988).

The principle of avoiding harm is particularly important when applied to health communication interventions conducted in a community or large-scale national setting because the effects of the communication on different segments of the audience can be difficult to gauge. Special care should be taken to ensure that information and messages do not confuse and/or offend populations. For example, information that is presented in a tentative way or with caveats may be perceived as confusing, culturally inappropriate, and even culturally irrelevant. Words, concepts, and terms that are meaningful to one audience may have entirely different connotations for another. Moreover, because health messages disseminated through mass media must deal with complex social or medical topics in an extremely short time frame, they must provide a simplified distillation that can lead to incomplete or inaccurate understanding.

In developing health messages for specific populations, care should be taken to avoid stereotyping and underscoring disadvantages. For example, developers of communication interventions intended for populations with limited literacy skills should be aware of the potential to embarrass their intended audience with text messages (Davis et al., 1998). In another example, the positive application of a belief through cultural message themes can contribute to a positive feeling of self-determination and cultural pride as well as being effective in achieving behavior change. Also, positive themes can promote notions of responsibility and benefit. However, using these beliefs in a way that detaches them from their original meaning may be perceived as demeaning. This appropriation may offend groups that may not want their cultural symbols used in a particular way, even in health communication efforts, out of concern that such use will have a stereotyping effect (López, 1997).

Audience selection can raise concerns about equity of benefits. One approach is to focus on relatively large segments of the population. The rationale for this approach is that even modest health-related changes (for example, modifying diet to lead to reductions in blood cholesterol levels or systolic blood pressure) in large populations will produce substantial changes in overall morbidity and mortality (Rose, 1985). These efforts can have a positive effect on those with easy-to-modify behavior—but those whose behaviors are most difficult to change may be shortchanged. The population approach is valuable because it represents an efficient use of resources, it avoids stigmatizing effects, and it may do some degree of good in reaching those with hard-to-modify behaviors (Beauchamp, 1988). However, health communication initiatives should not overlook harder to reach groups, and sponsors may wish to dedicate at least a portion of their resources to these individuals.

In terms of gauging social equality, all health promotion campaigns can be guided by a consideration of the following questions. How is the relationship between the behavior and the adverse health outcome framed? Is the behavior portrayed as a sufficient cause (or preventive measure) for the health effect? Do people, particularly members of socially or culturally disadvantaged populations, have a choice of whether to engage or not engage in the recommended health practice? Do they fully understand the relationship between the behavior and potential adverse health outcomes? Do people engage in the potentially hazardous behavior only for their own personal gratification? Finally, to what extent should health promotion messages be framed in a way that reinforces a perception of responsibility for the behaviors and outcomes of others?

THE SOCIOCULTURAL ENVIRONMENT

The fields of social epidemiology, psychology, anthropology, sociology, and economics are converging in the development of theories and methodologies, helping us to understand factors underlying health disparities. Levine and his colleagues set the stage for this convergence, especially with the *Handbook of Medical Sociology* (Freeman and Levine, 1989). Recent reviews by Yen and Syme (1999) and *Social Studies in Health and Medicine* (Albrecht, Fitzpatrick, and Scrimshaw, 2000) are among many recent analyses dealing with these complex issues. The recent Institute of Medicine report, *Promoting Health* (2000), advances our understanding of health behavior and health disparities. Some common themes from these sources give directions to the underlying factors contributing to health disparities, as follows:

- Disparate access to prevention and treatment services;
- Differences in patterns of use of services;
- Differences in behaviors in response to illness;
- Differences in environmental and occupational risks;
- Differences in health promotion and disease prevention behaviors;
- Differences in community factors such as stress, societal support, and community cohesion; and
- Genetic factors that come into play for individuals, but seldom for groups.

The Centers for Disease Control and Prevention Task Force on the *Guide to Community Preventative Services* developed an organizing logic framework for looking at many of these themes (see Figure 7-1). The Task Force was charged with developing evidence-based guidelines for community public health practice (Truman et al., 2000; Centers for Disease Control and Prevention, 2000b). Other topics in the guide include major risk behaviors such as smoking, sex, drugs, injury, nutrition, and exercise, and some diseases, such as cancer and diabetes. The discussion of the

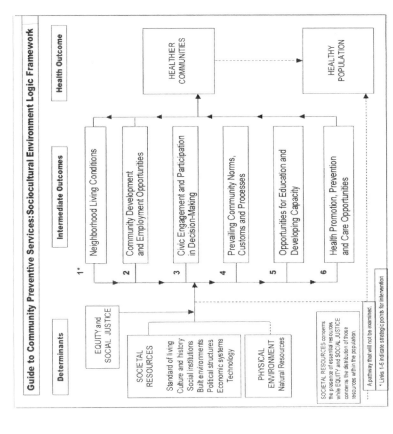

FIGURE 7-1 Guide to community preventive services: Sociocultural environment logic framework.

sociocultural environment looks at underlying contextual issues related to health status. The framework includes six areas of potential interventions, with the outcomes being healthier communities and a healthier population. The six areas are:

- Neighborhood living conditions;
- Community development and employment opportunities;
- Civic engagement and participation in decision making;
- Prevailing community norms, customs, and processes;
- Opportunities for education and developing capacity; and
- Health promotion, prevention, and care opportunities.

Any communication efforts to change health behavior should understand these contextual factors and their influences on both reception of communication efforts and the ability of individuals to change behaviors.

SUMMARY AND CONCLUSIONS

All bases for categorizing humans are socially derived, change over time, and have bounded situational relevance. Powerful social forces, such as the desires to advance political agendas or to obtain resources, lead to an emphasis on differences among groups. Health communication efforts must recognize these social realities, but not be driven by them without careful consideration on the part of the communicators of their impact on a given message.

For health communication purposes, the way we divide this real-world complexity should reflect an understanding of relevant dynamic social and cultural processes. Diversity has been conceptualized in terms of broad "ethnic" and/or "racial" categories. These categories, which reflect shared group and life experiences, have been useful in identifying disparities in health status and may be useful in developing effective health communication strategies.

A focus on ethnoracial groups tends to confuse culture with ethnicity, risks, and stereotyping, and creates a view of culture as static and of groups as more homogeneous than they really are.

This view of culture deflects attention from a richer understanding of the diverse social and cultural processes that are meaningful for the development of effective health communication strategies. Cultural processes are dynamic, embedded in social context, and therefore influenced by social factors such as immigration or discrimination as well as by interactive social processes and cultural products like music, food, and language.

The consideration of the proximal social and cultural processes, as opposed to group categories, facilitates the translation of theory-based strategies to reflect the life experiences of targeted communities. For example, to develop a health communication strategy for the population age 80 and up requires the identification of factors in their daily lives that are related to the message and specific health behavior under consideration. Their lives may be impacted by a lack of economic resources, limited accessibility of health care services, deaths of significant others, or decreasing physical and cognitive capabilities.

The concept of self-identity allows us to look at individuals in the context of their life experiences and realities. Knowledge of the relevant experiences that individuals are likely to share allows health communicators to package the theoretical constructs of attitudes, norms, and efficacy beliefs in ways that are meaningful to the targeted group—and therefore will result in more effective health communication.

RECOMMENDATIONS

Based on its consideration of the various issues related to diversity, the committee offers the following recommendations:

1. Demographic factors are useful in epidemiological studies to understand whether health benefits are distributed equally and to identify intergroup differences. Policy makers and program planners should continue to use demographic factors to understand whether health benefits are equally distributed and to identify intergroup differences. Where there are existing disparities, it will

be important to monitor trends in gap opening and closing according to these categories.

2. However, because demographic groupings are limited and crude categories with relatively little explanatory power, they should be avoided as markers for designing health communication strategies or developing health messages. Instead, researchers and practitioners should identify and operationalize the particulars associated with a group's life experiences, attitudes, and behaviors in designing and assessing health communication strategies.

3. Health communication strategies focusing on demographically diverse populations must be based on a recognition that demographic groupings represent a constellation of individuals with shared and unique life experiences, social processes, and cultural artifacts, and that the examination of these particulars as they impact individuals is important to understanding the context for health communication.

4. Health communication strategies and health messages must be informed by an understanding of the sociocultural environment of individuals within populations to be reached. Economic contexts, discrimination, and community resources such as access to health services are some of the important aspects of the sociocultural environment. These contextual factors have implications for the commonly held attitudes, norms, efficacy beliefs, and practices pertinent to the health issue in question.

5. We recommend that greater support be provided for qualitative research that examines the historical, social, and cultural contexts of communities' health behavior. Such research should be designed to result in greater understanding of the implications of cultural factors and processes on effective health communications, and lead to more efficient ways of assessing relevant cultural processes in health communication interventions. A focus on qualitative ethnographic studies is likely to be required to identify cultural processes relevant to health communication, but it is also important to develop strategies that permit those processes to be reflected in large-scale health communication interventions.

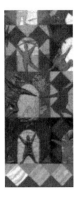

8

Findings and Recommendations

INTRODUCTION

The Committee on Communication for Behavior Change in the 21st Century: Improving the Health of Diverse Populations accepted its charge in the context of three assumptions: Communication interventions to affect health behaviors are an increasingly important strategy for improving the health of the American people. Evidence shows that some of these communication interventions have affected health behavior. At the same time, there is evidence that disparities in some health outcomes are associated with identifiable characteristics of individuals, including race/ethnicity, socioeconomic status, gender, and age.

This charge led to the central question for this volume: What is the performance and the promise of health communication interventions in the context of diversity? This question includes the following subquestions: Have current communication interventions effectively served diverse populations? Is there added benefit for reducing disparities in using communication strategies that take account of diverse populations in one way or another? What do communication programs do now to serve the diverse audiences they must address? How might what they do be improved?

In the process of examining this central question, the committee addressed a series of closely related questions:

- What is the role of theory in the construction of communication programs in the context of diversity? In particular, is there a need to modify theory for different subgroups of the population?
- Given concerns about diversity, do special ethical issues arise in health communication?
- Is the promise of communication and diversity different according to the health behavior(s) and disease process addressed? Is there evidence that targeting or tailoring messages for different cultural groups makes a difference in the effects of these messages on behavior change? The committee contrasted two important cases to help us consider this issue. Mammography was chosen to represent a discrete behavior that is recommended to occur every year or two for women age 40 and over; it is relevant to a large segment of the healthy population. Diabetes was selected as a contrast. Its treatment requires a complex set of continuing behaviors that is responsive to an evolving illness and relevant to those who have the illness and those around them.
- Large-scale communication campaigns are widely used as a mechanism for affecting the behaviors of broad populations when risk is widespread. Thus, as a third area of focus, the committee considered evidence from such large-scale campaigns. What is known about the best ways of constructing such programs in the context of diversity?
- The application of newer communication technologies to the problems of health promotion has an extraordinary dynamism. What are the implications of the rapid development of new technology-based health behavior interventions for the health of diverse audiences?
- How helpful are the conventional categories of diversity in constructing communication interventions? Are there other, more useful, approaches to thinking about diversity?

This chapter takes each of these questions in turn, summarizing the committee's findings with regard to the question, then presenting the recommendations that come from those findings.

OVERALL FINDINGS AND RECOMMENDATIONS

1. The review makes it clear that researchers, program planners, and managers quite often take diversity into account when they construct their communication programs. This was true both for communication interventions addressing mammography and for those that were examined in the review of large-scale campaigns. The committee found few examples of communication programs that addressed diabetes. Three broad diversity-respecting strategies emerged from the rich variety of approaches described in the literature:

- They construct a unified communication program, but look for a common-denominator message that will be relevant across most populations.
- They construct a unified communication program, but systematically vary message executions to make them appeal to different segments, while retaining the same fundamental message strategy.
- They develop distinct message strategies and/or distinct interventions for each target segment.

2. Despite the efforts to take diversity into account, the evidence base is quite thin about differential effects of interventions according to diversity subgroups. Some of those programs have been successful in changing behavior, including that of the diversity subgroups of particular interest in this volume. However, the available data do not effectively address the focus question for this volume: is there added benefit in addressing the behaviors associated with health disparities by using communication that takes diversity into account?

In some cases, there are data about comparative trend lines for subgroups with regard to a health outcome or health behavior. (Most often the subgroups examined are defined by race/ethnicity, but sometimes they are reported by other conventional diversity categories.) These tend to show parallel trends among subgroups, although that varies. However, even if such comparative trend line data were available in more cases, it would not adequately address the question. Comparative trend lines do not deal with whether more or less diversity-respecting campaigns have differential effects. Few studies address the relative effectiveness of communication interventions across relevant diverse groups, and none were found that systematically compare the various approaches to addressing diversity, or compare those approaches with efforts that ignore diversity altogether. This does not mean there are no diversity-respecting programs. Rather, where such programs exist, they do not provide direct evidence about the interaction of communication programs and subgroup status. In general, the evidence does not indicate whether the efforts to take diversity into account were worthwhile, or which approaches were worthwhile and under what circumstances. Overall, the committee was surprised by the lack of published comparative effectiveness evidence.

Overall Recommendation 1: There is a need to undertake comparative effectiveness research in each of the following ways:

• *Secondary analysis of evidence already collected from existing communication programs.* The committee assumes there is a substantial store of data that has already been collected, but not analyzed to examine diversity-related effectiveness issues. The committee encourages systematic analysis comparing subgroups with regard to trends in disparities in the target health outcomes, while simultaneously documenting specific diversity strategies that were employed at particular times.

• *Ongoing effectiveness evaluations of new and ongoing programs.* Evaluations of larger scale communication programs should collect appropriate data so they can complement overall conclusions about effectiveness with conclusions about important subgroups of the population. These analyses should be reported in the context of systematic descriptions of diversity implementation strategies.

• *Field tests of alternative diversity strategies.* Where feasible, systematic comparative studies should be undertaken in which equivalent groups of the general population and of focus subgroups are assigned to different communication treatments reflecting alternative diversity strategies. These may be undertaken either in the context of ongoing communication programs, or as separately mounted field experiments.

The National Institutes of Health (NIH) and other agencies that are funding communication interventions should provide special funding to evaluation staff or other researchers willing to pursue this research agenda. This recommendation is consistent with regulations that require researchers to include adequate numbers of men and women and diverse populations in funded research.

Overall Recommendation 2: Until more convincing evidence is available pro or con, the committee believes it is sensible for many existing programs to continue to pay attention to diversity, particularly when diversity is associated with substantial disparities in health status and outcomes. However, this recommendation is subject to some limitations:

• The most important categories of diversity may not be the conventional ones. In this volume, there is some discussion of the tradeoff between relying on the conventional categories of diversity (e.g., race and ethnicity) and focusing on alternative characteristics that are closely tied to the focus health behavior and to susceptibility to communication interventions. It is appropriate to consider alternatives to conventional categories, including attending to the life experiences and contextual settings of the population. This issue is discussed further in this chapter.

• Communication interventions should be targeted to specific subgroups only when evidence from program research suggests that important differences exist in health behavior or in the antecedents of health behavior or when there is a strong hypothesis that such differences exist. Otherwise, a reasonable approach will be to design communication interventions based on common features among groups/people.

THEORIES OF COMMUNICATION AND
HEALTH BEHAVIORS

1. A substantial body of literature addresses many aspects of theory relevant to communication interventions. These include theories of behavior and behavior change focusing on the structural, social, and psychological factors that influence behavior, and theories of communication or persuasion that underlie approaches to influencing change in those factors. Substantial research underpins the theories of behavior, and there is substantial research on persuasive processes and some research on communication effects models.

2. The committee considered the argument that current theories were inappropriately applied to some subgroups of the population—that is, theories of behavior change or theories of communication, for example, were developed with general population samples, and might not apply in important aspects to culturally distinct subpopulations. The committee found no evidence base for this claim, however. On the contrary, although subgroups may differ on the particular beliefs or social factors that affect their behaviors, this was not a challenge to existing theory. Relevant theory, in the committee's assessment, does not assert causal preeminence for any particular belief or social influence or skill; it does not indicate which persuasion processes will be most effective for a particular audience; rather, theory suggests what the important categories of influence and important alternative influence processes might be. Therefore, most of the major theoretical frameworks are consistent with the possibility of variation across diver-

sity groups in the constructs that matter in a particular circumstance. Moreover, if theories are used appropriately, researchers and program planners alike will obtain population-specific data for planning purposes.

3. Theory is highly relevant to the construction of communication programs in the context of diversity. Theory can drive the investigation of differences among diverse subgroups with regard to what influences on behavior are relevant and thus what factors should be addressed in a communication program.

4. In its limited review of cases, the committee found great variation in the use of theory as an underpinning to implementation decisions. Some programs saw themselves as implementing certain theoretical principles and did so using theoretical constructs to guide intervention development; some made reference to theory as a justification for their implementation decisions, but outside observers found it difficult to match theory and implementation; and some programs made no theoretical claims at all.

5. The committee recognizes that the research base for the translation of these theoretical notions into operational programs is less strong than the underlying theoretical research itself.

Theory Recommendation 1: Theory has an important place in the construction of communication programs in general and for diverse populations. The committee encourages program developers and implementers to use theory in a more consistent and aggressive way in developing implementation plans. This implies each of the following:

• Whenever possible, program planners should use evidence-based programs that are grounded in theory.
• Implementing groups may want to develop formal training opportunities for their staffs to develop the skills in turning relevant theory into implementation when new programs are required.
• Agencies funding such programs should give strong priority to potential implementers who have a track record in applying

theory successfully, or who have provided proposals that establish their full understanding of relevant theory and of the practical implications of theory for implementation.

• Reports about communication research should specify clearly the theory that was used and indicate how the underlying theoretical constructs were applied and measured.

Theory Recommendation 2: Additional research is needed about the translational process of moving from theory to implementation. The committee recommends that more attention be given to how behavior change theories are translated into effective practice and implemented in health communication interventions; that is, how the theoretical principles are applied in practice. This would include:

• *Case studies.* Documentation is needed on the theoretical basis for particular interventions, and the particular ways that theory was implemented in practice. These narratives might include discussion of the operational difficulties of translating theory into practice, and evidence that expected theoretical processes mediated observed changes in outcomes.

• *Research on translational programs.* There is a need to develop and test transfer and implementation models for health promotion using communication.

ETHICS

1. A number of ethical principles should be considered in the development and implementation of health communication for diverse populations. These include avoidance of harm, maximizing benefit, respecting an individual's autonomy to make choices, and treating groups and individuals justly and equitably. Many ethicists argue that direct incorporation of representatives of affected groups in decision making increases the likelihood that the rights of and benefit to those groups will be respected.

2. Ethical principles are easily endorsed, but not always easily achieved. Implementing ethical principles can be complicated by developers' needs to consider tradeoffs among efficiency, cost, and improving the health of those most in need versus benefiting a broader range of persons. A communication strategy may have to choose between maximizing benefit for one segment of the population versus another. Also, there is always the opportunity for unintended consequences, even with the most well-intentioned and well-executed health communication interventions. This risk may be heightened in the context of reaching heterogeneous audiences with a common message. Risks include confusion about the meaning of the message, unwarranted anxiety resulting from implying individual culpability, or the stigmatizing of certain cultural practices. The recommendation for the incorporation of relevant group representatives may be complex to implement in practice, given the need to choose among potential representatives and the possible tension between technical "expertise" and beneficiary preferences.

3. Many intervention programs may not explicitly consider ethical issues and tensions as they make implementation decisions, and they may not avoid problematic ethical dilemmas. Approaches for translating ethical principles into practical recommendations are not well established in health communication.

Ethics Recommendation 1: Health communication programs should explicitly consider ethical guidelines in their decisions about implementation. This process is likely to be helped if:

• NIH convenes a workshop to assist in the development of an ethical framework and operational guidelines for implementing the framework.

Ethics Recommendation 2: Programs are encouraged to involve individuals and communities affected as active participants in decision making and not only as passive respondents. There is now a growing literature on participatory research that may be helpful.

• NIH may wish to commission a review of the alternative mechanisms that programs have used to incorporate representatives of recipients in their decision making, including some evaluation of the success of those mechanisms.

COMMUNICATION CAMPAIGNS

1. The findings stated previously in the overall findings section apply specifically to communication campaigns: There are many such campaigns, and many address issues of diversity in their plans and their implementation; there is credible evidence for the overall positive effects of some of these programs; there is sometimes evidence available about differential trends with regard to target outcomes for different demographic groups, but there is little evidence available as to whether diversity strategies contribute to success, or as to which strategies are more and less effective.

2. Sophisticated public health communication programs pay close attention to the heterogeneity of their audiences, recognizing that their audiences are different with regard to the behaviors they are currently undertaking; the psychological, social, and structural factors that influence those behaviors; the channels through which they can be reached; and the types of message executions to which they will respond. They follow the lead of commercial marketers who "segment" the audience into more homogeneous groups, choosing to focus attention on only some segments, or addressing multiple segments with different communication strategies. Sometimes these segments correspond to the conventional diversity categories based on demographic characteristics. Sometimes there is much less correspondence. In these situations, relying on the conventional categories to segment the audience can be unproductive. Recently, some programs have used tailored approaches designed to customize interventions for individuals. In this case, the factors relevant to an individual can be used as the basis for messages.

3. Successful public communication programs have met certain conditions. These include a strong science base for recommended behaviors, a realistic possibility that recommendations can be implemented by the population, coordination with other programs addressing related issues, enough resources available for the development and particularly the transmission of messages so that the intended audience sees them at needed frequency, and often the resources to maintain the campaign over time if the pace of change is slow.

4. Communication programs may be particularly effective if they are an integral part of a multicomponent intervention. Examples include interventions that complement or facilitate access to services—such as improved local mammography availability—with a variety of communication strategies such as television advertisements, telephone reminders, and personal letters. Similarly, a television series focused on smoking cessation can offer a toll-free telephone number that viewers can call for referral to quit-smoking programs.

5. Communication campaigns operate at a distance from their audiences. Therefore, they require extensive and virtually continuous gathering of "tracking" data about their target population's awareness of messages, changes in relevant beliefs, social expectations and self-efficacy with regard to recommended behaviors, as well as measures of those behaviors themselves. This need is magnified in the context of programs that address heterogeneous audiences, when tracking research has to allow estimation of differential trends across important population subgroups.

6. Communication campaign effects can be magnified if the exposure to messages achieved by the direct buying of media time (e.g., through purchases of broadcast time for TV ads) is complemented by other diffusion of messages. This may involve stimulating coverage of a particular health issue by newspapers or by broadcast news or talk shows, or inclusion of supportive messages in entertainment programming (or discouragement of modeling of problematic behaviors in entertainment programming). From the opposite perspective, some campaigns have been successful in the

context of media coverage of related events (e.g., Rock Hudson's death from AIDS). Prohealth messages transmitted by programs may receive a better hearing in the context of such coverage. Also, programs may be able to encourage journalists to write about events to reinforce prohealth messages. In general, the presence of social environmental changes, such as policy initiatives supporting healthy behaviors, can provide fertile ground for communication campaigns.

The committee addressed the urgent need for research about diversity and communication program effects in Overall Recommendation 1. The judicious use of existing subgroups was the focus of Overall Recommendation 2. Both of those are specifically relevant to communication campaigns. In addition, each of the following recommendations addresses the additional findings presented here.

Communication Campaign Recommendation 1: Underresourced campaigns are unlikely to be effective and may deflect researchers from employing the most appropriate strategies. Campaigns are appropriately an attractive strategy to a health agency anxious to influence population behavior change. However, if the minimum conditions for successful public communication programs are not met—and often they are not, particularly with regard to resources needed to obtain high levels of exposure to messages—then the campaign is not an appropriate strategy. This concern is magnified in the context of a campaign that intends to address multiple diverse segments, when resource demands are even higher. Agencies should not initiate communication campaigns unless they are able to satisfy these conditions.

Communication Campaign Recommendation 2: The committee recommends that practitioners employ evidence-based multicomponent programs that integrate communication with access to services, where feasible, and especially where the appropriateness for diverse populations has been demonstrated. The Centers for Disease Control and Prevention's *Guide to Community Preventative Services* is an important source of information about evidence-based programs (http:/www.the communityguide.org).

Communication Campaign Recommendation 3: NIH Institutes that are considering mounting communication programs in high-priority public health areas, such as diabetes, that have not been systematically addressed by communications in the past should fund additional exploratory research to examine the suitability of communication approaches before developing full-scale campaigns.

Communication Campaign Recommendation 4: The committee recommends that agencies undertaking campaigns incorporate ongoing tracking studies.

• These should be conducted in a timely manner to monitor the process and effects of the campaign (intended and unintended) and to refine and adjust campaign strategies and executions.

• They should be sensitive to potential differences among important subgroups of the population.

• The Office of Management and Budget (OMB) Paper Reduction Act and its complex and extended research approval process makes the undertaking of such tracking studies more difficult because, by their nature, tracking studies, like the campaigns they follow, are constantly evolving and need to respond to changing circumstances. There is a need to negotiate with OMB for an appropriate exception or an expedited process for such monitoring research.

• The results of these studies, which are likely to be relevant to other implementation planning, should be made available to the scientific and practitioner communities.

NEW COMMUNICATION TECHNOLOGY

1. The application of new communication technology in health programs is occurring at a rapid pace. These include programs to individualize messages as well as those that permit interactive involvement by users. Moreover, Internet-based programs offer opportunities not only to tailor content to diversity issues, but to provide social support and create communities of interest. The committee found good evidence that a variety of communication technologies, including those based on older (e.g., telephone) and newer (e.g., wireless computer devices) technologies, have been used effectively to influence behavior.

2. The impressive growth of new communication technologies offers significant opportunities to integrate mass and micro communication strategies, allowing more effective and efficient population reach while permitting segmentation and even tailoring to diverse populations. Some of these technologies depend on active engagement by individuals, such as searching for information on the Internet. Although there has been a dramatic increase in the reach of the Internet, little is known about how diverse populations use the Internet for behavior change. Some people will be interested in the Internet, some will lose interest, others will be interested but lack access, and still others will have interest and access, but lack the skills to obtain the information they need. Nevertheless, the menu of communication choices is expanding rapidly, and we must be prepared to use those options, where appropriate, for health communication.

Technology Recommendation 1: Investments are needed in research, training, and delivery of technology-based communication interventions to improve the health of diverse populations. In many cases, new technology should be combined with established communication strategies, such as face-to-face contact and telephone counseling. New applications such as "live help" may be useful in this regard. Research methods are needed to estimate untapped potential and costs of communication technology used to improve health care for diverse populations.

DIVERSITY

1. Diversity frequently is defined for policy and research purposes by broad social demographic categories such as race, ethnicity, and socioeconomic status as well as gender and age. This has some advantages. These characteristics are apparent and are often easily measured, and thus comparisons between groups are facilitated. Also, for many health behaviors and health outcomes, researchers using these categories have located important disparities. This evidence has allowed groups with poor health outcomes and their advocates to make a strong moral claim for redress and reallocation of resources. Also, groups organized around these identities have forged political bonds, and that has given them some power and ability to make additional claims on resources.

2. At the same time, these diversity categories may have more political relevance than substantive relevance in the construction of communication programs. There is often as much heterogeneity with regard to a behavior and its determinants within a specified group as between groups. Also, the use of such categories to report disparities may reinforce stigma, a sense that a disadvantaged group is incapable of helping itself. This may be a particular concern when race and ethnicity are used as the criterion for diversity.

3. There are alternative ways to describe heterogeneity in the population that do not rely on these categories.

• It is argued in Chapter 7 that programs need to focus on cultural processes, on understanding the life experiences of the communities and individuals being served, and on the sociocultural environment of individuals within the populations to be reached. This includes multiple dimensions ranging from economic contexts and community resources such as access to health services to commonly held attitudes, norms, efficacy beliefs, and practices pertinent to the health issue in question. Researchers and practitioners should identify and operationalize the particulars associated with a given group's life experiences in designing and assessing health communication strategies.

• This concern reflects much current research by anthropologists, sociologists, and psychologists. At the same time, it reflects the applied wisdom of sophisticated social marketers and communication campaign planners, who are making the same argument. As already described, their research is designed to segment audiences according to behavior and factors related to behavior. They suggest partitioning the audience on characteristics relevant to their behavior, not on irrelevant characteristics. This also applies to tailored programs.

Diversity Recommendation 1: Policy makers and program planners should continue to use demographic factors to understand whether health benefits are equally distributed and to identify intergroup differences. Where there are existing disparities, it will be important to monitor trends in gap opening and closing according to these categories.

Diversity Recommendation 2: At the same time, program planners need to recognize that other measures such as life experiences and cultural processes are needed to understand within-group variations and to understand their association with health behaviors. Actual planning of health communication programs will rarely be well served by an assumption of homogeneity within any of these categories. This may also require efforts to more systematically educate policy makers about the relevant domains of diversity for purposes of communication interventions.

Diversity Recommendation 3: We recommend that greater support be provided for qualitative, ethnographic research that examines the historical, social, and cultural contexts of diverse communities' health behavior.

INFRASTRUCTURE

1. The field of public health communication relies on the contribution of many disciplines. Skilled communicators and interventionists are central to successful communication programs, but they depend on expertise from many other fields. Public health communication requires theories about behavior and behavior change; deep understanding of its audiences, their cultural experience, and their social and structural circumstances; and understanding of the health infrastructure around the health concern and its medical nature. Increasingly, public health communication requires technical expertise with new communication technologies. Some programs need the expertise of marketers and others need informatics expertise. Too often, resource constraints and routine work processes mean that practitioners are not able to bring these other skills and insights to their work; they are isolated from the public health and medical expertise; the social science expertise of psychologists, sociologists, and anthropologists; and the marketers and informatics experts who might help.

2. Communication programs often are proposed, and sometimes even developed, when there is no likelihood that the resources will be available to operate a full-scale program. Research and resources are often lacking to permit the appropriate scale-up required to take evidence-based communication strategies from research or demonstration settings to larger scale implementation with assessment of impact. More attention to and resources for dissemination of evidence-based communication programs are essential.

Infrastructure Recommendation 1: If advances are to be made in communication for diverse populations, the field of public health communication should be strengthened. This requires not only investment in research and training, but the active participation and collaboration of people from many disciplines. Interdisciplinary teams to design and implement communication strategies in diverse populations should be encouraged by funding agencies.

Infrastructure Recommendation 2: National campaigns to address major health priorities require the mustering of substantial resources and, often, coordinated efforts of multiple agencies if national audiences are to be reached and effects are to be sustained over time. They cannot be undertaken successfully without such commitment. A national strategy and the infrastructure for prioritizing and implementing such large-scale campaigns are needed.

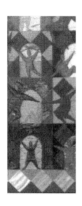

References

Abrams, D.B. 1999. Transdisciplinary paradigms for tobacco prevention research. *Nicotine and Tobacco Research* 1(Suppl 1):S15-23.

Acton, K., S. Valway, S. Helgerson, J. Huy, K. Smith, V. Chapman, and D. Gohdes. 1993. Improving diabetes care for American Indians. *Diabetes Care* 16(1):372-375.

Adler, M. 1999. Milk Matters Spanish-Language Adaptation: Observations and Recommendations Based on Focus Group Results. Unpublished manuscript (December 15).

Ahdieh, L., and R.A. Hahn. 1996. Use of the terms "race," "ethnicity," and "national origins": A review of articles in the *American Journal of Public Health*, 1980-1989. *Ethnicity and Health* 1(1):95-98.

Ajzen, I. 1985. From intentions to actions: A theory of planned behavior. Pp. 11-39 in *Action Control: From Cognition to Behavior*, J. Kuhl and J. Bechmann, eds. New York: Springer-Verlag.

Ajzen, I. 1988. *Attitudes, Personality and Behavior*. Chicago: Dorsey.

Ajzen, I. 1991. The theory of planned behavior. *Organizational Behavior and Human Decision Processes* 50:179-211.

Ajzen, I., and M. Fishbein. 1980. *Understanding Attitudes and Predicting Social Behavior*. Englewood Cliffs, NJ: Prentice-Hall.

Ajzen, I., and T.J. Madden, T.J.. 1986. Prediction of goal-directed behavior: Attitudes, intentions, and perceived behavioral control. *Journal of Experimental Social Psychology* 22:453-474.Albrecht, G.L., R. Fitzpatrick, and S.C. Scrimshaw, eds.

Albrecht, G.L., R. Fitzpatrick, and S.C. Scrimshaw, eds. 2000. *Handbook of Social Studies in Health and Medicine*. London: Sage.

Alemi, F., R.C. Stephens, R.G. Javalghi, H. Dyches, J. Butts, and A. Ghadiri. 1996. A randomized trial of a telecommunications network for pregnant women who use cocaine. *Medical Care* 34(10 Suppl):OS10-20.

Allen, M. 1998. Comparing the persuasive effectiveness one- and two-sided message. Pp. 87-98 in *Persuasion: Advances Through Meta-Analysis*, M. Allen and R.W. Preiss, eds. Cresskill, NJ: Hampton Press.

American Cancer Society. 2001. *Facts and Figures, 2001.* Atlanta, GA: American Cancer Society.

American Diabetes Association. 2000. Diabetes Facts and Figures [Online]. Available at <http://www.diabetes.org/ada/facts.asp#toll>. Accessed February 25, 2000.

American Heart Association. 1998-1999. *Heart and Stroke Statistical Update.* Dallas, TX: American Heart Association.

Andersen, M.R., Y. Yasui, H. Meischke, A. Kuniyuki, R. Etzioni, and N. Urban. 2000. The effectiveness of mammography promotion by volunteers in rural communities. *American Journal of Preventive Medicine* 18(3):199-207.

Andreasen, A.A. 1995. *Marketing Social Change: Changing Behavior to Promote Health, Social Development, and the Environment.* San Francisco: Jossey-Bass.

Atkin, C.K., and V. Freimuth. 1989. Formative evaluation research in campaign design. Pp. 131-150 in *Public Communication Campaigns* (Second Edition), R.E. Rice, and C.K. Atkin, eds. Newbury Park, CA: Sage Publications.

Atkinson, N.L., and R.S. Gold. 2001. Online research to guide knowledge management planning. *Health Education Research* 16(6):747-764.

Baier, A.C. 1993. What do women want in moral theory? Pp. 19-32 in *An Ethic of Care: Feminist and Interdisciplinary Perspectives*, M.J. Larrabee, ed. New York: Routledge.

Balas, E.A., F. Jaffrey, G.J. Kuperman, S.A. Boren, G.D. Brown, F. Pinciroli, and J.A. Mitchell. 1997. Electronic communication with patients. Evaluation of distance medicine technology. *Journal of the American Medical Association* 278:152-159.

Bandura A. 1977. Self-efficacy: Toward a unifying theory of behavioral change. *Psychological Review* 84:191-215.

Bandura A. 1986. *Social Foundations of Thought and Action: A Social Cognitive Theory.* Englewood Cliffs, NJ: Prentice-Hall

Bandura A. 1991. Self-efficacy mechanism in physiological activation and health-promoting behavior. Pp. 229-269 in *Neurobiology of Learning, Emotion and Affect*, J. Madden, ed. New York: Raven.

Bandura A. 1994. Social cognitive theory and exercise of control over HIV infection. Pp. 25-29 in *Preventing AIDS: Theories and Methods of Behavioral Interventions*, R.J. DiClemente and J.L. Peterson, eds. New York: Plenum Press.

Bandura A. 1997a. *Self-efficacy: The Exercise of Control.* New York: W.H. Freeman and Co, Publishers.

Bandura A. 1997b. The anatomy of stages of change. *American Journal of Health Promotion* 12(1):8-10.

Bandura A. 2000. Exercise of human agency through collective efficacy. *Curr Dir Psychol Sci* 9:75-78.

Bandura A. 2001. Social cognitive theory: An agentic perspective. Pp. 1-26 in *Annual Review of Psychology* (Volume 52). Palo Alto, CA: Annual Reviews.

Bandura A. 2002a. Social cognitive theory of mass communications. In *Media Effects: Advances in Theory and Research* (Second Edition), J. Bryant and D. Zillman, eds. Hillsdale, NJ: Lawrence Erlbaum Associates.

Bandura A. 2002b. Growing primacy of human agency in adaptation and change in the electronic era. *Eur Psychol* 7(1):

Bass, D.M., M.J. McClendon, P.F. Brennan, and C. McCarthy. 1998. The buffering effect of a computer support network on caregiver strain. *Journal of Aging and Health* 10(1):20-43.

Bauman, K.J. 1995. *Extended Measures of Well-Being: Meeting Basic Needs. Household Economic Studies.* Current Population Reports, U.S. Bureau of the Census. Washington, DC: U.S. Government Printing Office.

Bayer, R. 1996. AIDS prevention: Sexual ethics and responsibility. *New England Journal of Medicine* 334(23):1540-1542.

Beauchamp, D. 1976. Public health as social justice. *Inquiry* 12:3-14.

Beauchamp, D.E. 1988. *The Health of the Republic: Epidemics, Medicine, and Moralism as Challenges to Democracy.* Philadelphia, PA: Temple University Press.

Beauchamp, T.L. (1994). Ethical theory and bioethics. In T.L. Beauchamp and J.F. Childress (Eds.), Principles of biomedical ethics (4th edition. pp. 1-43). New York: Oxford University Press.

Becker, M.H. 1974.The health belief model and personal health behavior. *Health Education Monographs* 2:324-508.

Becker, M.H. 1988. AIDS and behavior change. *Public Health Reviews* 16:1-11.

Becona, E., and F.L. Vazquez. 2001. Effectiveness of personalized written feedback through a mail intervention for smoking cessation: A randomized-controlled trial in Spanish smokers. *Journal of Consulting and Clinical Psychology* 69(1):33-40.

Behavioral Risk Surveillance System (BRFSS). 2000. Survey data [online]. Available at <http://www.cdc.gov.brfss.ti.surveydata2000.htm>.

Bennett, C.E., and B. Martin. 1995. The Asian and Pacific Islander population. Pp. 48-49 in *Population Profile of the United States: 1995.* U.S. Bureau of the Census, Current Population Reports, Series P23-189. Washington DC: U.S. Government Printing Office.

Bennett, J. 2001. Crittenton links patients to Web: Wireless tablets used for e-mail and research. *Detroit Free Press*. October 26. Available at <http://www.freep.com/money/tech/critt26_20011026.htm>.

Bental, D.S., A. Cawsey, and R. Jones. 1999. Patient information systems that tailor to the individual. *Patient Education and Counseling* 36(2):171-180.

Bernhardt, J.M. 2000. Health education and the digital divide: Building bridges and filling chasms [editorial]. *Health Education Research* 15:527-531.

Berry, D. 1998. Benefits and risks of screening mammography for women in their forties: A statistical appraisal. *Journal of the National Cancer Institute* 90:1431-1439.

Bichakjian, C.K., J.L. Schwartz, T.S. Wang, J.M. Hall, T.M. Johnson, and J.S. Biermann. 2002. Melanoma information on the Internet: Often incomplete—A public health opportunity? *Journal of Clinical Oncology* 20(1):134-141.

Bird, J.A., S.J. McPhee, N.T. Ha, B. Le, T. Davis, and C.N. Jenkins. 1998. Opening pathways to cancer screening for Vietnamese-American women: Lay health workers hold a key. *Preventive Medicine* 27:821-829.

Black, S.A. 2002. Diabetes, diversity, and disparity: What do we do with the evidence? *American Journal of Public Health* 92(4):543-547.

Blalock, S.J., B.M. DeVellis, C.C. Patterson, M.K. Campbell, D.R. Orenstein, and M.A. Doolery. 2002. Effects of an osteoporosis prevention program incorporating tailored educational materials. *American Journal of Health Promotion* 16(3):146-156.

Blanchard, M.C., L.E. Rose, J. Taylor, M.A. McEntee, and L.L. Latchaw. 1999. Using a focus group to design a diabetes education program for an African American population. *Diabetes Educator* 25(6):917-924.

Bluman, L.G., B.K. Rimer, D.A. Berry, N. Borstelmann, J.D. Iglehart, K. Regan, J. Schildkraut, and E.P. Winer. 1999. Attitudes, knowledge, and risk perceptions of women with breast and/or ovarian cancer considering testing for BRCA1 and BRCA2. *Journal of Clinical Oncology* 17(3):1040-1046.

Boberg, E.W., D.H. Gustafson, R.P. Hawkins, E. Bricker, S. Pingree, F. McTavish, M. Wise, B. Owens, and R. Botta. 1997. CHESS: The Comprehensive Health Enhancement Support System. In *Information Networks for Community Health*, P.F. Brennan, S.J. Schneider, and E. Tornquist, eds. Berlin: Springer-Verlag.

Bock, B.C., B.H. Marcus, and B.M. Pinto. 2001. Maintenance of physical activity following an individualized motivationally tailored intervention. *Annals of Behavioral Medicine* 23(2):79-87.

Bonfill, X., M. Marzo, M. Pladevall, J. Marti, and J.I. Emparanza. 2001. Strategies for increasing women's participation in community breast cancer screening. *Cochrane Database Systems Review* 1(1):CD002943.

Bonham, G.S., and D.B. Brock. 1985. The relationship of diabetes with race, sex, and obesity. *The American Journal of Clinical Nutrition* 41(4):776-83.

Bosworth, K., D.H. Gustafson, and R.P. Hawkins. 1994. The BARN system: Use and impact of adolescent health promotion via computer. *Computers in Human Behavior* 10(4):467-482.

Bosworth, K., D. Espelage, T. DuBay, L.L. Dahlberg, and G. Daytner. 1996. Using multimedia to teach conflict-resolution skills to young adolescents. *American Journal of Preventive Medicine* 12(Suppl 2):65-74.

Boule, N.G., E. Haddad, and G.P. Kenny. 2001. Effects of exercise on glycemic control and body mass in type 2 diabetes mellitus. *Journal of the American Medical Association* 286(10):1218-1227.

Bowen, D.J., N. Tomoyasu, M. Anderson, M. Carney, and A. Kristal. 1992. Effects of expectancies and personalized feedback on fat consumption, taste, and preference. *Journal of Applied Sociology and Psychology* 22:1061-1079.

Brancati, F.L., P.K. Whelton, L.H. Kuller, and M.J. Klag. 1996. Diabetes mellitus, race, and socioeconomic status: A population-based study. *Annals of Epidemiology* 6(1):67-73.

Breen, N., and L. Kessler. 1994. Changes in the use of screening mammography: Evidence from the 1987 and 1990 National Health Interview Surveys. *American Journal of Public Health* 84:62-67.

Breen, N., D.K. Wagener, M.L. Brown, W.W. Davis, and R. Ballard-Barbash. 2001. Progress in cancer screening over a decade: Results of cancer screening from the 1987, 1992, and 1998 National Health Interview Surveys. *Journal of the National Cancer Institute* 93(22):1704-1713.

Brennan, P.F., S.M. Moore, G. Bjornsdottir, J. Jones, C. Visovsky, and M. Rogers. 2001. HeartCare: An Internet-based information and support system for patient home recovery after coronary artery bypass graft (CABG) surgery. *J Adv Nurs* 35:699-708.

Brinberg, D., and M.L. Axelson. 1990. Increasing the consumption of dietary fiber: A decision theory analysis. *Health Education Research* 5:409-420.

Brown, R.H., D.J. Barram, E.M. Ehrlich, and M.F. Riche. 1996. *Population Projections of the United States by Age, Sex, Race, and Hispanic Origian: 1995-2050.* Current Population Reports, U.S. Bureau of the Census. Washington, DC: U.S. Government Printing Office.

Brown, S., and M. Nightingale. 2000. Development, implementation, and evaluation of programs of the Campaign to Prevent Teen Pregnancy. Personal communication, July 5.

Brown, S.J., D.A. Lieberman, B.A. Gemeny, Y.C. Fan, D.M. Wilson, and D.J. Pasta. 1997. Educational video game for juvenile diabetes: Results of a controlled trial. *Medical Informatics* 22(1):77-89.

Brownlee, S., E.A. Leventhal, and H. Leventhal. 2000. Regulation, self regulation and regulation of the self in maintaining physical health. Pp. 369-

416 in *Handbook of Self-Regulation*, M. Boekartz, P.R. Pintrich, and M. Zeidner, eds. San Diego, CA: Academic Press.

Brug, J., I. Steenhuis, P. van Assema, and H. de Vries. 1996. The impact of a computer-tailored nutrition intervention. *Preventive Medicine* 25(3):236-242.

Brug, J., K. Glanz, P. van Assema, G. Kok, and G.J.P. van Breukelen. 1998. The impact of computer-tailored feedback and iterative feedback on fat, fruit, and vegetable intake. *Health Education and Behavior* 25(4):517-531.

Bruner, J. 1996. *The Culture of Education*. Cambridge, MA: Harvard University Press.

Brushin, B., M. Gonzalez, and R. Payne. 1997. *Exploring Cultural Attitudes to Breast Cancer: Towards the Development of Culturally Appropriate Information Resources for Women from Greek, Italian, Arabic and Polish Speaking Backgrounds*. Woolloomooloo (NSW): NHMRC National Breast Cancer Centre.

Bruyère, J., and L.C. Garro. 2000. He walks in the body: Nêhinaw (Cree) understandings about diabetes. *Canadian Nurse* 96:25-28.

Buchanan, B.G., J.D. Moore, D.E. Forsythe, G. Carenini, S. Ohlsson, and G. Banks. 1995. An intelligent interactive system for delivering individualized information to patients. *Artificial Intelligence in Medicine* 7(2):117-154.

Bull, F.C., K. Jamrozik, and B.A. Blanksby. 1999a. Tailored advice on exercise: Does it make a difference? *American Journal of Preventive Medicine* 16(3):230-239.

Bull, F.C., M.W. Kreuter, and D.P. Scharff. 1999b. Effects of tailored, personalized and general health messages on physical activity. *Patient Education and Counseling* 36:181-192.

Burack, R.C., and J. Liang. 1989. The acceptance and completion of mammography by older black women. *American Journal of Public Health* 79(6):721-726.

Burack, R.C., P.A. Gimotty, J. George, M.S. Simon, P. Dews, and A. Moncrease. 1996. The effect of patient and physician reminders on use of screening mammography in a health maintenance organization. Results of a randomized controlled trial. *Cancer* 78:1708-1721.

Burack, R.C., P.A. Gimotty, J. George, W. Stengle, L. Warbasse, and A. Moncrease. 1994. Promoting screening mammography in inner-city settings: A randomized controlled trial of computerized reminders as a component of a program to facilitate mammography. *Medical Care* 32:609-624.

Burnett, K.F., C.B. Taylor, and W.S. Agras. 1985. Ambulatory computer-assisted therapy for obesity: a new frontier for behavior therapy. *Journal of Consulting and Clinical Psychology* 53(5):698-703.

Cain, M.M., J. Sarasohn-Kahn, and J.C. Wayne. 2000. August. Health e-People: The onlineconsumer experience—Five-year forecast. California

Health Foundation. Institute for the Future for the California HealthCare Foundation. Available at <http://www.informatics-review.com/thoughts/chf.html>.

Calle, E.E., W.D. Flanders, M.J. Thun, and L.M. Martin. 1993. Demographic predictors of mammography and Pap smear screening in U.S. women. *American Journal of Public Health* 83:53-60.

Cameron, L.D., and H. Leventhal. In press. *The Self-Regulation of Health and Illness Behavior.* New York: Harwood Academic.

Campbell, M.K., B.M. DeVellis, V.J. Strecher, A.S. Ammerman, R.F. DeVellis, and R.S. Sandler. 1994. Improving dietary behavior: The effectiveness of tailored messages in primary care settings. *American Journal of Public Health* 84:783-787.

Campbell, M.K., J.M. Bernhardt, M. Waldmiller, B. Jackson, D. Potenziani, B. Weathers, and S. Demissie. 1999. Varying the message source in computer-tailored nutrition education. *Patient Education and Counseling* 36(2):157-169.

Campbell, M.K., I Tessaro, B. DeVellis. S. Benedit, K. Kelsey, L. Belton, and A. Sanhueza. 2002. Effects of a tailored health promotion program for female blue-collar workers: Health works for women. *Preventive Medicine* 34:313-323.

Campinha-Bacote, J. 1994. *The Process of Cultural Competence in Health Care: A Culturally Competent Model of Care* (pp. 1-37). Transcultural C.A.R.E. Associates.

Caplan, L.S., D.S. May, and L.C. Richardson. 2000. Time to diagnosis and treatment of breast cancer: Results from the National Breast and Cervical Cancer Early Detection Program, 1991-1995. *American Journal of Public Health* 90(1):130-134.

Cappella, J.N., M. Fishbein, R. Hornik, R.K. Ahern, and S. Sayeed. 2001. Using theory to select messages in antidrug media campaigns: reasoned action and media priming. In *Public Communication Campaigns* (Third Edition), R. Rice and C. Atkin, eds. Thousand Oaks, CA: Sage.

Carter, J.S., J.A. Pugh, and A. Monterrosa. 1996. Non-insulin-dependent diabetes mellitus in minorities in the United States. *Annals of Internal Medicine* 125(3):221-232.

Carter, J., R. Horowitz, R. Wilson, S. Sava, P. Sinnock, and D. Gohdes. 1989. Tribal differences in diabetes: Prevalence among American Indians in New Mexico. *Public Health Reports* 104(6):665-669.

Cassell, M.M., C. Jackson, and B. Cheuvront. 1998. Health communication on the Internet: An effective channel for health behavior change? *Journal of Health Communication* 3:71-79.

Cassileth, B.R. 2001. Enhancing doctor-patient communication. *Journal of Clinical Oncology* 9(18 Suppl):61S-63S.

Centers for Disease Control and Prevention. 1993. Use of race and ethnicity in public health surveillance. Summary of the CDC/ATSDR Workshop. *Morbidity and Mortality Weekly Report.* 42 (No. RR-10). Available online at: <http://www.cdc.gov/mmwr//preview/mmwrhtml/00021729. htm>.

Centers for Disease Control and Prevention. 1999. Progress in reducing risky infant sleeping positions—13 States, 1996-1997. *Morbidity and Mortality Weekly Review* 48(39):878-882.

Centers for Disease Control and Prevention. 2000a. Diabetes Public Health Resource. Publications and Products National Diabetes Fact Sheet [Online]. Available at <http://www.cdc.gov/diabetes/pubs/facts98.htm>. Accessed April 20, 2000.

Centers for Disease Control and Prevention. 2000b. Guide to community preventive services. *Morbidity and Mortality Weekly Report* 49(12).

Centers for Disease Control and Prevention. 2001. *Loving Support Campaign*. Washington, DC.

Chaffee, S.H.. 1982. Mass media and interpersonal channels: Competitive, convergent or complementary? In *Inter/Media: Interpersonal Communication in a Media World*, G. Gumpert and R. Cathcart, eds. New York: Oxford University Press.

Chamberlain, M.A. 1996. Health communication: Making the most of new media technologies—an international overview. *Journal of Health Communication* 1:43-50.

Chen, X., and L.L. Siu. 2001. Impact of the media and the Internet on oncology: Survey of cancer patients and oncologists in Canada. *Journal of Clinical Oncology* 19(23):4291-4297.

Chewning, B., P. Mosena, D. Wilson, H. Erdman, S. Potthoff, A. Murphy, and K.K. Kuhnen. 1999. Evaluation of a computerized contraceptive decision aid for adolescent patients. *Patient Education and Counseling* 38(3):227-239.

Children's Partnership. 2000. (March). Online content for low-income and underserved Americans: The digital divide's new frontier. Available at <http://www.childrenspartnership.org>.

Clemow, L., M.E. Costanza, W.P. Haddad, R. Luckmann, M.J. White, D. Klaus, and A.M. Stoddard. 2000. Underutilizers of mammography screening today: Characteristics of women planning, undecided about, and not planning a mammogram. *Annals of Behavioral Medicine* 22:80-88.

Cline, R.J.W., and K.M. Haynes. 2001. Consumer health information seeking on the Internet: The state of the art. *Health Education Research* 116(6):671-692.

Colditz, G.A., K.A.Atwood, K. Emmons, R.R. Monson, W.C. Willett, D. Trichopoulos, and D.J. Hunter. 2000. Harvard report on cancer prevention. Volume 4: Harvard Cancer Risk Index. *Cancer Causes and Control* 11:477-488.

Collins, F.S., and M.K. Mansoura. 2001. The human genome project. *Cancer* 91(S1):221-225.

Connolly, G.N. 2001. Smokes and cyberspace: A public health disaster in the making [editorial]. *Tobacco Control* 10:299.

Cooke, A. 1999. Quality of health and medical information on the Internet. *Clinical Performance and Quality Health Care* 1999;7(4):178-85.

Cooper, R.S., C.N. Rotimi, S.L. Altman, D.L. McGee, O. Babatunde, S. Kadri, M. Walenjom, S. Kingue, H. Fraser, T. Forrester, F. Bennett, and R. Wilks. 1997. Hypertension prevalence in seven populations of African origin. *American Journal of Public Health* 87(2):160-168.

Coreil, J., and J.S. Levin. 1984. A critique of the life style concept in public health education. *International Quarterly of Community Health Education* 5:103-114.

Coughlin, S.S., and R.J. Uhler. 2002. Breast and cervical cancer screening practices among Hispanic women in the United States and Puerto Rico, 1998-1999. *Preventive Medicine* 34:242-251.

Cross, T.L., B.J. Bazron, K.W. Dennis, and M.R. Isaacs. 1989. *Towards a Culturally Competent System of Care: A Monograph on Effective Services for Minority Children Who Are Severely Emotionally Disturbed, Volume* 1. Washington, DC: CASSP Technical Assistance Center and Georgetown University Child Development Center.

Cruz, M.G. 1998. Explicit and implicit conclusions in persuasive messages. Pp. 217-230 in *Persuasion: Advances Through Meta-Analysis*, M. Allen and R.W. Preiss, eds. Cresskill, NJ: Hampton Press.

Cruz, T.H., and A.D. Mickalide. 2000. The National Safe Kids Campaign Child Safety Seat Distribution Program: A strategy for reaching low-income, underserved, and culturally diverse populations. *Health Promotion Practice* 1(2):148-158.

Cultural Access Group. 2001. Ethnicity in the electronic age: Looking at the Internet through multicultural lens. Access Worldwide Communications. January. Available at <http://www.accesscag.com/internet%20 report%20v.pdf>.

Curry, S.J., C. McBride, L.C. Grothaus, D. Louie, and E.H. Wagner. 1995. A randomized trial of self-help materials, personalized feedback, and telephone counseling with nonvolunteer smokers. *Journal of Consulting and Clinical Psychology* 63(6):1005-1014.

Cyber Dialogue. 2000a. (August) Cyber Dialogue releases Cybercitizen Health 2000 (press release). Available at <http://www.cyberdialogue. com/news/releases/index.html>.

Cyber Dialogue. 2000b. (December 5). Internet industry challenged to provide physicians with valuable online applications (press release). Available at <http://www.cyberdialogue.com/news/releases/index.html>.

Dalaker, J., and B. Proctor. 2000. *Poverty in the United States, 1999*. Current Population Reports, U.S. Bureau of the Census. Washington, DC: U.S. Government Printing Office.

Daniel, M., L.W. Green, S.A. Marion, D. Gamble, C.P. Gerbert, C. Hretzman, and S.B. Sheps. 1999. Effectiveness of community-directed diabetes pre-

vention and control in a rural Aboriginal population in British Colum-
    bia, Canada. *Social Science and Medicine* 48(6):815-832.
Daniels, N. 1985. *Just Health Care.* New York: Cambridge University Press.
Davidoff, I. 1998. Depression Awareness, Recognition, and Treatment (D/
    ART) Program, A Record of Achievement: 1985-1997. National Insti-
    tute of Mental Health, Division of Services and Intervention Research.
    Unpublished manuscript, January.
Davis, F.J. 1991. *Who Is Black?: One Nation's Definition.* University Park,
    PA: The Pennsylvania State University Press.
Davis, T.C., R. Michielutte, E.N. Askov, M.V. Williams, and B.D. Weiss.
    1998. Practical assessment of adult literacy in health care. *Health Educa-
    tion and Behavior* 25(5):613-624.
Dean, L., I.H. Meyer, K. Robinson, R.L. Sell, R. Sember, V.M.B. Silenzio,
    D.J. Bowen, J. Bradford, E. Rothblum, Scout, J. White, P. Dunn, A.
    Lawrence, D. Wolfe, and J. Xavier. 2000. Lesbian, gay, bisexual, and
    transgender health: Findings and concerns. *Journal of the Gay and Les-
    bian Medical Association* 4(3):101-151.
Dearing, J.W., and E.M. Rogers. 1994. *Agenda Setting.* Newbury Park, CA:
    Sage.
De Bourdeaudhuij, I., and J. Brug. 2000. Tailoring dietary feedback to reduce
    fat intake: An intervention at the family level. *Health Education Research*
    15(4):449-462.
DeBusk, R.F., N.H. Miller, H.R. Superko, C.A. Dennis, R.J. Thomas, H.T.
    Lew, W.E. Berger, III, R.S. Heller, J. Rompf, D. Gee, et al. 1994. A case
    management system for coronary risk factor modification after acute
    myocardial infarction. *Archives of Internal Medicine* 120:721-729.
DeGuzman, M.A., and M.W. Ross. 1999. Assessing the application of HIV
    and AIDS related education and counselling on the Internet. *Patient Edu-
    cation and Counseling* 36:209-228.
DeJong, W., and J.A. Winsten. 1998. The Media and the Message: Lessons
    Learned from Past Public Service Campaigns (Summary). National Cam-
    paign to Prevent Teen Pregnancy.
Delgado, M. 1983. Hispanics and psychotherapeutic groups. *International
    Journal of Group Psychotherapy* 33(4):507-520.
Delichatsios, H.K., M.K. Hunt, R. Lobb, K. Emmons, and M.W. Gillman.
    2001. EatSmart: Efficacy of a multifaceted preventive nutrition interven-
    tion in clinical practice. *Preventive Medicine* 33:91-98.
de Vries, H., and J. Brug. 1999. Computer-tailored interventions motivating
    people to adopt health promoting behaviours: Introduction to a new
    approach. *Patient Education and Counseling* 36(2):99-105.
The Diabetes Control and Complications Trial. 2000. Retinopathy and neph-
    ropathy in patients with type 1 diabetes four years after a trial of inten-
    sive therapy.   The Diabetes Control and Complications Trial/
    Epidemiology of Diabetes Interventions and Complications Research
    Group. *New England Journal of Medicine* 342(6):381-389.

Diabetes Prevention Program Research Group. 2001. Reduction in the incidence of Type 2 diabetes with lifestyle intervention or metformin. *New England Journal of Medicine* 346:393-403.

Dibble, S.L., J.M. Vanoni, and C. Miaskowski. 1997. Women's attitudes toward breast cancer screening procedures: Different by ethnicity. *Women's Health Issues* 7(1):47-54.

Dijkstra, A., and H. de Vries. 1999. The development of computer-generated tailored interventions. *Patient Education and Counseling* 36(2):193-203.

Dijkstra, A., H. de Vries, and J. Roijackers. 1998a. Long-term effectiveness of computer-generated tailored feedback in smoking cessation. *Health Education Research* 13(2):207-214.

Dijkstra, A., H. de Vries, and J. Roijackers. 1999. Targeting smokers with low readiness to change with tailored and nontailored self-help materials. *Preventive Medicine* 28:203-211.

Dijkstra, A., H. de Vries, J. Roijackers, and G. van Breukelen. 1998b. Tailoring information to enhance quitting in smokers with low motivation to quit: Three basic efficacy questions. *Health Psychology* 17(6):513-519.

Dini, E.F., R.W. Linkins, and J. Sigafoos. 2000. The impact of computer-generated messages on childhood immunization coverage. *American Journal of Preventive Medicine* 18(2):132-139.

Dirkin, G. 1994. Technological supports for sustaining exercise. In *Advances in Exercise Adherence*, R.K. Dishman, ed. Champaign, IL: Human Kinetics.

Dolan, N.C., M.M. McDermott, M. Morrow, L. Venta, and G.J. Martin. 1999. Impact of same-day screening mammography availability: Results of a controlled clinical trial. *Archives of Internal Medicine* 159:393-398.

Dressler, W.W. 1990. Lifestyle, stress, and blood pressure in a southern black community. *Psychosomatic Medicine* 52(2):182-198.

Dressler, W.W. 1991. Social support, lifestyle incongruity, and arterial blood pressure in a southern black community. *Psychosomatic Medicine* 53(6):608-620.

Drossaert, C.H.C., H. Boer, and E.R. Seydel. 1996. Health education to improve repeat participation in the Dutch breast cancer screening programme: Evaluation of a leaflet tailored to previous participants. *Patient Education and Counseling* 28:121-131.

DuBois-Arber, F., et al. 1997. Increased condom use without other major changes in sexual behavior among the general population in Switzerland. *American Journal of Public Health* 87(4):558-566.

Dubos, R. 1959. *Mirage of Health*. New York: Harper and Row.

Dunham, P.J., A. Hurshman, E. Litwin, J. Gusella, C. Ellsworth, and P.W.D. Dodd. 1998. Computer-mediated social support: Single young mothers as a model system. *American Journal of Community Psychology* 26(2):281-306.

Duranti, A. 1997. *Linguistic Anthropology*. Cambridge: Cambridge University Press.

Eagley, A.H., and S. Chaiken. 1993. *The Psychology of Attitudes.* New York: Harcourt, Brace, Jovanovich.

Earp, J.A., E. Eng, M.S. O'Malley, M. Altpeter, G. Rauscher, L. Mayne, H.F. Mathews, K.S. Lynch, and B. Qaqish. 2002. Increasing use of mammography among older, rural African American women: Results from a community trial. *Amreican Journal of Public Health* 92(4):646-654.

Eastman, P. 1997. NCI adopts new mammography screening guidelines for women. *Journal of the National Cancer Institute* 89:538-539.

Edwards, A., and G. Elwyn. 1999. How should effectiveness of risk communication to aid patients' decisions be judged? A review of the literature. *Medical Decision Making* 19:428-434.

Edwards, B.K., H.L. Howe, L.A.G. Ries, M.J. Thun, H.M. Rosenberg, R. Yancik, P.A. Wingo, A. Jemal, and E G. Feigal. 2002. Annual report to the nation on the status of cancer (1973 through 1999). *Cancer* 94(10):2766-2792.

Ellison, R.C., A.L. Capper, R.J. Goldberg, J.C. Witschi, and F.J. Stare. 1989. The environmental component: Changing school food service to promote cardiovascular health. *Health Education Quarterly* 16(2):285-297.

Eng, T.R., A. Maxfield, K. Patrick, M.J. Deering, S.C. Ratzan, and D.H. Gustafson. 1998. Access to health information and support: a public highway or a private road? *Journal of the American Medical Association* 280:1371-1375.

Erwin, D.O., T.S. Spatz, R.C. Stotts, and J.A. Hollenberg. 1999. Increasing mammography practice by African American women. *Cancer Practice* 7:78-85.

Etter, J.F., and T.V. Perneger. 2001. Effectiveness of a computer-tailored smoking cessation program. *Archives of Internal Medicine* 161:2596-2601.

Eveland, W.P., Jr, and S. Dunwoody. 2000. Examining information processing on the World Wide Web: Using think aloud protocols. *Media Psychology* 3:219-244.

Eysenbach, G. 2000. Consumer health informatics. *British Medical Journal* 320(7251):1713-1716.

Eysenbach, G., and A.R. Jadad. 2001. Evidence-based patient choice and consumer health informatics in the Internet age. *Journal of Medical Internet Research* 3(2):e19.

Eysenbach, B., and C. Kohler. 2002. How do consumers search for and appraise health information on the World Wide Web? Qualitative study using focus groups, usability tests, and in-depth interviews. *British Medical Journal* 324:573-577.

Eysenbach, G., G. Yihune, K. Lampe, P. Cross, and D. Brickley. 2000. MedCERTAIN: Quality management, certification and rating of health information on the Net. *Proceedings/AMIA, Annual Symposium* 230-234.

Facione, N.C., C. Giancarlo, and L. Chan. 2000. Perceived risk and help-seeking behavior for breast cancer. A Chinese-American perspective. *Cancer Nursing* 23(4):258-267.

Fallowfield, L.. 2001. Participation of patients in decisions about treatment for cancer. *British Medical Journal* 323(7322):1144.

Farrell, M.A., P.A. Quiggins PA, J.D. Eller, P.A. Owle, K.M. Miner, and E.S. Walkingstick. 1993. Prevalence of diabetes and its complications in the Eastern band of Cherokee Indians. *Diabetes Care* 16(1):253-256.

Ferguson, S.D. 1999. *Communication Planning: An Integrated Approach.* Thousand Oaks, CA: Sage Publications.

Fernandez, M.A., G. Tortolero-Luna, and R.S. Gold. 1998. Mammography and Pap test screening among low-income foreign-born Hispanic women in USA. *Cad Saude Publica* 14(Suppl 3):133-147.

Festinger, L. 1957. *A Theory of Cognitive Dissonance.* Evanston, IL: Row, Peterson.

Fieler, V.K., and A. Borch. 1996. Results of a patient education project using a touch-screen computer. *Cancer Practices* 4(6):341-345.

Fiore, M.C., W.C. Bailey, S.J. Cohen, S.F.Dorfman, M.G. Goldstein, E.R. Gritz, et al. 2000. *Treating Tobacco Use and Dependence. Clinical Practice Guideline.* Public Health Service. Rockville, MD: U.S. Department of Health and Human Services.

Fishbein, M. 1995. Developing effective behavior change interventions: Some lessons learned from behavioral research. Pp. 246-261 in *Reviewing the Behavioral Sciences Knowledge Base on Technology Transfer* (NIDA Research Monograph No. 155, NIH Publication No. 95-4035), T.E. Backer, S.L. David, and G. Soucy, eds. Rockville, MD: National Institute on Drug Abuse.

Fishbein, M. 2000. The role of theory in HIV prevention. *AIDS Care* 12(3):273-278.

Fishbein M, and I. Ajzen. 1975. *Belief, Attitude, Intention, and Behavior: An Introduction to Theory and Research.* Reading, MA: Addison-Wesley.

Fishbein, M., S.E. Middlestadt, and P.J. Hitchcock. 1991. Using information to change sexually transmitted disease-related behaviors: An analysis based on the theory of reasoned action. Pp. 243-257 in *Research Issues in Human Behavior and Sexually Transmitted Diseases in the AIDS Era,* J.N. Wasserheit, S.O. Aral, and K.K. Holmes, eds. Washington, DC: American Society for Microbiology.

Fisher, J.D., and W.A. Fisher. 1992. Changing AIDS-risk behavior. *Psychological Bulletin* 111:455-474.

Fishman, P., S. Taplin, D. Meyer, and W. Barlow. 2000. Cost-effectiveness of strategies to enhance mammography use. *Effective Clinical Practice* 4:213-220.

Flegal, K., T. Ezzati, M. Harris, S. Haynes, R. Juarez, W. Knowler, E. Perez-Stable, and M. Stern. 1991. Prevalence of diabetes in Mexican Americans, Cubans and Puerto Ricans from the Hispanic Health and Nutritional Examination Survey, 1982-1984. *Diabetes Care* 14:628-638.

Fletcher, S.W., R.P. Harris, J.J. Gonzalez, D. Degnan, D.R. Lannin, V.J. Strecher, C. Pilgrim, D. Quade, J.A. Earp, and R.L. Clark. 1993. Increasing mammography utilization: a controlled study. *Journal of the National Cancer Institute* 85:112-120.

Flood, A.B., J.W. Wennberg, R.F. Nease, Jr., F.J. Fowler, Jr., J. Ding, and L.M. Hynes. 1996. The importance of patient preference in the decision to screen for prostate cancer. *Journal of General Internal Medicine* 11(6):342-349.

Florida Department of Health. 2000a. (March 1) 2000 Florida Youth Tobacco Survey results. *Florida Youth Tobacco Survey* 3(1):1-12.

Florida Department of Health. 2000b. (January 7). Tobacco use among Florida's diverse populations, 1998-1999. *Florida Youth Tobacco Survey* 2(5):1-12.

Fox, S.A., and R.G. Roetzheim. 1994. Screening mammography and older Hispanic women. *Cancer* 74(7 Suppl):2028-2033.

Fox, S.A., P.J. Murata, and J.A. Stein. 1991. The impact of physician compliance on screening mammography for older women. *Archives of Internal Medicine* 151:50-56.

Fox, S.A., R.G. Roetzheim, and R.S. Kington. 1997. Barriers to cancer prevention in the older person. Cancer in the elderly: Part I. *Clinics in Geriatric Medicine* 13(1):79-95.

Fox, S..A, J.A. Stein, R.E. Gonzalez, M. Farrenkopf, and A. Dellinger. 1998. A trial to increase mammography utilization among Los Angeles Hispanic women. *Journal of Health Care for the Poor and Underserved* 9:309-321.

Freeman, H.E., and S. Levine, eds. 1989. *Handbook of Medical Sociology* (Fourth Edition). Pp. 1-13. Englewood Cliffs, NJ: Prentice Hall.

Freeman, W.L., G.M. Hosey, P. Diehr, and D. Gohdes. 1989. Diabetes in American Indians of Washington, Oregon, and Idaho. *Diabetes Care* 1989 12(4):282-288.

Frosch, D.L., and R.M. Kaplan. 1999. Shared decision making in clinical medicine: Past research and future directions. *American Journal of Preventive Medicine* 17(4):285-294.

Fujimoto, W.Y., R.W. Bergstrom, E.J. Boyko, J.L. Kinyoun, D.L. Leonetti, L.L. Newell-Morris, L.R. Robinson, W.P. Shuman, W.C. Stolov, C.H. Tsunehara, et al. 1994. Diabetes and diabetes risk factors in second- and third-generation Japanese Americans in Seattle, Washington. *Diabetes Research and Clinical Practice* 24 Suppl:S43-52.

Gaillard, T.R., D.P. Schuster, B.M. Bossetti, P.A. Green, and K. Osei. 1997. Do sociodemographics and economic status predict risks for type II diabetes in African Americans? *The Diabetes Educator* 23(3):291-300.

Gamson, W.A. 1989. News as framing: Comments on Graber. *American Behavioral Scientist* 33(2):157-162.

Gardner, L.I., Jr., M.P. Stern, S.M. Haffner, S.P. Gaskill, H.P. Hazuda, J.H. Relethford, and C.W. Eifler. 1984. Prevalence of diabetes in Mexican Americans. Relationship to percent of gene pool derived from Native American sources. *Diabetes* 33(1):86-92.

Gargiully, P., P.A. Wingo, R.J. Coates, and T.D. Thompson. 2002. Recent trends in mortality rates for four major cancers, by sex and race/ethnicity—United States, 1990-1998. *Morbidity and Mortality Weekly Review* 51(03):49-53.

Garro, L.C. 1990. Continuity and change: The interpretation of illness in an Anishinaabe (Ojibway) community. *Culture, Medicine and Psychiatry* 14:417-454.

Garro, L.C. 1995. Individual or societal responsibility? Explanations of diabetes in an Anishinaabe (Ojibway) community. *Social Science and Medicine* 40:37-46.

Garro, L.C. 1996. Intracultural variation in causal accounts of diabetes: A comparison of three Canadian Anishinaabe (Okubway) communities. *Culture, Medicine and Psychiatry* 20:381-420.

Garro, L.C. 2000. Remembering what one knows and the construction of the past: A comparison of cultural consensus theory and cultural schema theory. *Ethos* 28:275-319.

Garro, L.C. 2001. The remembered past in a culturally meaningful life: Remembering as cultural, social and cognitive process. Pp. 105-147 in *The Psychology of Cultural Experience*, C. Moore and H. Mathews, eds. Cambridge: Cambridge University Press.

Garro, L.C. In press. Cultural, social and self processes in narrating troubling experiences. In *Narrative and Society*, C. Mattingly and U. Jensen, eds. Aarhus, Denmark: University of Aarhus Press.

Garruto, R.M., M.A. Little, G.D. James, and D.E. Brown. 1999. Natural experimental models: The global search for biomedical paradigms among traditional, modernizing and modern populations. *Proceedings of the National Academy of Sciences* 96:10536-10543.

Gbadegesin, S. 1998. Bioethics and cultural diversity. Pp. 24-31 in *A Companion to Bioethics*, H. Kuhse and P. Singer, eds. Oxford: Blackwell.

Geertz, C. 1973. The impact of the culture concept on the concept of man. P. 3354 in author's *Interpretations of Culture*. New York: Basic Books.

Geronimus, A.T., J. Bound, T.A. Wardman, M.M. Hillemeier, and P.B. Burns. 1996. Excess mortality among Blacks and Whites in the United States. *New England Journal of Medicine* 335(21):1552-1558.

Gerrard, M., F.X., Gibbons, and B.J. Bushman. 1996. Relation between perceived vulnerability to HIV and precautionary sexual behavior. *Psychological Bulletin* 119:390-409.

Glanz, K., and R.M. Mullis. 1988. Environmental interventions to promote healthy eating: A review of models, programs, and evidence. *Health Education Quarterly* 15(4):395-415.

Glanz, K., F.M. Lewis, and B.K. Rimer. 1997. *Health Behavior and Health Education: Theory, Research and Practice*, Second Edition. San Francisco: Jossey-Bass Publishers.

Glanz, K., B. Rimer, and F. Lewis. In press. *Health Behavior and Health Education: Theory, Research, and Practice.* San Francisco, CA: Jossey-Bass.

Glanz, K., B. Lankenau, S. Forester, S. Temple, R. Mullis, and T. Schmid. 1995. Environmental and policy approaches to cardiovascular disease prevention through nutrition: Opportunities for state and local action. *Health Education Quarterly* 22(4):512-527.

Gohdes, D., S. Rith-Najarian, K. Acton, and R. Shields. 1996. Improved diabetes care in a primary health setting. The Indian Health Service experience. *Annals of Internal Medicine* 124(1 Pt. 2):149-152.

Gollwitzer, P.M. 1999. Implementation intentions: Strong effects of simple plans. *American Psychologist* 54(7):493-503.

Gollwitzer, P.M., and G. Oettingen. 1998. The emergence and implementation of health goals. *Psychology and Health* 13:687-715.

Good, B.J., and M.J.D. Good. 1981. The meaning of symptoms: A cultural hermeneutic model for clinical practice. Pp. 165-196 in *The Relevance of Social Science for Medicine*, L. Eisenberg and A. Kleinman, eds. Dordecht, Holland: Reidel.

Goodman, A.H. 2001. Biological diversity and cultural diversity: From race to radical bioculturalism. Pp. 29-49 in *Cultural Diversity in the United States*, I. Susser and T.C. Patterson, eds. Malden, MA: Blackwell.

Goodman, N. 2000. Development, implementation, and evaluation of programs of the National Cancer Institute's "Not Just Once But for a Lifetime" Campaign. Personal communication, August.

Graber, M.A., C.M. Roller, and B. Kaeble. 1999. Readability levels of patient education material on the World Wide Web. *Journal of Family Practice* 48(1):58-61.

Green, L., and J. Raiburn. 1990. Contemporary developments in health promotion: Definitions and challenges. Pp. 29-44 in *Health Promotion at the Community Level*, N. Bracht, ed. Newbury Park, CA: Sage.

Greist, J., L. Baer, I. Marks, et al. 1999. Multi-site RCT of computer-aided treatment for OCD. Presented at the American Psychiatric Association, Washington, DC, May.

Grelen, A.C. 2001. Injury and violence prevention: A primer. *Patient Education and Counseling* 46(3):163-168.

Grunig, J.E. 1989. Publics, audiences and market segments: Segmentation principles for campaigns. In *Information Campaigns: Balancing Social Values and Social Change*, C.T. Salmon, ed. Newbury Park, CA: Sage Publications.

Gustafson, D., R. Hawkins, S. Pingree, F. McTavish, N. Arora, J. Salmer, J. Stewart, J. Mendenhall, R. Cella, R. Serlin, and F. Apenteko. 2000. Effect of Computer Support on Younger Women With Breast Cancer. The

Center for Health Systems Research and Analysis, University of Wisconsin-Madison.

Gustafson, D.H., R. Hawkins, E. Boberg, S. Pingree, R.E. Serlin, F. Graziano, and C.L. Chan. 1999. Impact of a patient-centered, computer-based health information/support system. *American Journal of Preventive Medicine* 16(1):1-9.

Guttman, N. 2000. *Public Health Communication Interventions: Values and Ethical Dilemmas*. Thousand Oaks, CA: Sage Publications.

Haffner, S.M., H.P. Hazuda, M.P. Stern, J.K. Patterson, W.A.J. Van Heuven, and D. Fong. 1989. Effect of socioeconomic status on hyperglycemia and retinopathy levels in Mexican Americans with NIDDM. *Diabetes Care* 12(2):128-134.

Hahn, R. 1992. The state of federal health statistics on racial and ethnic groups. *Journal of the American Medical Association* 267(2):268-271.

Hahn, R.A. 1999. Why race is differentially classified on U.S. birth and infant death certificates: An examination of two hypotheses. *Epidemiology* 19(2):108-111.

Hahn, R.A., and D.F. Stroup. 1994. Race and ethnicity in public health surveillance: Criteria for the scientific use of social categories. *Public Health Reports* 109(l):7-15.

Hall, H.I., R.J. Uhler, S.S. Coughlin, and D.S. Miller. 2002. Breast and cervical cancer screening among Appalachian women. *Cancer Epidemiology, Biomarkers and Prevention* 11:137-142.

Hallstein, L.O. 1999. A postmodern caring: Feminist standpoint theories, revisioned caring, and communication ethics. *Western Journal of Communication* 63(1):32-56.

Hamman, R.F., J.A. Marshall, J. Baxter, L.B. Kahn, E.J. Mayer, M. Orleans, J.R. Murphy, and D.C. Lezotte. 1989. Methods and prevalence of non-insulin-dependent diabetes mellitus in a biethnic Colorado population. *American Journal of Epidemiology* 129(2):295-311.

Hanis, C.L., R.E. Ferrell, S.A. Barton, L. Aguilar, A. Garza-Ibarra, B.R. Tulloch, C.A. Garcia, and W.J. Schull. 1983. Diabetes among Mexican Americans in Starr County, Texas. *American Journal of Epidemiology* 118(5):659-672.

Harpole, L.H., C. McBride, T. Strigo, and D. Lobach. 2000. Feasibility of a tailored intervention to improve preventive care use in women. *Preventive Medicine* 31:440-446.

Harris, E.L., S. Feldman, C.R. Robinson, S. Sherman, and A. Georgopoulos. 1993. Racial differences in the relationship between blood pressure and risk of retinopathy among individuals with NIDDM. *Diabetes Care* 16(5):748-54.

Harris Interactive. 2001. (January 8). Study reveals big potential for Internet to improve doctor-patient relations (press release). Available at <http://www.harrisinteractive.com/news/index.asp?NewsID=215&H1_ election =All>.

Harris, M. 1990. Noninsulin-dependent diabetes mellitus in black and white Americans. *Diabetes/Metabolism Reviews* 6(2):71-90.

Harris, M.I. 1991. Epidemiological correlates of NIDDM in hispanics, whites, and blacks in the U.S. population. *Diabetes Care* 14(7):639-648.

Harris, M.I., K.M. Flegal, C.C. Cowie, M.S. Eberhardt, D.E. Goldstein, R.R. Little, H. Wiedmeyer, and D.D. Byrd-Holt. 1998. Prevalence of diabetes, impaired fasting glucose, and impaired glucose tolerance in U.S. adults. *Diabetes Care* 21(4):518-525.

Hedlund, N. 1988. In *Communication in Mental Health Psychiatric Nursing: A Holistic Lifecycle Approach*, C.K. Beek, R.P. Rawlins, and S. Williams, eds. St. Louis: CV Mosby.

HeliosHealth.com. 2000. <http://www.helioshealth.com/diabetes_full/diabetes_01.html>

Hendrick, R.E., R.A. Smith, J.H. Rutledge, III, and C.R. Smart. 1997. Benefit of screening mammography in women aged 40-49: A new meta-analysis of randomized controlled trials. *Journal of the National Cancer Institute, Monographs* 22:87-92.

Hendricks, R.T., and L.B. Haas. 1991. Diabetes in minority populations. *Nurse Practitioner Forum* 2(3):199-202.

Hiatt, R.A., and R.J. Pasick. 1996. Unsolved problems in early breast cancer detection: Focus on the underserved. *Breast Cancer Research and Treatment* 40:37-51.

Hiltz, S.R., and M. Turoff. 1978. *The Network Nation: Human Communication Via Computer*. Reading, MA: Addison-Wesley.

Hoare, T., C. Thomas, A. Biggs, M. Booth, S. Bradley, and E. Friedman. 1994. Can the uptake of breast screening by Asian women be increased? A randomized controlled trial of a linkworker intervention [see comments]. *Journal of Public Health Medicine* 16:179-185.

Homer, C., O. Susskind, H.R. Alpert, M.S. Owusu, L. Schneider, L.A. Rappaport, and D.H. Rubin. 2000. An evaluation of an innovative multimedia educational software program for asthma management: Report of a randomized, controlled trial. *Pediatrics* 106(1 Pt 2):210-215.

Hornik, R. 1989. Channel effectiveness in development communication programs. In *Public Communication Campaigns* (Second Edition), R. Rice and C. Atkin, eds. Beverly Hills, CA: Sage.

Hornik, R. 1997. Public health education and communication as policy instruments for bringing about changes in behavior. Pp. 45-60 in *Social Marketing: Theoretical and Practical Perspectives*, M. Goldberg, M. Fishbein, S. Middlestadt, eds. Hillsdale, NJ: Lawrence Erlbaum.

Hornik, R., ed.. 2002. *Public Health Communication: Evidence for Behavior Change*. Mahwah, NJ: Lawrence Erlbaum.

Hornik, R., and K.D. Woolf. 1999. Using cross-sectional surveys to plan message strategies. *Social Marketing Quarterly* 5:34-41.

Hornung, R.L., P.A. Lennon, J.M.Garrett, R.F. DeVellis, P.D. Weinberg, and V.J. Strecher. 2000. Interactive computer technology for skin cancer prevention targeting children. *American Journal of Preventive Medicine* 18(1):69-76.

House, J.S., and D.R. Williams. 2000. Understanding and reducing socioeconomic and racial/ethnic disparities in health. Pp. 81-124 in *Promoting Health: Intervention Strategies from Social and Behavioral Research*, B. Smedley and L. Syme, eds. Committee on Capitalizing on Social Science and Behavioral Research to Improve the Public's Health, Division of Health Promotion and Disease Prevention, Institute of Medicine. Washington, DC: National Academy Press.

Hovland, C.I., I.L. Janis, and H.H. Kelley. 1953. *Communication and Persuasion: Psychological Studies of Opinion Change*. New Haven, CT: Yale University Press.

Hovland, C.I., A.A. Lumsdaine, and F.D. Sheffield. 1949. *Experiments on Mass Communication*. Princeton, NJ: Princeton University Press.

Hoy, W., A. Light, and D. Megill. 1995. Cardiovascular disease in Navajo Indians with type 2 diabetes. *Public Health Reports* 110(1):87-94.

Hoy, W.E., D.M. Megill, and M.D. Hughson. 1987. Epidemic renal disease of unknown etiology in the Zuni Indians. *American Journal of Kidney Disease* 9(6):485-496.

Huang, B., B.L. Rodriguez, C.M. Burchfiel, P. Chyoa, J.D. Curb, and K. Yano. 1996. Acculturation and prevalence of diabetes among Japanese-American men in Hawaii. *American Journal of Epidemiology* 144(7):674-681.

Hunt, L.M., M.A. Valenzuela, and J.A. Pugh. 1998. Porque me toco a mi? Mexican American diabetes patients' causal stories and their relationship to treatment behaviors. *Social Science and Medicine* 46(8):959-969.

Hutchins, E. 1980. *Culture and Inference*. Cambridge, MA: Harvard University Press.

Institute for the Future. 1999. Household Survey. Menlo Park, California.

Institute of Medicine. 1999a. *Lesbian Health: Current Assessment and Directions for the Future*. Committee on Lesbian Health Research Priorities, Neuroscience and Behavioral Health Program, Health Sciences Section. Washington, DC: National Academy Press.

Institute of Medicine. 1999b. *Networking for Health*. Committee on Enhancing the Internet for Health Applications. Washington, DC: National Academy Press.

Institute of Medicine. 1999c. *The Unequal Burden of Cancer: An Assessment of NIH Research and Programs for Ethnic Minorities and the Medically Underserved*, M.A. Haynes and B.D. Smedley, eds. Committee on Cancer Research Among Minorities and the Medically Underserved. Washington, DC: National Academy Press.

Institute of Medicine. 2000. *Promoting Health: Intervention Strategies from Social and Behavioral Research*, B.D. Smedley and S.L. Syme, eds. Committee on Capitalizing on Social Science and Behavioral Research to Improve the Public's Health, Division of Health Promotion and Disease Prevention. Washington, DC: National Academy Press.

Institute of Medicine. 2001. *Health and Behavior: The Interplay of Biological, Behavioral, and Societal Influences.* Committee on Health and Behavior: Research, Practices and Policy, Board on Neuroscience and Behavioral Health. Washington, DC: National Academy Press.

Internet Healthcare Coalition. 2000. e-Health Ethics Initiative. Available at <http://www/ihealthcoalition.org/ethics/ethics.html>.

Iyengar, S. 1991. *Is Anyone Responsible?* Chicago, IL: University of Chicago Press.

Jadad, A.R. 1999. Promoting partnerships: Challenges for the Internet age. *British Medical Journal* 319:761-764.

James, S.A., A.Z. LaCroix, D. G. Kleinbaum, and D.S. Strogatz. 1984. John Henryism and blood pressure differences among black men. II. The role of occupational stressors. *Journal of Behavioral Medicine* 7(3):259-275.

Janis, I.L. 1967. Effects of fear arousal on attitude change: Recent developments in theory and experimental research. *Advances in Experimental Social Psychology* 3:166-224.

Janz , N.K., and M.H. Becker. 1984. The Health Belief model: A decade later. *Health, Education Quarterly* 11:1-47.

Johnson, L.G., and K. Strauss. 1993. Diabetes in Mississippi Choctaw Indians. *Diabetes Care* 16(1):250-252.

Johnston, L.D., P.M. O'Malley, and J.G. Bachman. 2001. *Demographic Subgroup Trends for Various Licit and Illicit Drugs: 1975-2000.* Institute for Social Research. Ann Arbor, MI: University of Michigan.

Jones, J.K., M.A. Dragone, P.J. Bush, and S. Kamani. 2000. An interactive CD-ROM to provide information on leukemia to children and their families. *Patient's Network* 5(3):19-20.

Journal of the Mississippi State Medical Association. 2000. MSMA joins Medem to provide members and their patients with authoritative and secure online information and communications. *Journal of the Mississippi State Medical Association* 41(9):736-737.

Kahn, H.A., and R. Hiller. 1974. Blindness caused by diabetic retinopathy. *American Journal of Ophthalmology* 78(1):58-67.

Kang, S.H., and J.R. Bloom. 1993. Social support and cancer screening among older black Americans. *Journal of the National Cancer Institute* 85:737-742.

Kang, S.H., J.R. Bloom, and P.S. Romano. 1994. Cancer screening among African-American women: their use of tests and social support. *American Journal of Public Health* 84:101-103.

Kaplan, B., and P.F. Brennan. 2001. Consumer informatics supporting patients as co-producers of quality. *Journal of the American Medical Informatics Association* 8:309-316.

Karter, A.J., A. Ferrara, J.Y. Liu, H.H. Moffet, L.M. Ackerson, and J.V. Selby. 2002. Ethnic disparities in diabetic complications in an insured population. *Journal of the American Medical Association* 287(19):2519-2527.

Kassirer, J.P. 2000. Medicine at the turn of the century. *The Annals of Thoracic Surgery* 70(2):351-353.

Kelly, A.W., M. Fores Chacori, P.C. Wollan, et al. 1996. A program to increase breast and cervical cancer screening for Cambodian women in a midwestern community. *Mayo Clinic Proceedings* 71(5):437-444.

Kelly, J.A. 1994. HIV prevention among gay and bisexual men in small cities. Pp. 297-317 in *Preventing AIDS: Theories and Methods of Behavioral Interventions*, R.J. DiClemente and J.L. Peterson, eds. New York: Plenum Press.

Kelly, J.A., J.S. St. Lawrence, L.Y. Stevenson, A.C. Hauth, S.C. Kalichman, Y.E. Diaz, T.L. Brasfield, J.J. Koob, and M.G. Morgan. 1992. Community AIDS/HIV risk reduction: The effects of endorsements by popular people in three cities. *American Journal of Public Health* 82:1483-1489.

Kiefe, C.I., S.V. McKay, A. Halevy, and B.A. Brody. 1994. Is cost a barrier to screening mammography for low-income women receiving Medicare benefits? A randomized trial. *Archives of Internal Medicine* 154:1217-1224.

King, E., B.K. Rimer, A. Balshem, E. Ross, and J. Seay. 1993. Mammography-related beliefs of older women: A survey of an HMO population. *Journal of Aging and Health Behavior* 5:82-100.

King, E.S., B.K. Rimer, J. Seay, A. Balshem, and P.F. Engstrom. 1994. Promoting mammography use through progressive interventions: Is it effective? *American Journal of Public Health* 84(1):104-106.

King, E.S., E. Ross, J. Seay, A. Balshem, and B. Rimer. 1995. Mammography interventions for 65- to 74-year-old HMO women. *Journal of Aging and Health* 7:529-551.

King, E., B.K. Rimer, T. Benincasa, C. Harrop, K. Amfoh, G. Bonney, P. Kornguth, W. Denmark-Wahnefried, T. Strigo, and P. Engstrom. 1998. Strategies to encourage mammography use among women in senior citizens' housing facilities. *Journal of Cancer Education* 13:108-115.

Kirkwood, W.G., and D. Brown. 1995. Public communication about the causes of disease: The rhetoric of responsibility. *Journal of Communication* 45(1):55-76.

Kleinman, A. 1980. *Patients and Healers in the Context of Culture*. Berkeley, CA: University of California Press.

Kleinman, A. 1986. *Social Origins of Distress and Disease*. New Haven, CT: Yale University Press.

Kleinman, A. 1988. *The Illness Narratives: Suffering, Healing, and the Human Condition*. New York: Basic Books.

Knowles, J.H. 1977. The responsibility of the individual. In *Doing Better and Feeling Worse: Health in the United States*, J.H. Knowles, ed. New York: Norton.

Kothari, V., R.J. Stevens, A.I. Adler, I.M. Stratton, S.E. Manley, H.A.W. Neil, and R.R. Holman. 2002. UKPDS 60 risk of stroke in Type 2 diabetes estimated by the UKPDS risk engine. *Stroke* 33:1776-1781.

Kreher, N.E., J.M. Hickner, M.T. Ruffin, IV, and C.S. Lin. 1995. Effect of distance and travel time on rural women's compliance with screening mammography: An UPRNet study. Upper Peninsula Research Network. *Journal of Family Practice* 40:143-147.

Kretch, D., R. Crutchfield, and E. Ballachey. 1962. *Individual and Society*. New York: McGraw-Hill.

Kreuter, M.W., and C.L. Holt. 2001. How do people process health information? Applications in an age of individualized communication. *Current Directions in Psychological Science* 10(6):1-4.

Kreuter, M.W., and C.S. Skinner. 2000. Tailoring: What's in a name? *Health Education Research* 15(1):1-4.

Kreuter, M.W., and V.J. Strecher. 1996. Do tailored behavior change messages enhance the effectiveness of health risk appraisal? Results from a randomized trial. *Health Education Research* 11(1):97-105.

Kreuter, M.W., S.G. Chheda, and F.C. Bull. 2000a. How does physician advice influence patient behavior? *Archives of Family Medicine* 9:426-433.

Kreuter, M.W., E. Vehige, and A.G. McGuire. 1996. Using computer-tailored calendars to promote childhood immunization. *Public Health Reports* 111(12):176-178.

Kreuter, M.W., F.C. Bull, E.M. Clark, and D.L. Oswald. 1999. Understanding how people process health information: A comparison of tailored and nontailored weight-loss materials. *Health Psychology* 18(5):487-494.

Kreuter, M., D. Farrell, L. Olevitch, and L. Brennan. 2000b. *Tailoring Health Messages, Customizing Communication With Computer Technology*. Mahway, NJ: Lawrence Erlbaum Associates.

Kreuter, M.W., S.N. Lukwago, D.B. Bucholtz, and E.M. Clark. In press. Achieving cultural appropriateness in health promotion programs: Targeted and tailored approaches. *Health Education and Behavior*.

Krieger, N. 2000. Discrimination and health. Pp 36-75 in *Social Epidemiology*, L.F. Berkman and I. Kawachi, eds. New York: Oxford University Press.

Krieger, N., and S. Sidney. 1996. Racial discrimination and blood pressure: The CARDIA study of young black and white adults. *American Journal of Public Health* 86(10):1370-1378.

Krishna, S., E.A. Balas, D.C. Spencer, J.Z. Griffin, and S.A. Boren. 1997. Clinical trials of interactive computerized patient education: implications for family practice. *Journal of Family Practice* 45(1):25-33.

Kristal, A.R., S.J. Curry, A.L. Shattuck, Z. Feng, and S. Li. 2000. A randomized trial of a tailored, self-help dietary intervention: The Puget Sound eating patterns study. *Preventive Medicine* 31(4):380-389.

Kukafka, R., Y.A. Lussier, V.L. Patel, and J.J. Cimino. 2001. Developing tailored theory-based educational content for WEB applications: Illustrations from the MI-HEART project. *Medinfo* 19(Pt. 2):1474-1478.

Kumar, N.B., D.E. Bostow, D.V. Schapira, and K.M. Kritch. 1993. Efficacy of interactive, automated programmed instruction in nutrition education for cancer prevention. *Journal of Cancer Education* 8(3):203-211.

Lane, D.S., J. Zapka, N. Breen, C.R. Messina, and D.J. Fotheringham. 2000. A systems model of clinical preventive care: The case of breast cancer screening among older women. *Preventive Medicine* 31:481-493.

Lang, G.C. 1985. Diabetes and Health Care in a Sioux Community. *Human Organization* 44(3):251-260.

Lang, G.C. 1989. "Making Sense" about diabetes: Dakota narratives of illness. *Medical Anthropology* 11:305-327.

Lantz, P.M., L. Dupuis, D. Reding, M. Krauska, and K. Lappe. 1994. Peer discussions of cancer among Hispanic migrant farm workers. *Public Health Reports* 109:512-520.

Lantz, P.M., D. Stencil, M.T. Lippert, S. Beversdorf, L. Jaros, and P.L. Remington. 1995. Breast and cervical cancer screening in a low-income managed care sample: The efficacy of physician letters and phone calls [published erratum appears in *American Journal of Public Health* 1995 Aug;85(8 Pt 1):1063]. *American Journal of Public Health* 85:834-836.

LaPorte, R.E., M. Matushima, and Y.-F. Chang. 1995. Prevalence and incidence of insulin-dependent diabetes. In *Diabetes in America*. Bethesda, MD: National Diabetes Data Group (National Institutes of Health).

Lauver, D.R., and J. Kane. 1999. A motivational message, external barriers, and mammography utilization. *Cancer Detection and Prevention* 23:254-264.

Lebo, H. 2001 (November). *The UCLA Internet report 2001—Surveying the digital future: Year two.* UCLA Center for Communication. Available at <http://www.ccp.ucla.edu>.

Lee, M.M., F. Lee, S. Stewart, and S.J. McPhee. 1999. Cancer screening practices among primary care physicians serving Chinese Americans in San Francisco. *WJM* 170:148-155.

Legler, J., H.I. Meissner, C. Coyne, N. Breen, V. Chollette, and B.K. Rimer. 2002. The effectiveness of interventions to promote mammography among women with historically lower rates of screening. *Cancer Epidemiology, Biomarkers and Prevention* 11:59-71.

LeGrow, G., and J. Metzger. 2001. (November). E-Disease management. First Consulting Group for the California HealthCare Foundation. Available at <http://ehealth.chcf.org/view.cfm?section=Industry&itemID=4637>.

Lenhart, A. 2000. (September 21). *Who's not online: 57% of those without Internet access say they do not plan to log on. The Pew Internet & American Life Project.* Available at <http://www.pewinternet.org/reports/toc.asp?Report=21>.

Lennox, A.S., L.M. Osman, E. Reiter, R. Robertson, J. Friend, K. McCan, D. Skatun, and P.T.Donna. 2001. Cost effectiveness of computer tailored and on-tailored smoking cessation letters in general practice: Randomised controlled trial. *British Medical Journal* 322(7299):1396.

Leo, R.J., C. Sherry, and A.W. Jones. 1999. Referral patterns and recognition of depression among African-American and Caucasion patients. *General Hospital Psychiatry* 29(3):175-182.

Leventhal, H. 1970. Findings and theory in the study of fear communications. *Advances in Experimental Social Psychology* 5:119-186.

Leventhal, H., M. Diefenbach, and E.A. Leventhal. 1992. Illness cognition: Using common sense to understand treatment adherence and affect cognition interactions. *Cognitive Therapy and Research* 16:143-163.

Leventhal, H., S. Hudson, and C. Robitaille. 1997. Social comparison and health: A process model. Pp. 411-432 in *Health, Coping and Well Being: Perspectives from Social Comparison Theory*, B. Buunk and F.X. Gibbons, eds. Hillsdale, NJ: Lawrence Erlbaum.

Leventhal, H., R.P. Singer, and S. Jones. 1965. Effects of fear and specificity of recommendations upon attitudes and behavior. *Journal of Personality and Social Psychology* 2:20-29.

Leventhal, H., C. Rabin, E. A. Leventhal, and E. Burns. 2001. Health/risk behaviors and aging. Pp. 186-214 in *Handbook of the Psychology of Aging, Fifth Edition*, R. Birren and W. Schaie, eds. CA: Academic Press.

Leventhal, H., I. Brissette, and E.A. Leventhal. In press. The common-sense model of self-regulation of health and illness. In *The Self-Regulation of Health and Illness Behavior*. New York: Harwood Academic.

Leventhal, H., D. Meyer, and D. Nerenz. 1980. The common sense representation of illness danger. Pp. 7-30 in *Contributions to Medical Psychology*, Volume II, S. Rachman, ed. New York: Pergamon Press.

Lewis, D. 1999. Computer-based approaches to patient education: A review of the literature. *Journal of the American Medical Informatics Association* 6(4):272-282.

Libman, I., and S.A. Arslanian. 1999. Type II diabetes mellitus: No longer just adults. *Pediatric Annals* 28(9):589-593.

Libman, I.M., R.E. LaPorte, D. Becker, J.S. Dorman, A.L. Drash, and L. Kuller. 1998. Was there an epidemic of diabetes in nonwhite adolescents in Allegheny County, Pennsylvania? *Diabetes Care* 21(8):1278-1281.

Liburd, L.C., L.A. Anderson, T. Edgar, and L. Jack, Jr. 1999. Body size and body shape: Perceptions of black women with diabetes. *Diabetes Education* 25(3):382-388.

Lieberman, A., and S. Chaiken. 1992. Defensive processing of personally relevant health messages. *Personality and Social Psychology Bulletin* 18:669-679.

Lieberman, D.A. 2000. Using interactive media in communication campaigns for children and adolescents. In *Public Communication Campaigns* (Third Edition), R.E. Rice and C.K. Atkin, eds. Thousand Oaks, CA: Sage Publications.

Lieninger, N. 1978. *Transcultural Nursing: Concepts, Theories and Practices.* New York: John Wiley & Sons. (Reprinted in 1995 by McGraw-Hill, Columbus, OH.)

Lindenbaum, S., and M. Lock, eds. 1993. *The Biopolitics of Postmodern Bodies: Determinations of Self in Immune System Discourse. Knowledge, Power, and Practice: The Anthropology of Medicine and Everyday Life.* Berkeley: University of California Press.

Lipkus, I.M., B.K. Rimer, and T.S. Strigo. 1996. Relationships among objective and subjective risk for breast cancer and mammography stages of change. *Cancer Epidemiology, Biomarkers, and Prevention* 15(2):1005-1011.

Lipkus, I.M., P.R. Lyna, and B.K. Rimer. 1999. Using tailored interventions to enhance smoking cessation among African-Americans at a community health center. *Nicotine and Tobacco Research* 1:77-85.

Lipkus, I.M., B.K. Rimer, S. Halabi, and T.S. Strigo. 2000. Can tailored interventions increase mammography use among HMO women? *American Journal of Preventive Medicine* 18(1):1-10.

Lipton, R.B., Y. Liao, G. Cao, R.S. Cooper, and D. McGee. 1993. Determinants of incident non-insulin-dependent diabetes mellitus among blacks and whites in a national sample. The NHANES I Epidemiologic Follow-up Study. *American Journal of Epidemiology* 138(10):826-839.

Livingstone, F.B. 1962. On the non-existence of human races. *Current Anthropology* 3:279-381.

Long, A., S.C.M. Scrimshaw, and N. Hernandez. 1992. Transcultural epilepsy services. In *Rapid Assessment Procedures: Qualitative Methodologies for Planning and Evaluation of Health Related Programmes*, N.S. Scrimshaw and G.R. Gleason, eds. Boston: International Nutrition Foundation for Developing Countries.

López, S.R. 1997. Cultural competence in psychotherapy: A guide for clinicians and their supervisors. Pp. 570-588 in *Handbook of Psychotherapy Supervision*, C.E. Watkins, Jr., ed. New York: John Wiley and Sons.

Lorig, K.R., D.S. Sobel, A.L. Stewart, B.W. Brown, Jr., A. Bandura, P. Ritter, V.M. Gonzalez, D.D. Laurent, and H.R. Holman. 1999. Evidence suggesting that a chronic disease self-management program can improve health status while reducing hospitalization: A randomized trial. *Medical Care* 37(1):5-14.

Lucky, R. 2000. The quickening of science communication. *Science* 289 (5477):259-264.

Lukwago, S.N., M.W. Kreuter, D.C. Bucholtz, C. Holt, and E. Clark. 2001. Development and validation of brief scales to measure collectivism, religiosity, racial pride, and time orientation in urban African American women. *Family and Community Health* 24(3):63-71.

Lukwago, S.N., M.W. Kreuter, C.L. Holt, K. Steger-May, D.C. Bucholtz, and C.S. Skinner. In press. Sociocultural correlates of breast cancer knowledge and screening in urban African-American women. *American Journal of Public Health*.

Lutz, S.F., A.S. Ammerman, J.R. Atwood, M.K. Campbell, R.F. DeVellis, and W.D. Rosamond. 1999. Innovative newsletter interventions improve fruit and vegetable consumption in healthy adults. *Journal of the American Dietetic Association* 99:705-709.

Lynch, J., and G. Kaplan. 2000. Socioeconomic position. In *Social Epidemiology*, L. Berkman and I. Kawachi, eds. New York: Oxford University Press.

MacDonald, K., J. Case, and J. Metzger. 2001. (November). E-Encounters. First Consulting Group for the California HealthCare Foundation. Available at <http://ehealth.chcf.org/view.cfm?section=Industry&itemID=4636>.

Mandelblatt, J.S., and K.R. Yabroff. 1999. Effectiveness of interventions designed to increase mammography use: a meta-analysis of provider-targeted strategies. *Cancer Epidemiology, Biomarkers and Prevention* 8:759-767.

Mandelblatt, J., M. Traxler, P. Lakin, L. Thomas, P. Chauhan, S. Matseoane, and P. Kanetsky. 1993. A nurse practitioner intervention to increase breast and cervical cancer screening for poor, elderly black women. *Journal of General Internal Medicine* 8:173-178.

Mandl, K.D., I.S. Kohane, and A.M. Brandt. 1998. Electronic patient-physician communication: problems and promise. *Archives of Internal Medicine* 129(6):495-500.

Mann, J.M. 1997. Medicine and public health, ethics and human rights. *Hastings Center Report* 27(3):6-13.

Marcus, B.H., C.R. Nigg, D. Riebe, and L.H. Forsyth. 2000. Interactive communication strategies: Implications for population-based physical-activity promotion. *American Journal of Preventive Medicine* 19(2):121-126.

Margolis, K.L., N. Lurie, P.G. McGovern, M. Tyrrell, and J.S. Slater. 1998. Increasing breast and cervical cancer screening in low-income women. *Journal of General Internal Medicine* 13:515-521.

Martin, L.M., E.E. Calle, P.A. Wingo, and C.W. Heath. 1996. Comparison of mammography and pap test use from the 1987 and 1992 National Health Interview Surveys: Are we closing the gaps? *American Journal of Preventive Medicine* 12:82-90.

Martinez, C.B., and K. Strauss. 1993. Diabetes in St. Regis Mohawk Indians. *Diabetes Care* 16(1):260-262.

Maryland Community and Public Health Administration. 2000. *Annual Report*. Pp. 14-16. Annapolis, MD: Author.

Massari, P. 2000. Research and evaluation of the National Truth Campaign. Personal communication, September.

Maxwell, A.E., R. Bastani, and U.S. Warda. 1997. Breast cancer screening and related attitudes among Filipino-American women. *Cancer Epidemiology, Biomarkers and Prevention* 6:719-726.

Maxwell, A.E., R. Bastani, and U.S. Warda. 1998a. Misconceptions and mammography use among Filipino- and Korean-American women. *Ethnicity and Disease* 8:377-384.

Maxwell, A.E., R. Bastani, and U.S. Warda. 1998b. Mammography utilization and related attitudes among Korean-American women. *Women's Health* 27:89-107.

McBride, C.M., and B.K. Rimer. 1999. Using the telephone to improve health behavior and health service delivery. *Patient Education and Counseling* 37(1):3-18.

McBride, C.M., L.A. Bastian, S. Halabi, L. Fish, I.M. Lipkus, H.B. Bosworth, B.K. Rimer, and I.C. Siegler. In press. Efficacy of a tailored intervention to aid decision-making about hormone replacement therapy. *American Journal of Public Health* McBride, C.M., G. Bepler, I.M. Lipkus, P. Lyna, G. Samsa, J. Albright, S. Datta, and B.K. Rimer

McBride, C.M., L.A. Bastian, S. Halabi, L. Fish, I.M. Lipkus, H.B. Bosworth, B.K. Rimer, and I.C. Siegler. 2002. Incorporating genetic susceptibililty feedback into a smoking cessation program for African-American smokers with low income. *Cancer Epidemiology, Biomarkers and Prevention* 11(6):

McCoombs, M., and D. Shaw. 1972. The agenda setting function of mass media. *Public Opinion Quarterly* 36:176-187.

McCroskey, J.C. 1970. The effects of evidence as an inhibitor of counter persuasion. *Speech Monographs* 37:188-194.

McDonald, P.A., D.D. Thorne, J.C. Pearson, and L.L. Adams-Campbell. 1999. Perceptions and knowledge of breast cancer among African-American women residing in public housing. *Ethnicity and Disease* 9:81-93.

McElroy, A., and M.A. Jezewski. 2000. Cultural variation in the experience of health and illness. In *Handbook of Social Studies in Health and Medicine*, G.L. Albrecht, R. Fitzpatrick, and S.C. Scrimshaw, eds. London: Sage.

McGinnis, J.M., and W.H. Foege. 1993. Actual causes of death in the United States. *Journal of the American Medical Association* 270:2207-2212.

McGuire, W.J. 1969. The nature of attitudes and attitude change. Pp. 136-314 in *The Handbook of Social Psychology* (Second Edition, Volume 3), G. Lindzey and E. Aronson, eds. Reading, MA: Addison-Wesley.

McKay, H.G., E.G. Feil, R.E. Glasgow, and J.E. Brown. 1998. Feasibility and use of an Internet support service for diabetes self-management. *Diabetes Educ* 24(2):174-179.

McNabb, W., M. Quinn, and J. Tobian. 1997. Diabetes in African American women: The silent epidemic. *Women's Health* 3(3-4):275-300.

McPhee, S.J., S. Stewart, K.C. Brock, J.A. Bird, C.N.H. Jenkins, and C.Q. Pham. 1997a. Factors associated with breast and cervical cancer screening practices among Vietnamese American women. *Cancer Detection and Prevention* 21:510-521.

McPhee, S.J., J.A. Bird, T. Davis, N.T. Ha, C.N. Jenkins, and B. Le. 1997b. Barriers to breast and cervical cancer screening among Vietnamese-American women. *American Journal of Preventive Medicine* 13:205-213.

Meissner, H.I., N. Breen, C. Coyne, J.M. Legler, D.T. Green, and B.K. Edwards. 1998. Breast and cervical cancer screening interventions: An assessment of the literature. *Cancer Epidemiology, Biomarkers and Prevention* 7:951-961.

Meldrum, P., D. Turnbull, H.M. Dobson, C. Colquhoun, W.H. Gilmour, and G.M. McIlwaine. 1994. Tailored written invitations for second round breast cancer screening: A randomised controlled trial. *Journal of Medical Screening* 1:245-248.

Meyer, D., H. Leventhal, and M. Gutmann. 1985. Common-sense models of illness: The example of hypertension. *Health Psychology* 4:115-135.

Mickey, R.M., J. Durski, J.K. Worden, and N.L. Danigelis. 1995. Breast cancer screening and associated factors for low-income African-American women. *Preventive Medicine* 24:467-476.

Middlestadt, S.E., K. Bhattacharyya, J. Rosenbaum, and M. Fishbein. 1996. The use of theory based semi-structured elicitation questionnaires: formative research for CDC's Prevention Marketing Initiative. *Public Health Reports*111(Supplement 1):18-27.

Milio, N. 1981. *Promoting Health Through Public Policy*. Philadelphia: F. A. Davis.

Miller, W.R., and S. Rollnick. 1991. *Motivational Interviewing: Preparing People to Change Addictive Behavior*. New York: Guilford Press.

Mills, C. 1959. *The Sociological Imagination*. New York: Oxford University Press.

Mishra, S.I., L.R. Chavez, J.R. Magana, P. Nava, R.B. Valdez, and F.A. Hubbell. 1998. Improving breast cancer control among Latinas: Evaluation of a theory-based educational program. *Health Education and Behavior* 25:653-670.

Mongeau, P.A. 1998. Another look at fear-arousing persuasive appeals. Pp. 53-68 in *Persuasion: Advances Through Meta-Analysis*, M. Allen and R.W. Preiss, eds. Cresskill, NJ: Hampton Press.

Morbidity and Mortality Weekly Report. 2000. End-stage renal disease attributed to diabetes among American Indians/Alaska Natives with diabetes—United States, 1990-1996. *MMWR* 49(42):959-962.

Morgan, C., E. Park, and D.E. Cortes. 1995. Beliefs, knowledge, and behavior about cancer among urban Hispanic women. *Journal of the National Cancer Institute, Monographs* 18:57-63.

Moyer, C.A., H. Lennartz, A.A. Moore, and J.A.L. Earp. 2001. Expanding the role of mammographers: A training strategy to enhance mammographer-patient interaction. *Breast Disease* 13:13-19.

Muneta, B., J. Newman, S. Wettall, and J. Stevenson. 1993. Diabetes and associated risk factors among Native Americans. *Diabetes Care* 16(12):1619-1620.

Murphy, N.J., C.D. Schraer, L.R. Bulkow, E.J. Boyko, and A.P. Lanier. 1992. Diabetes mellitus in Alaskan Yup'ik Eskimos and Athabascan Indians after 25 yr. *Diabetes Care* 15(10):1390-1392.

Murray, C.J.L., and A.D. Lopez, eds. 1996. *Summary: The Global Burden of Disease: A Comprehensive Assessment of Mortality and Disability from Diseases, Injuries, and Risk Factors in 1990 and Projected to 2020.* Published on behalf of the World Health Organization and the World Bank. Cambridge, MA: Harvard University Press.

Myers, R.E., G.W. Chodak, T.A. Wolf, D.Y. Burgh, G.T. McGrory, S.M. Marcus, J.A. Diehl, and M. Williams. 1999. Adherence by African American men to prostate cancer education and early detection. *Cancer* 86(1):88-104.

Nagourney, E. 2000. Words of warning to help stop SIDS. *The New York Times* [Online]. Available at <www.Nyt.Com>.

Nakamura, R.M. 1999. *Health in America: A Multicultural Perspective.* San Francisco: Benjamin Cummings.

Nansel, T., N. Weaver, M. Donlin, H. Jacobsen, M.W. Kreuter, and B. Simons-Morton. 2002. Baby, be safe: The effect of pediatric injury prevention tailored communications provided in a pediatric primary care setting. *Patient Education and Counseling* 46(3):175-190.

National Cancer Institute. 2002. Accessed on May 15. SEER (Surveillance, Epidemiology, and End Results). *SEER Cancer Statistics Review, 1973-1999*, L.A. G. Ries, M.P. Eisner, C.L. Kosary, B.F. Hankey, B.A. Miller, L. Clegg, and B.K. Edwards, eds. Available at <http://www.seer.cancer.gov/csr/1973_1999>. (Main Internet site page found at <http://www.seer.cancer.gov/>.)

National Center for Cultural Competence, G.U.C.D.C. 2000. (September 12). Sudden Infant Death Syndrome/Infant Death (SIDS/ID) Component: National Center for Cultural Competence [Online]. Available at. <http://www.dml.georgetown.edu/depts/pediatrics/gucdc/nccc5.html>.

National Center for Health Statistics. 2000. Health, United States, 2000, with Adolescent Health Chartbook [Online]. Available at <http://www.cdc.gov/nchs/products/pubs/pubd/hus/hus.htm>. Hyattsville, MD: U.S. Department of Health and Human Services. Accessed August 2, 2000.

National Cholesterol Education Program. 2001. *Live Healthier, Live Longer.* Bethesda, MD: National Heart, Lung, and Blood Institute.

National Diabetes Education Program. 2002. Internet site located at <http://ndep.nih.gov/>. Accessed May 21.

National Heart, Lung, and Blood Institute. 2000. National High Blood Pressure Education Program: Program Description [Online]. Available at <http://www.nhlbi.nih.gov/about/nhbpep/nhbp_pd.htm>. Accessed May 22, 2000.

National Institute of Child Health and Human Development (NICHD). 1998. NIH News Alert: SIDS Rate Drops as More Babies are Placed to Sleep on their Backs or Sides [Online]. July 21. Available at: <http://www.nichd.nih.gov/new/releases/Sidsrate.htm>.

National Institute of Child Health and Human Development (NICHD). 2000. (April 28) To Reduce SIDS Risk, Doctor's Advice Most Important in

Choice of Placing Infants to Sleep on Their Backs. *NIH News Alert* [Online]. Available at <http://www.nichd.nih.gov/nre/releases/bts.htm>.

National Insititutes of Health. 1998. Clinical Guidelines on the Identification, Evaluation, and Treatment of Overweight and Obesity in Adults: The Evidence Report. Bethesda, MD: National Institutes of Health, NHLBI.

National Institutes of Health Consensus Development Panel. 1997. National Institutes of Health Consensus Development Conference Statement: Breast Cancer Screening for Women Ages 40-49, January 21-23, 1997. *Journal of the National Cancer Institute* 89(14):1015-1026.

National Safe Kids Campaign. 2000 (accessed August 28). "Get in the Game." <http://www.safekids.org>.

National Youth Anti-Drug Media Campaign. 1998. <http://www.mediacampaign.org/publications/>

Navarro, A.M., K.L. Senn, R.M. Kaplan, L. McNicholas, M.C. Campo, and B. Roppe. 1998. Por La Vida Intervention Model for Cancer Prevention in Latinas. *Journal of the National Cancer Institute, Monographs* 18:137-145.

Nelson, R.G., and P.H. Bennett. 1989. Diabetic renal disease in Pima Indians. *Transplant Proceedings* 21(6):3913-3915.

Neufeld, N.D., L.J. Raffel, C. Landon, Y.D.I. Chen, and C.M. Vadhein. 1998. Early presentation of type 2 diabetes in Mexican-American youth. *Diabetes Care* 21(1):80-86.

Nichter, M. 1981. Negotiation of the illness experience: Ayurvedic therapy and the psychosocial dimension of illness. *Culture, Medicine and Psychiatry* 5(1):5-24.

Niebuhr, H.R. 1978. *The Responsible Self*. New York: Harper and Row.

Nobles, M. 2000. History counts: A comparative analysis of racial/color categorization in U.S. and Brazilian censuses. *American Journal of Public Health* 90:1738-1745.

Nodding, N. 1990. Ethics from the standpoint of women. Pp. 370-390 in *Women and Values: Reading in Recent Feminist Philosophy* (Second Edition), M. Pearsall, ed. Belmont, CA: Wadsworth.

Norris, S.L., M.M. Engelgau, and K.M. Narayan. 2001. Effectiveness of self-management training in type 2 diabetes: A systematic review of randomized controlled trials. *Diabetes Care* 24:561-587.

Novelli, W.D. 1984. Developing marketing programs. In *Marketing Health Behavior: Principles, Techniques, and Applications*, L.W. Frederiksen, L.J. Soloman, and K.A. Brehony, eds. New York: Plenum Press.

O'Brien, T.R., W.D. Flanders, P. Decoufle, C.A. Boyle, F. DeStefano, and S. Teutsch. 1989. Are racial differences in the prevalence of diabetes in adults explained by differences in obesity? *Journal of the Amerian Medical Association* 262(11):1485-1488.

O'Connor, A.M., C.J. Griffiths, M.R. Underwood, and S. Eldridge. 1998. Can postal prompts from general practitioners improve the uptake of breast screening? A randomised controlled trial in one east London general practice. *Journal of Medical Screening* 5:49-52.

Oenema, A., J. Brug, and L. Lechner. 2001. Web-based tailored nutrition education: Results of a randomized controlled trial. *Health Education Research* 16(6):647-660.

Oermann, M.H., and F.L. Wilson. 2000. Quality of care information for consumers on the Internet. *J Nurs Care Qual* 14(4):45-54.

Office of Management and Budget. 1997a. Revisions to the standards for the classification of Federal data on race and ethnicity. *Federal Register* 62(210):58781-58790.

Office of Management and Budget. 1997b. *Statistical Programs of the United States Government: Fiscal Year 1997*. Washington, DC: U.S. Government Printing Office.

Office of National Drug Control Policy. 2000. Evaluation of the National Youth Anti-Drug Media Campaign: Campaign Exposure and Baseline Measurement of Correlates of Illicit Drug Use from November 1999 through May 2000. Available online at <http://www.mediacampaign.org/publications/index.html>.

Olsen, O., and P.C. Gatzsche. 2001. Cochrane review on screening for breast cancer with mammography. *Lancet* 358:1340-1342.

O'Malley, A.S., J. Kerner, A.E. Johnson, and J. Mandelblatt. 1999. Acculturation and breast cancer screening among Hispanic women in New York City. *American Journal of Public Health* 89:219-227.

O'Malley, M.S., J.A.L. Earp, S.T. Hawley, M.J. Schell, H.F. Mathews, and J. Mitchell. 2001. The association of race/ethnicity, socioeconomic status, and physician recommendation for mammography: who gets the message about breast cancer screening? *American Journal of Public Health* 91:49-54.

Orleans, C.T., N.R. Boyd, E. Noll, L. Crosette, and B. Glassman. 2000. Computer-tailored intervention for older smokers using transdermal nicotine. *Tobacco Control* 9(Suppl 1):i53.

Ossip-Klein, D.J., G.A. Giovino, N. Megahed, P.M. Black, S.L. Emont, J. Stiggins, E. Shulman, and L. Moore. 1991. Effects of a smokers hotline: Results of a 10-county self-help trial. *Journal of Consulting and Clinical Psychology* 59(2):325-332.

Ostbye, T., and P. Hurlen. 1997. The electronic house call. Consequences of telemedicine consultations for physicians, patients, and society. *Archives of Family Medicine* 6(3):266-271.

Palmgreen, P., L. Donohew, E.P. Lorch, M. Rogus, D. Helm, and N. Grant. 1991. Sensation seeking, message sensation value, and drug use as mediators of PSA effectiveness. *Health Communication* 3:217-227.

Paperny, D.M.N., and V.A. Hedberg. 1999. Computer-assisted health counselor visits: A low-cost model for comprehensive adolescent preventive services. *Archives of Pediatrics and Adolescent Medicine* 153:63-67.

Parker, J.G. 1994. The lived experience of Native Americans with diabetes within a transcultural nursing perspective. *Journal of Transcultural Nursing* 6(1):5-11.

Paskett, E.D., C.M. Tatum, R. D'Agostino, J. Rushing, R. Velez, R. Michiellutte, and M. Dignan. 1999. Community-based interventions to improve breast and cervical cancer screening: Results of the Forsyth County Cancer Screening (FoCaS) Project. *Cancer Epidemiology, Biomarkers and Prevention* 5:453-459.

Patel, A.M. 2001. Using the Internet in the management of asthma. *Current Opinion in Pulmonary Medicine* 7:39-42.

Patrick, K., T.N. Robinson, F. Alemi, and T.R. Eng. 1999. Policy issues relevant to evaluation of interactive health communication applications. *American Journal of Preventive Medicine* 16(1):35-42.

Peachmann, C, and D.W. Stewart. 1990. The effects of comparative advertising on attention, memory, and purchase intentions. *Journal of Consumer Research* 17(2):180-191.

Pellegrino, E.D. 1985. The virtuous physician, and the ethics of medicine. Pp. 243-255 in *Virtue and Medicine: Exploration in the Character of Medicine* (Philosophy and Medicine Series No. 17), E.E. Shelp, ed. Dordrecht, the Netherlands: D Reidel Publishing.

Pellegrino, E.D. 1993. The metamorphosis of medical ethics: A 30-year retrospective. *Journal of the American Medical Association* 269(9):1158-1162.

Pennbridge, J., R. Moya, and L. Rodrigues. 1999. Questionnaire survey of California consumers' use and rating of sources of health care information including the Internet. *The Western Journal of Medicine* 171:302-305.

Petraitis, J., B.R. Flay, and T.Q. Miller. 1995. Reviewing theories of adolescent substance use: Organizing pieces of the puzzle. *Psychological Bulletin* 117(1):67-86.

Petrie, K.J., and J.A. Weinman. 1997. *Perceptions of Health and Illness.* Amsterdam: Harwood Academic.

Petty, R.E., and J.T. Cacioppo. 1979a. Issue involvement can increase or decrease persuasion by enhancing message-relevant cognitive responses. *Journal of Personality and Social Psychology* 37:1915-1926.

Petty, R.E., and J.T. Cacioppo. 1979b. Effects of message repetition and position on cognitive response, recall, and persuasion. *Journal of Personality and Social Psychology* 37(1):97-109.

Pew Internet & American Life Project. 2000a. (October 22). African-Americans and the Internet. Available at <http://www.pewinternet.org/reports/toc.asp?Report=25>.

Pew Internet & American Life Project. 2000b. (November 26). Online health care revolution: How the Web helps Americans take better care of themselves. Available at <http://www.pewinternet.org/reports/toc.asp?Report=26>.

Pew Internet & American Life Project. 2002. (March 3). Getting serious online. Available at <http://www.pewinternet.org/reports/toc.asp?Report=55>.

Pierce, J.P., S. Emery, and E. Gilpin. 2002. The California Tobacco Control Program: A long term health communication project. In *Public Health Communication: Evidence for Behavior Change*, R. Hornik, ed. Mahwah, NJ: Lawrence Erlbaum Associates.

Pierce, J. P., and E.A. Giplin. 1995. A historical analysis of tobacco marketing and the uptake of smoking by youth in the United States: 1890-1977. *Health Psychology* 14:500-508.

Piette, J.D. 1997. Moving diabetes management from clinic to community: Development of a prototype based on automated voice messaging. *The Diabetes Educator* 23(6):672-680.

Piette, J.D. 1999. Patient education via automated calls: A study of English and Spanish speakers with diabetes. *American Journal of Preventive Medicine* 17(2):138-141.

Piette, J.D. 2000. Interactive voice response systems in the diagnosis and management of chronic disease. *The American Journal of Managed Care* 6(7):817-827.

Piette, J.D., S.J. McPhee, M. Weinberger, C.A. Mah, and F.B. Kraemer. 1999. Use of automated telephone disease management calls in an ethnically diverse sample of low-income patients with diabetes. *Diabetes Care* 22(8):1302-1309.

Pinhas-Hamiel, O., L.M. Dolan, S.R. Daniels, D. Standiford, P.R. Khoury, and P. Zeitler. 1996. Increased incidence on non-insulin-dependent diabetes mellitus among adolescents. *Journal of Pediatrics* 128:608-615.

Pinhey, T.K., T.J. Iverson, and R.L.Workman. 1994. The influence of ethnicity and socioeconomic status on the use of mammography by Asian and Pacific island women on Guam. *Women's Health* 21:57-69.

Potts, H.W.W., and J.C. Wyatt. 2001. Survey of doctors' experience of patients using the Internet. *Journal of Medical Internet Research* 4(1):e5.

Prochaska, J.O., and C.C. DiClemente. 1983. Stages and processes of self-change in smoking: Towards an integrative model of change. *Journal of Consulting Clinical Psychology* 51:390-395.

Prochaska, J.O., and C.C. DiClemente. 1986. Toward a comprehensive model of change. Pp. 3-27 in *Treating Addictive Behaviors: Processes of Change*, in W.R. Miller, and N. Neather, eds. New York: Plenum Press.

Prochaska, J.O., and C.C. DiClemente. 1992. The transtheoretical approach. Pp. 300-334 (chapter) in *Handbook of Psychotherapy Integration*, J.C. Norcross and M.R. Goldfried, eds. New York: Basic Books, Inc.

Prochaska, J.O., C.C. DiClemente, and J.C. Norcross. 1992. In search of how people change: Applications to addictive behaviors. *American Psychologist* 47:1102-1114.

Prochaska, J.O., C.A. Redding, L.L. Harlow, J.S. Rossi, and W.F. Velicer. 1994. The transtheoretical model of change and HIV prevention: A review. *Health Education Quarterly* 21(4):471-486.

Prochaska, J.J., M.F. Zabinski, K.J. Calfas, J.F. Sallis, and K. Patrick. 2000. PACE+: Interactive communication technology for behavior change in clinical settings. *American Journal of Preventive Medicine* 19(2):127-131.

Prochaska, J.O., W.F. Velicer, J.L. Fava, L. Ruggiero, R.G. Laforge, J.S. Rossi, S.S. Johnson, and P.A. Lee. 2001. Counselor and stimulus control enhancements of a stage-matched expert system intervention for smokers in a managed care setting. *Preventive Medicine* 32:23-32.

Pugh, J.A., R.A. Medina, J.C. Cornell, and S. Basu. 1995. NIDDM is the major cause of diabetic end-stage renal disease. More evidence from a tri-ethnic community. *Diabetes* 1995 44(12):1375-1380.

Pugh, J.A., M.P. Stern, S.M. Haffner, C.W. Eifler, and M. Zapata. 1988. Excess incidence of treatment of end-stage renal disease in Mexican Americans. Review. *American Journal of Epidemiology* 127(1):135-44.

Purcell, G.P. 2002. The quality of health information on the Internet. *British Medical Journal* 324:557-558.

Puschel, P.K., B. Thompson, G.D. Coronado, L.C. Lopez, and A.M. Kimball. 2001. Factors related to cancer screening in Hispanics: A comparison of the perceptions of Hispanic community members, health care providers, and representatives of organizations that serve Hispanics. *Health Education and Behavior* 28:573-590.

Quiggins, P.A., and M.A. Farrell. 1993. Renal disease among the Eastern Band of Cherokee Indians. *Diabetes Care* 16(1):342-345.

Quinn, N., and D. Holland. 1987. Culture and Cognition. Pp. 3-40 in *Cultural Models in Language and Thought*, D. Holland and N. Quinn, eds. Cambridge: Cambridge University Press.

Quotromoni, P.A., M. Milbauer, B.M. Posner, N.P. Carballeira, M. Brunt, and S.R. Chipkin. 1994. Use of focus groups to explore nutrition practices and health beliefs of urban Caribbean Latinos with diabetes. *Diabetes Care* 17(8):869-873.

Rainie, L. 2002. The online health care revolution. The Pew Internet & American Life Project. Presented to the National Cancer Institute, Washington, DC, January.

Rakowski, W,. B. Ehrich, M.G. Goldstein, B.K. Rimer, D.N. Pearlman, M.A. Clark, W.F. Velicer, and H. Woolverton, III. 1998. Increasing mammography among women aged 40-74 by use of a stage-matched, tailored intervention. *Preventive Medicine* 27:748-756.

Ramelson, H.Z., R.H. Friedman, and J.K. Ockene. 1999. An automated telephone-based smoking cessation education and counseling system. *Patient Education and Counseling* 36:131-144.

Raymond, E. 1999. *The Cathedra and the Bazaar: Musings on Linux and Open Source by an Accidental Revolutionary*. Sebastopol, CA: O'Reilly and Associates.

Resnicow, K., T. Baranowski, J. Ahluwalia, and R. Braithwaite. 1999. Cultural sensitivity in public health: Defined and demystified. *Ethnicity and Disease* 9:10-21.

Revere, D., and P.J. Dunbar. 2001. Review of computer-generated outpatient health behavior interventions: Clinical encounters "in Absentia." *Journal of the American Medical Informatics Association* 8:62-79.

Rhodes, F., M. Fishbein, and J. Reis. 1997. Using behavioral therapy in computer-based health promotion and appraisal. *Health Education and Behavior* 24(1):20-34.

Ribisl, K.M., A.E. Kim, and R.S. Williams. 2001. Web sites selling cigarettes: How many are there in the USA and what are their sales practices? *Tobacco Control* 10:352-359.

Rice, R.E., and C.K. Atkin, eds. 1989. *Public Communication Campaigns* (Second Edition). Newbury Park, CA: Sage Publications.

Rice, R.E., and C.K. Atkin, eds. 2001. *Public Communication Campaigns* (Third Edition). Thousand Oaks, CA: Sage Publications.

Rimer, B., H. Meissner, N. Breen, J. Legler, and C. Coyne. 2000a. Social and behavioral interventions to increase breast cancer screening. In *Integrating Behavioral and Social Sciences With Public Health*, N. Schneiderman, M.A. Speers, J.M. Silva, H. Tomes, and J.H. Gentry, eds. Washington, DC: American Psychological Association.

Rimer, B.K. 1994. Mammography use in the U.S.: Trends and the impact of interventions. *Annals of Behavioral Medicine* 16:317-326.

Rimer, B.K., and B. Glassman. 1999. Is there a use for tailored print communications in cancer risk communication? *Journal of the National Cancer Institute, Monographs* 25:140-148.

Rimer, B.K., E. Ross, A. Balshem, and P.F. Engstrom. 1993. The effect of a comprehensive breast screening program on self-reported mammography use by primary care physicians and women in a health maintenance organization. *Journal of the American Board of Family Practice* 6:443-451.

Rimer, B.K., M. Conaway, P. Lyna, B. Glassman, K.S.H. Yarnall, I. Lipkus, and L.T. Barber. 1999. The impact of tailored interventions on a community health center population. *Patient Education and Counseling* 37(2):125-140.

Rimer, B.K., S. Halabi, C.S. Skinner, I.M. Lipkus, T.S. Strigo, E.B. Kaplan, and G.P. Samsa. 2002. Effects of a mammography decision-making intervention at 12 and 24 months. *American Journal of Preventive Medicine* 22(4):247-257.

Rimer, B.K., M.R. Conaway, P.R. Lyna, W. Rakowski, C.T. Woods-Powell, I. Tessaro, K. Yarnall, and L.T. Barber. 1996. Cancer screening practices among women in a community health center population. *American Journal of Preventive Medicine* 12:351-357.

Rimer, B.K., S. Halabi, C.S. Skinner, E.B. Kaplan, Y. Crawford, G.P. Samsa, T.S. Strigo, and I.M. Lipkus. 2000b. The short-term impact of tailored mammography decision-making interventions. *Patient Education and Counseling* 43(3):271-287.

Rimer, B.K., N. Resch, E. King, E. Ross, C. Lerman, A. Boyce, H. Kessler, and P.F. Engstrom. 1992. Multistrategy health education program to increase mammography use among women ages 65 and older. *Public Health Reports* 107:369-380.

Rippletoe, P.A., and R.W. Rogers. 1987. Effects of components of protection motivation theory on adaptive and maladaptive coping with a health threat. *Journal of Personality and Social Psychology* 52:596-604.

Risendal, B., D. Roe, J. DeZapien, M. Papenfuss, and A. Giuliano. 1999. Influence of health care, cost, and culture on breast cancer screening: Issues facing urban American Indian women. *Preventive Medicine* 29(6 Pt 1):501-509.

Rith-Najarian, S.J., S.E. Valway, and D.M. Gohdes. 1993. Diabetes in a Northern Minnesota Chippewa tribe. *Diabetes Care* 16(1):266-270.

Roccella, E.J. 2002. The contributions of public health education toward the reduction of cardiovascular disease mortality: Experience from the National High Blood Pressure Education Program. In *Public Health Communication: Evidence for Behavior Change*, R. Hornik, ed. Mahwah, NJ: Lawrence Erlbaum Associates.

Rocereto, L. 1981. Selected health beliefs of Vietnamese refugees. *The Journal of School Health* 51(1):63-64.

Rogers, E. 2000. Information, Globalization and Privatization in the News Millennium. Presented at Communication Beyond 2000: Technology, Industry and the Citizen in the Age of Globalization. International Association for Mass Communication Research Conference, Singapore, July 17.

Rogers, E.M. 1995. *Diffusion of Innovations* (Fourth Edition). New York: Free Press.

Rogers, E.M., and J.D. Storey. 1987. Communication campaigns. Pp. 817-846 in *Handbook of Communication Science*, C.R. Berger and S.H. Chaffee, eds. Beverly Hills, CA: Sage.

Rogers, R.W. 1983. Cognitive and physiological processes in fear appeals and attitude change: A revised theory of protection motivation. Pp. 153-176 in *Social Psychophysiology: A Sourcebook*, J.T. Cacioppo and R.E. Petty, eds. New York: Guilford Press.

Roper, W.L. 1993. Health communication takes on new dimensions at CDC. *Public Health Reports* 108(March-April):179-183.

Rose, G. 1985. Sick individuals and sick populations. *International Journal of Epidemiology* 14(1):32-38.

Rosenbloom, A.L., J.R. Joe, R.S. Young, and W.E. Winter. 1999. Emerging epidemic of type 2 diabetes in youth. *Diabetes Care* 22(2):345-352.

Rosenstock, I.M. 1974. The health belief model and preventive health behavior. *Health Education Monographs* 2:354-386.

Rosenstock, I.M., V.J. Strecher, and M.H. Becker. 1994. The health belief model and HIV risk behavior change. Pp. 5-24 in *Preventing AIDS: Theo-*

ries and Methods of Behavioral Interventions, R.J. DiClemente and J.L. Peterson, eds. New York: Plenum Press.

Rubel, A.J., and L.C. Garro. 1992. Social and cultural factors in the successful control of tuberculosis. *Public Health Reports* 107(6):626-636.

Rubel, A.J., C.W. O'Nell, and R. Collado-Ardon. 1984. *Susto: A Folk Illness.* Berkeley, CA: University of California Press.

Ryan, C. 1991. *Prime Time Activism.* Boston, MA: South End Press.

Ryan, G.L., C.S. Skinner, D. Farrell, and V.L. Champion. 2001. Examining the boundaries of tailoring: The utility of tailoring versus targeting mammography interventions for two distinct populations. *Health Education Research* 16(5):555-566.

Saaddine, J.B., M.M. Engelgau, G.L. Beckles, E.W. Gregg, T.J. Thompson, and K.M.V. Narayan. 2002. A diabetes report card for the United States: Quality of care in the 1990s. *Annals of Internal Medicine* 136(8):565-574.

Sadler, G.R., A.G. Thomas, J.Y. Yen, et al. 2000. Breast cancer education program based in Asian grocery stores. *Journal of Cancer Education* 15(3):173-177.

Salmon, C.T. 1989. Campaigns for social "improvement": An overview of values, rationales and impacts. Pp. 19-53 in *Information Campaigns: Balancing Social Values and Social Change*, C.T. Salmon, ed. Newbury Park, CA: Sage Publications.

Samet, J.M., D.B. Coultas, C.A. Howard, B.J. Skipper, and C.L. Hanis. 1988. Diabetes, gallbladder disease, obesity, and hypertension among hispanics in New Mexico. *American Journal of Epidemiology* 128(6):1302-1311.

San Francisco Examiner. 1999. (April 14). State Spending Big Bucks to Tell Us What to Do [Online]. Available at <http://www.aros.net/~hempower/drugwar/cost/990414.html>. Accessed on December 6, 2000.

Sapir, E. 1985 [1932]. Cultural anthropology and psychiatry. Pp. 509-521 in *Edward Sapir: Selected Writings*, D.G. Mandelbaurn, ed. Berkeley: University of California Press.

Schneider, S.J., M.D. Schwartz, and J. Fast. 1995. Computerized, telephone-based health promotion: I. Smoking cessation program. *Computers in Human Behavior* 11:135-148.

Schooler, C., S.H. Chaffee, J.A. Flora, and C. Roser. 1998. Health campaign channels: Trade-offs among reach, specificity, and impact. *Human Communication Research* 24(3):410-432.

Schraer, C.D., A.P. Lanier, E.J. Boyko, D. Gohdes, and N.J. Murphy. 1988. Prevalence of diabetes mellitus in Alaskan Eskimos, Indians, and Aleuts. *Diabetes Care* 11(9):693-700.

Schrage, M. 2000. Open for Business. *Strategy & Business* 21:101-107.

Schulmeister, L., and D.S. Lifsey. 1999. Cervical cancer screening knowledge, behaviors, and beliefs of Vietnamese women. *Oncology Nursing Forum* 26(5):879-887.

Schur, C.L., L.A. Leigh, and M.L. Berk. 1995. Health care use by Hispanic adults: Financial vs. non-financial determinants. *Health Care Financial Review* 17(2):71-88.

Schwab, T., J. Meyer, and R. Merrell. 1994. Measuring attitudes and health beliefs among Mexican American with diabetes. *The Diabetes Education* 20(3):221-227.

Science Panel on Interactive Communication and Health. 1999. *Wired for Health and Well-Being: The Emergence of Interactive Health Communication*, T.R. Eng and D.H. Gustafson, eds. Office of Public Health and Science. Washington, DC: U.S. Department of Health and Human Services.

Scott, C.R., J.M. Smith, M.M. Cradock, and C. Pihoker. 1997. Characteristics of youth-onset noninsulin-dependent diabetes mellitus and insulin-dependent diabetes mellitus at diagnosis. *Pediatrics* 100(1):84-91.

Segura, J.M., X. Castells, M. Casamitjana, F. Macia, M. Porta, and S.J. Katz. 2001. A randomized controlled trial comparing three invitation strategies in a breast cancer screening program. *Preventive Medicine* 33:325-342.

Selnow G. 2000. The Internet: The soul of democracy. *Vital Speeches of the Day* 67(2):58-60.

Serxner, S., and C.S. Chung. 1992. Trend analysis of social and economic indicators of mammography use in Hawaii. *American Journal of Preventive Medicine* 8:303-308.

Shaw, B.R., F. McTavish, R. Hawkins, D.H. Gustafson, and S. Pingree. 2000. Experiences of women with breast cancer: Exchanging social support over the CHESS computer network. *Journal of Health Communication* 5(2):135-159.

Sheeran, P., C. Abraham, and S. Orbell. 1999. Psychosocial correlates of heterosexual condom use: A meta-analysis. *Psychological Bulletin* 125(1):90-132.

Sheppard, B.H., J. Hartwick, and P.R. Warshaw. 1988. The theory of reasoned action: A meta-analysis of past research with recommendations for modifications and future research. *Journal of Consumer Research* 15:325-343.

Siegel, M, and L. Biener. 2000. The impact of an antismoking media campaign on progression to established smoking: Results of a longitudinal youth study. *American Journal of Public Health* 90(3):380-386.

Siero, F.W., J. Broer, W.J.E. Bemelmans, and B.M. Meyboom-de Jong. 2000. Impact of group nutrition education and surplus value of Prochaska-based stage-matched information on health-related cognitions and on Mediterranean nutrition behavior. *Health Education Research* 15(5):635-647.

Sin, J.P., and A.S. St. Legler. 1999. Interventions to increase breast cancer screening uptake: Do they make any difference? *Journal of Medical Screening* 6:170-181.

Singer, E., and P.M. Endreny. 1993. *Reporting on Risk: How the Mass Media Portray Accidents, Diseases, Disasters, and Other Hazards.* New York: Russell Sage Foundation.

Skaer, T.L., L.M. Robison, D.A. Sclar, and G.H. Harding. 1996. Financial incentive and the use of mammography among Hispanic migrants to the United States. *Health Care for Women International* 17:281-291.

Skelton, J.A., and R.T. Croyle. 1991. *Mental Representation in Health and Illness.* New York: Springer-Verlag.

Skinner, C.S., C.L. Arfken, and B. Waterman. 2000. Outcomes of the Learn, Share and Live breast cancer education program for older urban women. *American Journal of Public Health* 90:1229-1234.

Skinner, C.S., V.J. Strecher, and H. Hospers. 1994. Physicians' recommendations for mammography: Do tailored messages make a difference? *American Journal of PublicHealth* 84(1):43-49.

Skinner, C.S., M.K. Campbell, B.K. Rimer, S. Curry, and J.O. Prochaska. 1999. How effective is tailored print communication? *Annals of Behavioral Medicine* 21(4):290-298.

Skinner, H., M. Morrison, K. Bercovitz, D. Haans, M.J. Jennings, L. Magdenko, J. Plozer, L. Smith, and N. Weir. 1997. Using the Internet to engage youth in health promotion. *Int J Health Prom Educ* 4:23-25.

Skinner, C.S., J.M. Schildkraut, D. Berry, B. Calingaert, P.K. Marcom, J. Sugarman, E.P. Winer, J.D. Iglehart, P.A. Futreal, and B.K. Rimer. In press. Pre-counseling education materials for BRCA testing: Does tailoring make a difference? *Genetic Testing.*

Slater, M.D., D. Rounr, K. Murphy, F. Beauvais, J. Van Leuven, and M.D. Rodriguez. 1996. Adolescent responses to TV beer ads and sports content/context: Gender and ethnic differences. *Journalism and Mass Communication Quarterly* Spring 74(1):108-115.

Slater, J.S., C.N. Ha, M.E. Malone, P. McGovern, S.D. Madigan, J.R. Finnegan, A.L. Casey-Paal, K.L. Margolis, and N. Lurie. 1998. A randomized community trial to increase mammography utilization among low-income living in public housing. *Preventive Medicine* 27:862-870.

Slovic, P. 1987. Perception of risk. *Science* 236:280-285.

Slovic, P., D. MacGregor, and N.N. Kraus. 1987. Perception of risk from automobile safety defects. *Accident Analysis and Prevention* 19(5):359-73.

Sly, D.F., R.S. Hopkins, E. Trapido, and S. Ray. 2001. Influence of a counteradvertising media campaign on initiation of smoking: The Florida "Truth" Campaign. *American Journal of Public Health* 91(2):233-238.

Smaglik, P., R.P. Hawkins, S. Pingree, D.H. Gustafson, E. Boberg, and E. Bricker. 1998. The quality of interactive computer use among HIV infected individuals. *Journal of Health Communication* 3(1):53-68.

Snell, J.L., and E.L. Buck. 1996. Increasing cancer screening: A meta-analysis. *Preventive Medicine* 25:702-707.

Soet, J.E., and C.E. Basch. 1997. The telephone as a communication medium for health education. *Health Education and Behavior* 24(6):759-772.

Solovitch, S. 2001. (September). The citizen scientists. Wired. Available at <http://www.wired.com/wired/archive/9.09/disease.html>.

Songer, T.J., and P.Z. Zimmet. 1995. Epidemiology of Type 11 diabetes: An international perspective. *Pharmacoeconomics* 8(Supp 1):1-11.

Spielberg, A.R. 1998. On call and online: Sociohistorical, legal, and ethical implications of e-mail for the patient-physician relationship. *Journal of the American Medical Association* 280(15):1353-1359.

Stahn, R.M., D. Gohdes, and S.E. Valway. 1993. Diabetes and its complications among selected tribes in North Dakota, South Dakota, and Indian Hospital, Rapid City, South Dakota 57702. *Diabetes Care* 16(1):244-247.

Steckler, A., A. Farel, J.B. Bontempi, K. Umble, B. Polhamus, and A.Trester. 2001. Can health professionals learn qualitative evaluation methods on the World Wide Web? A case example. *Health Education Research* 16(6):735-746.

Stein, J.A., and S.A. Fox. 1990. Language preference as an indicator of mammography use among Hispanic women. *Journal of the National Cancer Institute* 82:1715-1716.

Stephenson, M.T. 1999. Message sensation value and sensation seeking as determinants of message processing. Unpublished doctoral dissertation, University of Kentucky, Lexington.

Stern, M.P., S.P. Gaskill, H.P. Hazuda, L.I. Gardner, and S.M. Haffner. 1983. Does obesity explain excess prevalence of diabetes among Mexican Americans? results of the San Antonio heart study. *Diabetologia* 24:272-277.

Stoner, T.J., B. Dowd, W.P. Carr, G. Maldonado, T.R. Church, and J. Mandel. 1998. Do vouchers improve breast cancer screening rates? Results from a randomized trial. *Health Services Research* 33:11-28.

Stout, P.A., J. Villegas, and H. Kim. 2001. Enhancing learning through use of interactive tools on health-related websites. *Health Education Research* 16(6):721-734.

Strecher, V.J. 1999. Computer-tailored smoking cessation materials: A review and discussion. *Patient Education and Counseling* 36:107-117.

Strecher, V., and I.M. Rosenstock. 1996. The Health Belief Model. In *Health Behavior and Health Education: Theory, Research, and Practice* (Second Edition), K. Glanz, F.M. Lewis, and B.K. Rimer, eds. San Francisco: Jossey Bass.

Suarez, L., R.A. Roche, L. Pulley, N.S. Weiss, D. Goldman, and D.M. Simpson. 1997. Why a peer intervention program for Mexican-American women failed to modify the secular trend in cancer screening. *American Journal of Preventive Medicine* 13:411-417.

Suárez-Orozco, M. 2000. Everything you ever wanted to know about assimilation but were afraid to ask. *Daedalus* 129:1-30.

Sugarman, J., and C. Percy. 1989. Prevalence of diabetes in a Navajo Indian community. *American Journal of Public Health* 79(4):511-513.

Summerson, J.H., J.C. Konen, and M.B. Dignan. 1992. Race-related differences in metabolic control among adults with diabetes. *Southern Medical Journal* 85(10):953-956.

Sung, J.F.C., D.S. Blumenthal, R.J. Coates, J.E. Williams, E. Alema-Mensah, and J.M. Liff. 1997. Effect of a cancer screening intervention conducted by lay health workers among inner-city women. *American Journal of Preventive Medicine* 13:51-57.

Sutton, S., G. Balch, and R.C. Lefebvre. 1995. Strategic questions for consumer-based health communications. *Public Health Reports* 110(November/December):725-733.

Taylor, H., and R. Leitman. 2001. The increasing impact of eHealth on consumer behavior. *Health Care News* 1(21):1-9.

Taylor, V., B. Thompson, D. Lessler, Y. Yasui, D. Montano, K.M. Johnson, J. Mahloch, M. Mullen, S. Li, G. Bassett, and H.I. Goldberg. 1999. A clinic-based mammography intervention targeting inner-city women. *Journal of General Internal Medicine* 14(2):104-111.

Taylor, V.M., S.M. Schwartz, J.C. Jackson, et al. 1999. Cervical cancer screening among Cambodian-American women. *Cancer Epidemiology, Biomarkers and Prevention* 8(6):541-546.

Thomas, R., J. Cahill, and L. Santilli. 1997. Using an interactive computer game to increase skill and self-efficacy regarding safer sex negotiation: Field test results. *Health Education and Behavior* 24(1):71-86.

Tirado, M. 1996. Tools for Measuring Cultural Competence in Health Care. January. Final project report to the Office of Planning and Evaluation, Health Resources and Services Administration. Washington, DC: Department of Health and Human Services.

Triandis H.C. 1972. *The Analysis of Subjective Culture.* New York: John Wiley and Sons.

Trock, B., B.K. Rimer, E. King, A. Balshem, C.S. Cristinzio, and P.F. Engstrom. 1993. Impact of an HMO-based intervention to increase mammography utilization. *Cancer Epidemiology, Biomarkers and Prevention* 2:151-156.

Trostle, J.A., and J. Sommerfeld. 1996. Medical anthropology and epidemiology. *Annual Review of Anthropology* 25:253-274.

Truman, B.I., C.K. Smith-Akin, A.R., Hinman, K.M. Gebbie, R. Brownson, L.F. Novick, R.S. Lawrence, M. Pappaioanou, J. Fielding, C.A. Evans, Jr., F. Guerra, M. Vogel-Taylor, C.S. Mahan, M. Fullilove, and S. Zaza. 2000. Task Force on Community Preventive Services. Developing the guide to community preventive services—Overview and rationale. *American Journal of Preventive Medicine* 18(1S):18-26.

Tucker, K.L., O.I. Bermudez, and C. Castaneda. 2000. Type 2 diabetes is prevalent and poorly controlled among Hispanic elders of Caribbean origin. *American Journal of Public Health* 90(7):1288-1293.

Tversky, A., and D. Kahneman. 1981. The framing of decisions and the psychology of choice. *Science* 211(4481):453-8.

Unger, J.B., L.A. Rohrbach, and K.M. Ribisl. 2001. Are adolescents attempting to buy cigarettes on the Internet? *Tobacco Control* 10:360-363.

U.S. Census Bureau. 1998. *Money Income in the United States: 1998*. Washington, DC: U.S. Government Printing Office. Available online at <http://www.census.gov/prod/www/abs/money.html>.

U.S. Census Bureau. 2000. *Census Brief. Women in the United States: A Profile*. Washington, DC: U.S. Government Printing Office.

U.S. Census Bureau. 2001. Census 2000 shows America's diversity. *United States Department of Commerce News*. [Online]. Available at <http://www.census.gov/Press-Release/www/2001/cb01cn61.html>. Accessed March 15, 2001.

U.S. Department of Commerce. 2000. *Falling Through the Net: Toward Digital Inclusion. A Report on Americans' Access to Technology Tools*. Economic and Statistics Administration, National Telecommunications and Information Administration. Washington, DC: U.S. Department of Commerce.

U.S. Department of Commerce. 2001. *Home Computers and Internet Use in the United States: August 2000*. Washington, DC: U.S. Census Bureau.

U.S. Department of Commerce. 2002. *A Nation Online: How Americans Are Expanding Their Use of the Internet*. National Telecommunications and Information Administration, Economics and Statistics Administration. Washington, DC: U.S. Department of Commerce.

U.S. Department of Health and Human Services. 1988a. Media Strategies for Smoking Control. January.

U.S. Department of Health and Human Services. 1988b. Understanding AIDS: A Message from the Surgeon General. Printed public service announcement.

U.S. Department of Health and Human Services. 1996. *Physical Activity and Health: A Report of the Surgeon General*. Centers for Disease Control and Prevention, National Center for Chronic Disease Prevention and Health Promotion. Atlanta GA: U.S. Department of Health and Human Services.

U.S. Department of Health and Human Services. 2000. *Tracking Healthy People 2010*. Washington, DC: U.S. Government Printing Office.

United States Renal Data System. 1993. Incidence and Causes of Treated ESRD: USRDS, 1993 Annual Report. *American Journal of Kidney Disease* 22(4 Suppl 2):30-37.

Valanis, B.G., R.E. Glasgow, J. Mullooly, T.M. Vogt, E.P. Whitlock, S.M. Boles, K.S. Smith, and T.M. Kimes. 2002. Screening HMO women overdue for both mammograms and Pap tests. *Preventive Medicine* 34:40-50.

Valdez, A., K. Banerjee, L. Ackerson, M. Fernandez, R. Otero-Sabogal, and C.P. Somkin. 2001. Correlates of breast cancer screening among low-income, low-education Latinas. *Preventive Medicine* 33:495-502.

Valway, S.E., R.W. Linkins, and D.M. Gohdes. 1993. Epidemiology of lower-extremity amputations in the Indian Health Service, 1982-1987. *Diabetes Care* Jan.16(1):349-53.

Van den Putte, B. 1991. 20 Years of the Theory of Reasoned Action of Fishbein and Ajzen: A Meta-Analysis. Unpublished manuscript, University of Amsterdam, The Netherlands.

Van Duyn, M.A. 2000. Development, implementation, and evaluation of programs of the National 5 A Day for Better Health Campaign. Personal correspondence.

Veatch, R.M. 1982. Health promotion: Ethical considerations. In *Health Promotion: Principles and Clinical Applications*, R.B. Taylor, J.R. Ureda, and J.W. Denham, eds. Norwalk, CT: Appleton Century-Crofts.

Velicer, W.F., J.O. Prochaska, J.L. Fava, R.G. Laforge, and J.S. Rossi. 1999. Interactive versus noninteractive interventions and dose-response relationships for stage-matched smoking cessation programs in a managed care setting. *Health Psychology* 18(1):21-28.

Vernon, S.W., E.A. Laville, and G.L. Jackson. 1990. Participation in breast screening programs: A review. *Social Sciences and Medicine* 30:1107-1118.

Volk, R.J., A.R. Cass, and S.J. Spann. 1999. A randomized controlled trial of shared decision making for prostate cancer screening. *Archives of Family Medicine* 8:333-340.

Wagner, T.H. 1998. The effectiveness of mailed patient reminders on mammography screening: A meta-analysis. *American Journal of Preventive Medicine* 14:64-70.

Wakefield. M, D. Banham, K. McCaul, J. Martin, R. Ruffin, N. Badcock, and L. Roberts. 2002. Effect of feedback regarding urinary continince and brief tailored advice on home smoking restrictions among low-income parents of children with asthma: A controlled trial. *Preventive Medicine* 34:58-65.

Wallack, L. 1994. Media advocacy: A strategy for empowering people and communities. *Journal of Public Health Policy* 15(4):420-436.

Wallack. L.M. 1989. Mass communication and health promotion: A critical perspective. Pp. 353-367 in *Public Communication Campaigns*, Second Edition, R.E. Rice and C.K. Atkin, eds. Newbury Park, CA: Sage.

Wallack, L., and L. Dorfman. 1996. Media advocacy: A strategy for advancing policy and promoting health. *Health Education Quarterly* 23(3):293-317.

Wallack, L., and R. Sciandra. 1990-91. Media advocacy and public education in the community trial to reduce heavy smoking. *International Quarterly of Community Health Education* 205-222.

Wallack, L., L. Dorfman, D. Jernigan, and M. Themba. 1993. *Media Advocacy and Public Health: Power for Prevention*. Newbury Park, CA: Sage Publications.

Wallack, L., K. Woodruff, L. Dorfman, and I. Diaz. 1999. *News for a Change. An Advocates Guide to Working with the Media.* Newbury Park, CA: Sage Publications.

Wang, C.Y., L. Abbott, A.K. Goodbody, W.T.Y. Hui, and C. Rausch. 1999. Development of a community-based diabetes management program for Pacific Islanders. *The Diabetes Educator* 25(5):738-746.

Ward, M. 2001. (July 18). Indian handheld to tackle digital divide. BBC News. <http://news.bbc.co.uk/hi/english/sci/tech/newsid_1442000/1442000.stm>.

Wasserman, M.P. 2001. Guide to community preventive services: State and local opportunities for tobacco use reduction. *American Journal of Preventive Medicine* 29(2 Suppl):8-9.

Weber, B.E., and B.M. Reilly. 1997. Enhancing mammography use in the inner city. A randomized trial of intensive case management. *Archives of Internal Medicine* 157:2345-2349.

Weinreich, N.D. 1999. *Hands-On Social Marketing: A Step-by-Step Guide.* Thousand Oaks, CA: Sage Publications.

Weller, S.C., R.D. Baer, L.M. Pachter, R.T. Trotter, M. Glazer, J. Garcia de Alba Garcia, and R.E. Klein. 1999. Latino beliefs about diabetes. *Diabetes Care* 22(5):722-728.

Wellings, K. 2002. Evaluating AIDS public education in Europe: A cross-national comparison. In *Public Health Communication: Evidence for Behavior Change.* Mahwah, NJ: Lawrence Erlbaum Associates.

Wellman, B. 1997. An electronic group is virtually a social network. In *Culture of the Internet*, S. Kielser, ed. Mahway, NJ: Lawrence Erlbaum Associates.

Wetterhall, S.F., D.R. Olson, F. DeStefano, J.M. Stevenson, E.S. Ford, R.R. German, J.C. Will, J.M. Newman, S.J. Sepe, and F. Vinicor. 1992. Trends in diabetes and diabetic complications, 1980-1987. *Diabetes Care* 15(8):960-967.

White, M., and S.M. Dorman. 2001. Receiving social support online: Implications for health education. *Health Education Research* 16(6):693-708.

Wiebe, D.J., and C. Korbel. In press. Defensive denial, affect, and the self-regulation of health threats. In *The Self-Regulation of Health and Illness Behavior,* L.D. Cameron and H. Leventhal, eds. New York: Harwood Academic.

Williams, D. 1990. Socioeconomic differences in health. *Social Psychology Quarterly* 14(1):11-25.

Willinger, M., C. Ko, H. Hoffman, R. Kessler, and M. Corwin. 2000. Factors associated with caregivers' choice of infant sleep position, 1994-1998: The National Infant Sleep Position Study. (Statistical data included.) *Journal of the American Medical Association* 283(16):2135.

Winett, L., and L. Wallack. 1996. Advancing public health goals through the mass media. *Journal of Health Communication* 1:173-196.

Wing, R.R., E. Venditti, J.M. Jakicic, B.A. Polley, and W. Lang. 1986. Behavioral self-regulation in the treatment of patients with diabetes mellitus. *Psychological Bulletin* 99:78-89.

Wing, R.R., E. Venditti, J.M. Jakicic, B.A. Polley, and W. Lang. 1998. Lifestyle intervention in overweight individuals with a family history of diabetes. *Diabetes Care* 21(3):350-359.

Wingo, P.A., E.E. Calle, and A. McTiernan. 2000. How does breast cancer mortality compare with that of other cancers and selected cardiovascular diseases at different ages in U.S. women? *Journal of Women's Health and Gender-Based Medicine* 9:999-1006.

Winzelberg, A.J., C. Barr Taylor, T. Sharpe, K.L. Eldredge, P. Dev, and P.S. Constantinou. 1998. Evaluation of a computer-mediated eating disorder intervention program. *International Journal of Eating Disorders* 24:339-349.

Winzelberg, A.J., D. Eppstein, K.L. Eldredge, D. Wilfley, R. Dasmahapatra, P. Dev, and C.B. Taylor. 2000. Effectiveness of an Internet-based program for reducing risk factors for eating disorders. *Journal of Consulting and Clinical Psychology* 68(2):346-350.

Wismer, B.A., J.M. Moskowitz, A.M. Chen, S.H. Kang, T.E. Novotny, K. Min, R. Lew, and I.B. Tager. 1998. Mammography and clinical breast examination among Korean American women in two California counties. *Preventive Medicine* 27:144-151.

Witte, K., and M. Allen. 2000. A meta-analysis of fear appeals: Implications for effective public health campaigns. *Health Education and Behavior* 27:591-615.

Worden, J.K., B.S. Flynn, L.J. Solomon, R.H. Secker-Walker, G.J. Badger, and J.H. Carpenter. 1996. Using mass media to prevent cigarette smoking among adolescent girls. *Health Education Quarterly* 23(4):453-68.

Wu, Z.H., S.A. Black, and K.S. Markides. 2001. Prevalence and associated factors of cancer screening: Why are so many older Mexican American women never screened? *Preventive Medicine* 33:268-273.

Yabroff, K.R., and J.S. Mandelblatt. 1999. Interventions targeted toward patients to increase mammography use. *Cancer Epidemiology, Biomarkers and Prevention* 8:749-757.

Yabroff, K.R., A. O'Malley, P. Mangan, and J. Mandelblatt. 2001. Inreach and outreach interventions to improve mammography use. *Journal of the American Medical Women's Association* 56(4):166-173, 188.

Yawn, B.P., P.J. Allgatt-Bergstrom, R.A. Yawn, P. Wollan, M. Greco, M. Gleason, and L. Markson. 2000. An in-school CD-ROM asthma education program. *The Journal of School Health* 70(4):153-159.

Yen, I.H., and S.L. Syme. 1999. The social environment of health: A discussion of the epidemiological literature. *Annual Review of Public Health* 20:287-308.

Young, J.C., and L.C. Garro. 1982. Variation in the choice of treatment in two Mexican communities. *Social Science and Medicine* 16:1453-1465.

Young, J.C., and L.C. Garro. 1994. *Medical Choice in a Mexican Village*. Prospect Heights, IL: Waveland Press. Reissue with changes of book by the same title by J.C. Young, published in 1981 by Rutgers University Press, New Brunswick, NJ.

Zajonc, R.B. 1998. Emotions. Pp. 591-632 in *The Handbook of Social Psychology, Volume 1* (Fourth Edition), D.T. Gilbert, S.T. Fiske, et al., eds. Boston, MA: McGraw-Hill.

Zaldivar, A., and J. Smolowitz. 1994. Perceptions of the importance placed on religion and folk medicine by non-Mexican-American hispanic adults with diabetes. *The Diabetes Educator* 20(4):303-306.

Zambrana, R.E., N. Breen, S.A. Fox, and M.L. Gutierrez-Mohamed. 1999. Use of cancer screening practices by Hispanic women: Analyses by subgroup. *Preventive Medicine* 29:466-477.

Zapka, J.G., D.R Harris, D. Hosmer, M.E. Costanza, E. Mas, and R. Barth. 1993. Effect of a community health center intervention on breast cancer screening among Hispanic American women. *Health Services Research* 28:223-235.

Zenner, W.P. 1996. Minorities in America. Pp. 291-299 in *Encyclopedia of Cultural Anthropology*, D. Levinson and M. Ember, eds. New York: Henry Holt and Company.

Zimicki, S., R.C. Hornik, C.C. Verzosa, J.R. Hernandez, E. De Guzman, M.Dayrit, A. Fausto, and M.B. Lee. 1994. Improving vaccination coverage in urban areas through a health communication campaign: The 1990 Philippines experience. *Bulletin of the World Health Organization* 72(3):409-422.

Appendixes

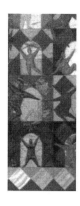

A

Consultants

Nina L. Agbayani, RN
BALANCE Program for
    Diabetes
Association of Asian Pacific
    Community Health
    Organizations
Oakland, CA

Rosie Sotelo Armijo
California Department of
    Health Services
Public Health Institute
Sacramento, CA

Desiree Backman, DrPH, MS
California Latino 5 A Day
    Campaign
Sacramento, CA

Ursula Bauer, PhD
Florida Department of Health
Tallahassee, FL

Brenda Bodily
Utah Diabetes Control
    Program
Salt Lake City, UT

Lois Book, EdD, RN
American Association of
    Diabetes Educators
Chicago, IL

John Ross Bradley, PhD
Behavioral Health Department
Northern Cheyenne Tribal
    Health
Lame Deer, Montana

James Coan
HCFA Multi-City
  Mammography Pilot
  Projects
Baltimore, MD

Ann Constance, MA, RD,
  CDE
Upper Peninsula Diabetes
  Outreach Network
Marquette, MI

Valerie Cook, PhD, CPNP
Diabetes Prevention Program
  for Children
Gila River Indian Community
Department of Public Health
Sacaton, AZ

Stephanie Craver
Buckle Up Program
National SAFE KIDS
  Campaign
Washington, DC

Richard Crespo, PhD
Marshall University School of
  Medicine
Huntington, WV

Lynne Dapice, MS, RN
Diabetes Control Program
Burlington, VT

Vanessa Duren-Winfield, MS
Wake Forest University School
  of Medicine
Public Health Sciences
Winston-Salem, NC

Kimberly Floyd, PhD
Virginia Department of Health
Division of Chronic Disease
  Prevention and Nutrition
Richmond, VA

Joanne Gallivan, MS, RD
National Institute of Diabetes,
  Digestive, and Kidney
  Diseases
National Institutes of Health
Bethesda, MD

Franklin Gilliam, PhD
Department of Political Science
University of California, Los
  Angeles
Los Angeles, CA

Willie-Ann Glenn
Local Health Department
Perry, FL

Nina Goodman, MHS, CHES
National Cancer Institute
National Institutes of Health
Bethesda, MD

Barbara Rose Gottlieb, MD
Brighams and Women's
    Hospital
Boston, MA

Sheldon Greenfield, MD
Diabetes PORT
Tufts Manages Care Institute
Boston, MA

Karen Gruebnau
National Air Bag and Seatbelt
    Safety Campaign
Washington, DC

David H. Gustafson, PhD
Department of Industrial
    Engineering
University of Wisconsin
Madison, WI

Nurit Guttman, PhD
Department of
    Communication
Faculty of Social Sciences
Tel Aviv University
Israel

Nancy Halpin, RN
Pike County Health
    Department
Pittsfield, IL

Richard F. Hamman, MD,
    DrPH
Department of Preventive
    Medicine and Biometrics
Denver, CO

Mimi Hartman, MA, RD,
    CDE
Idaho Diabetes Community
    Program
Boise, ID

Todd Harwell, MPH
Montana Diabetes Project
Helena, MT

David J Hill, PhD
Centre for Behavioural
    Research in Cancer
Anti-Cancer Council of
    Victoria
Australia

Theresa M. Hinman
New York State's Diabetes
    Control Programs
Albany, NY

Roland G. Hiss, MD
Demonstration and Education
    Division
Michigan Diabetes Research
    and Training Center
Ann Arbor, MI

Christine Hoak
National Safety Council
Washington, DC

Bette Iacino
National Breast Cancer
Awareness Month
Atlanta, GA

Linda J. Inglis
Best Start Social Marketing
Tampa, FL

Julie Kotzin Jacob
National Institute of Child
Health and Human
Development
National Institutes of Health
Bethesda, MD

Carolyn Jenkins, PhD, RN
REACH Program
Medical University of South
Carolina
Charleston, SC

Maria L. Jibaja, EdD
Department of Family and
Community Medicine
Baylor College of Medicine
Houston, TX

Joanie Jones, MA
Diabetes Control Program
Emergency Medical Services &
Prevention Division
Colorado Department of
Public Health and
Environment
Denver, CO

Marlene Kane, RN, BSN
Primary Care Clinician Plan
Commonwealth of
Massachusetts
Boston, MA

Aileen Kantor
Healthcare Writer
Bethesda, MD

Kimberly Kelker, MPH
Minnesota Department of
Health
Center for Health Promotion,
St. Paul, MN

Rachel Klugman
HCFA-NCI Medicare for
Mammography campaign
Chicago, IL

Terry Kruse, RN
Wisconsin Primary Health
Care Association
Madison, WI

Shiriki K. Kumanyika, PhD,
MPH
Center for Clinical
Epidemiology and
Biostatistics
University of Pennsylvania
School of Medicine
Philadelphia, PA

Barbara Larsen, MPH, RD
Utah Diabetes Control
Program
Utah Department of Health
Salt Lake City, UT

Janet Leiker, MPH
Medicare Quality
Improvement
Kansas Foundation for
Medical Care
Topeka, KS

Catherine J. Lewis
Lasting Education for Women,
Adults and Children of
WNY, Inc.
Buffalo, NY

Debra Lieberman, EdM, PhD
University of California, Santa
Barbara
Institute for Social, Behavioral,
and Economic Research
Santa Barbara, CA

Jackie Liro
Association of Asian Pacific
Community Health
Organizations
Oakland, CA

Mimi Lising, MPH
National Institute of Child
Health and Human
Development
National Institutes of Health
Bethesda, MD

Susan Lopez Mele
California Diabetes Control
Program
California Department of
Health Services
Sacramento, CA

Anne Lubenow, MPH, CHES
National Cancer Institute
National Institutes of Health
Bethesda, MD

Christine Macaluso
University of South Florida
Tampa, FL

Edward Maibach, MPH, PhD
Porter Novelli
Washington, DC

Elaine Massaro, MS, RN, CDE
Disease Management Programs
Elmhurst, IL

Maria M. Matias, MSW
Diabetes Multicultural
   Coalition
Rhode Island Department of
   Health
Providence, RI

Donald R. Mattison, MD
March of Dimes
White Plains, NY

**Mary Helen Mays, PhD,
MPH, MBA**
Texas Diabetes Institute
San Antonio, TX

Michael D. McDonald, DrPH
Global Health Initiatives, Inc.
Potomac, MD

Peter Messeri, PhD
American Legacy Foundation
Washington, DC

Angela Mickalide, PhD, CHES
National Safe Kids Campaign
Washington, DC

Tanya Monroe
Manager, National Folic Acid
   Campaign
March of Dimes
White Plains, NY

Timothy F. Murphy, PhD
Department of Medical
   Education
University of Illinois at
   Chicago
Chicago, IL

Chandana Nandi, MS, RD, LD
Diabetes Control Program
Illinois Department of Human
   Services
Springfield, IL

Anne Nettles, RN, MSN, CDE
Diabetes Careworks
Wayzata, MN

Marisa Nightingale
National Campaign to Prevent
   Teen Pregnancy
Washington, DC

Susan Nine, RN, MSN, CDE
Ebenezer Medical Outreach
Huntington, WV

Susan Norris, MD, MPH
CDC Diabetes Translation
   Center
Atlanta, GA

Kathleen Oberst, RN, MS
Taking on Diabetes Program
Michigan State University
East Lansing, MI

Casey Otis
Air Bag and Seat Belt Safety
    Campaign
Washington, DC

Sandra Parker, RD, CDE
TENDON
Diabetes Outreach Network
Grand Rapids, MI

John Pierce, PhD
Cancer Center
University of California, San
    Diego
San Diego, CA

Tommy B. Piggee Sr., MA,
    CHES
Arkansas Department of
    Health
Little Rock, AR

Elizabeth Pivonka, PhD, RD
Produce for Better Health
    Foundation
Wilmington, DE

Laurel Reger, MBA
Minnesota Diabetes Program
Minnesota Department of
    Health
St. Paul, MN

LaVerne Reid, PhD
North Carolina Central
    University
Durham, NC

Joelle Reizes, MA
Screening for Mental Health
Wellesley Hills, MA

Steven L. Reynolds, MPH
Division of Cancer Prevention
    and Control
Centers for Disease Control
    and Prevention
Atlanta, GA

Jeffrey M. Robbins, DPM
Cleveland VA Medical Center
Cleveland, OH

Ronald Sage, DPM
Department of Orthopedic
    Surgery and Rehabilitation
Loyola University Stritch
    School of Medicine
Maywood, IL

Charles T. Salmon, MA, PhD
College of Communication
    Arts and Sciences
Michigan State University
East Lansing, MI

Stephanie M. Santos, MPH
National SAFE KIDS
  Campaign
Washington, DC

Laura Shea
New York State Department
  of Health
Albany, NY

David F. Sly, PhD
Florida State University
Tallahassee, FL

David W. Smith, PhD, MPH
College of Public Health
University of Oklahoma
  Health Sciences Center
Oklahoma City, OK

E. Smith
Diabetes Education
  Empowerment Program
University of Illinois
Chicago, IL

Leslie B. Snyder, PhD
Department of
  Communication Sciences
University of Connecticut,
Storrs, CT

Suganya Sockalingam, PhD
National Center for Cultural
  Competence
Georgetown University Child
  Development Center
Washington, DC

Elizabeth Solan, RN, MPH
Diabetes Control Program
New Jersey Department of
  Health and Senior Services
Trenton, NJ

Eddie Staton
MAD DADS National
  Program
Omaha, NE

Ann Stys, RN, CDE
SouthEast Michigan Diabetes
  Outreach Network
Detroit, MI

**Mary Ann Van Duyn, PhD,
  MPH, RD**
National Cancer Institute
National Institutes of Health
Bethesda, MD

Carrie Vandyke
Freelance Writer and Video
  Producer
Indianapolis, IN

Andrew Winzelberg, PhD
Department of Psychiatry
Stanford University
Palo Alto, CA

Kimberlydawn Wisdom, MD,
MS
Center for Medical Treatment
Effectiveness Programs in
Diverse Populations,
Henry Ford Health System
Detroit, MI

Jamey Wise, MS
Division of Health Awareness
and Tobacco
Florida Department of Health
Tallahassee, FL

Clarissa K. Wittenberg
National Institute of Mental
Health
National Institutes of Health
Bethesda, MD

Faye L. Wong, MPH, RD
National Center for Chronic
Disease Prevention and
Health Promotion
Centers for Disease Control
and Prevention
Atlanta, GA

Elizabeth Woolfe
Education and Special Projects
National Alliance of Breast
Cancer Organizations
New York, NY

Stephanie Zaza, MD, MPH
Epidemiology Program Office
Centers for Disease Control
and Prevention
Atlanta, GA

David Zucker
Porter Novelli
New York, NY

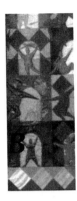

B

Biographical Sketches

SUSAN C. SCRIMSHAW, PHD (Chair), is Dean of the School of Public Health and Professor of Community Health Sciences and Anthropology at the University of Illinois at Chicago. Dr. Scrimshaw has extensive experience working with diverse populations in cross-cultural settings and in the fields of medical and applied anthropology, demography, culture change, and population health. An involved IOM member, Dr. Scrimshaw has served on the IOM Board on International Health and the IOM Panel on Cancer Research among Minorities and the Medically Underserved, among other IOM activities. She is a member of the Task Forces on Community Preventive Services and on Violence Prevention at the Centers for Disease Control and Prevention (CDC), and a member of the Executive Council of the Illinois Department of Public Health. Dr. Scrimshaw has worked extensively with city, state, governmental, national, and United Nations agencies. She has been honored by the American Anthropological Association and the Society for Applied Anthropology with the Margaret Mead Award for "outstanding achievement in bringing anthropology to a wider audience (public health, demography, and the general public)."

ALBERT BANDURA, PHD, is David Starr Jordan Professor of Social Sciences in Psychology at Stanford University. He is past president of the American Psychological Association, Western Psychological Association, and Honorary President of the Canadian Psychological Association. Throughout his career, Dr. Bandura has been honored with numerous honorary degrees and scientific awards, including the Distinguished Scientific Achievement Award from the American Psychological Association in 1972. He has served on the IOM Board on Neuroscience and Behavioral Health, as well as the IOM Committee on Preventing Nicotine Dependence in Children and Adolescents. Dr. Bandura was chair of the Board of Directors of both the American Psychological Association and the Western Psychological Association, and currently serves on the editorial boards of numerous psychological and behavioral journals, including the *Psychological Review, Cognitive Therapy and Research, Media Psychology, Social Behavior and Personality,* and *British Journal of Clinical Psychology.*

MARTIN FISHBEIN, PHD, is Harry C. Coles Jr. Distinguished Professor in Communication at the Public Policy Center, Annenberg School for Communication, University of Pennsylvania. He is past president of both the Society for Consumer Psychology and the Interamerican Psychological Society. Dr. Fishbein has served as guest researcher and acting chief of the Behavioral Intervention and Research Branch in the Division of STD Prevention at the Center for Disease Control and Prevention. Currently, he serves on the editorial boards of various journals, including *AIDS and Behavior*; the *Journal of Consumer Psychology*; *Psychology, Health and Medicine*; and the *Journal of Applied Social Psychology.*

LINDA C. GARRO, PHD, is Professor, Department of Anthropology, at the University of California at Los Angeles. Her work focuses on the following topics: the representation of cultural knowledge about illness; intracultural variation in such knowledge; how people make health care decisions; illness narratives and cultural knowledge; and remembering as a social, cultural, and cognitive process. Member of a number of Professional Societies, Dr. Garro has been elected to executive boards of the Society for Medical Anthropology and the Society for Psychological Anthropology. She has served on a number of editorial boards, including Culture, Medicine and Psychiatry and the book series for the Society for Psychological Anthropology. She has been a National Health Research Scholar in Canada and has received the Stirling Award for her contributions to psychological anthropology from the Society for Psychological Anthropology.

ROBERT C. HORNIK, PhD, is Wilbur Schramm Professor of Communication and Health Policy at the Annenberg School for Communication, University of Pennsylvania. He has a wide range of experience in public health communication evaluations, from AIDS education, and diarrhea treatment, immunization, and other child survival projects, to anti-drug and -domestic violence campaigns, at community, national, and international levels. He has won the Andreason Scholar award in social marketing, and the Fisher Mentorship award from the International Communication Association. Dr. Hornik has served as member of the IOM Committee on International Nutrition Programs, and as Consultant and Member of various Committees of the World Health Organization (WHO). He is scientific director for the evaluation of the National Youth Anti-drug Media Campaign. He is also consultant to other agencies such as the U.S. Agency for International Development, UNICEF, the Centers for Disease Control and Prevention, and the World Bank. Dr. Hornik serves on the editorial boards of several journals, including *Social Marketing Quarterly.*

HOWARD LEVENTHAL, PhD, is Board of Governor's Professor of Health Psychology at the Center for Research on Health and Behavior, and chair of the Division of Health at the Institute for Health, at Rutgers State University of New Jersey. Dr. Leventhal is a senior Member of the IOM and President of the APA, Division 38, which honored him with the Senior Investigator Award for

Outstanding Contributions to Health Psychology in 1987. He is co-chair of the Behavioral Sciences Program at the Cancer Institute of New Jersey, and is actively involved in Governing and Consulting Committees, including the National Heart Lung and Blood Institute Committee on Adherence to Medical and Lifestyle Interventions. Dr. Leventhal is editor of the *Journal of Health Psychology* and co-editor of *Psychology and Health*, and he serves on the editorial boards of numerous journals of applied psychology and education.

STEVEN R. LOPEZ, PHD, is professor in the Department of Psychology and Psychiatry, at the University of California, Los Angeles. Dr. Lopez has served as consultant to public mental health center staff, physicians, psychologists, and various clinical research and training units concerning the integration of cultural perspectives in training, research, and clinical practice. He is currently principal investigator of a project on Prosocial Family Factors, Culture, and Course of Schizophrenia, and was principal investigator and director of a research training program on Mental Disorders in Mexico. Dr. Lopez serves on the editorial boards of various psychological journals, such as *Journal of Psychopathology and Behavioral Assessment*, and recently served as one of the science editors for the Surgeon General's *Supplemental Report on Mental Health: Culture, Race, and Ethnicity*.

YOLANDA PARTIDA, MSW, MPA, is national program director for Hablamos Juntos, Improving patient-patient provider communication, an $18.5 million initiative to examine language barriers to health care for Latinos. Hablamos Juntos (We Speak Together) is funded by the Robert Wood Johnson Foundation and administered by Tomás Rivera Policy Institute based in the Claremont Graduate University. Dr. Partida has extensive experience in hospital and public health administration and in private consulting. In these settings she has been responsible for overseeing a variety of personal and public health programs, developing strategic plans, designing and conducting feasibility studies, and producing business case analyses, among other activities. She has worked with and on behalf of many different groups of underserved populations, including the uninsured, the U.S. Mexico border population, as well as the Latino community broadly and communities of other ethnic minority groups. Ms. Partida has served as Deputy Director of Health and Human Services, San Diego County HHSA, as Assistant Director of Ambulatory Care, Fresno County Health Services Agency and as senior manager with The Lewin Group, a private policy, research and management consulting firm. Dr. Partida is also the founder and executive director for The Partida Group, a health-focused research and management consulting firm specializing in diverse populations.

BARBARA K. RIMER, MPH, DRPH, is director of Cancer Control and Population Sciences at the National Cancer Institute. Her expertise lies in health promotion and disease prevention, particularly of cancer, through behavioral research and intervention. Dr. Rimer was honored with the American Society for Preventive Oncology's Distinguished Achievement Award and with the Mayhew Derryberry Award for her Contributions to Health Education Theory from the American Public Health Association. She has served on numerous advisory committees, including as chair of the National Cancer Advisory Board, and she currently serves on the Board of Directors of the American Family Life Assurance Corporation. Dr. Rimer is also is associate editor of *Preventive Medicine*, and serves on the editorial boards and as a reviewer of numerous medical and health education journals. Dr. Rimer is co-editor of one of the most widely-used textbooks for public health students: *Health Education and Health Behavior: Theory, Research and Practice* (with Drs. Karen Glanz and Francis Lewis).

EVERETT M. ROGERS, PHD, is Regents' Professor and Chair of the Department of Communication and Journalism at the University of New Mexico. Dr. Rogers' expertise lies in applied communication research, organizational aspects of health communication campaigns, intercultural communication, and agenda setting. His research examines HIV/AIDS prevention programs in San Francisco, the effects of an entertainment-education radio soap opera about HIV/AIDS prevention and family planning in Tanzania, and the effects of the Mothers Against Drunk Driver's Victim Impact Panels on drunk drivers in New Mexico. Dr. Rogers was also co-principal investigator of the Stanford Heart Disease Prevention Program, and he currently serves on the editorial board of the *Journal of Health Communication*.

GLORIAN SORENSEN, PhD, MPH, is Professor of Health and Social Behavior at the Harvard School of Public Health and Director of the Center for Community-Based Research at the Dana-Farber Cancer Institute. The core of Dr. Sorensen's research is randomized worksite- and community-based studies that test the effectiveness of theory-driven interventions targeting individual and organizational change. These interventions are designed particularly to be effective for low income, multiethnic populations, including blue-collar and service workers. These behavioral interventions are embedded in the social context or environments in which people live. Her research has focused on a range of community settings, including worksites and labor unions. Dr. Sorensen was a Member of the IOM Committee on Capitalizing on Social Sciences and Behavioral Research to Improve the Public's Health, and now serves on the IOM Committee on the Health and Safety Needs of Older Workers.

SHARYN MALLAMAD SUTTON, PhD, is president of Sutton Group and research professor at the School of Communication, American University. Dr. Sutton does innovative work in social marketing and effective consumer-based health communications, much of which has involved diverse or special populations. Dr. Sutton has acted as executive vice president of Research and Strategic Planning at Porter/Novelli, branch chief at the National Institutes of Health, directing the National Cancer Institute's Public and Patient Information Program, and director of Nutrition Marketing and Education for the U.S. Department of Agriculture. She has directed the research, strategic planning, and execution of award-winning public service campaigns such as "5 a Day for Better Health," "Do the Right Thing," "Mammography: Once a Year . . . for a Lifetime," and "Team Nutrition," which won the Silver Anvil Award of Excellence for "advancing public understanding of a social issue—child nutrition." Dr. Sutton has served on a number of national advisory panels, including the Expert Panel on National Anti-Tobacco Public Education Campaign for the Campaign for Tobacco Free Kids. As president of Sutton Social Marketing, she provides social marketing expertise to non-profit and advocacy groups, foundations, and government agencies to create successful communication programs for behavior change, and currently serves on the editorial board of *The Social Marketing Quarterly*.

LAWRENCE WALLACK, MS, MPH, DrPH, is director and professor at the School of Community Health at Portland State University and emeritus professor of Public Health at the University of California, Berkeley. Dr. Wallack's research has examined the presentation and policy implications of the framing of public health issues in the news and entertainment media. Most recently, he has explored the implications for public health communication strategies emerging from research linking social inequality, social capital, and health inequality. He was the principal investigator of the California site of the Community Intervention Trial for Smoking Cessation (COMMIT), and founding director of both the Prevention Research Center at the Pacific Institute for Research and Evaluation (funded by the National Institute on Alcohol Abuse and Alcoholism) and the Berkeley Media Studies Group, Western Consortium for Public Health. Dr. Wallack has served as a consultant to numerous local, state, national, and international agencies, including the World Health Organization and the Office of Technology Assessment (U.S. Congress), among others, and has testified before the U.S. Senate and House on the regulation of alcohol advertising.

A. EUGENE WASHINGTON, MD, MPH, MSc, is professor of Gynecology, Epidemiology and Health Policy in the School of Medicine at the University of California, San Francisco (UCSF). He is chair of the Department of Obstetrics, Gynecology and Reproductive Sciences, Director of the Medical Effectiveness Research Center for Diverse Populations at UCSF, and Director of the UCSF-Stanford Evidenced-based Practice Center. Dr. Washington has published extensively on topics in his major areas of research, which include effectiveness of reproductive health services, prevention of diseases in women, and explaining and eliminating racial/ethnic health disparities. He is the principal investigator of a program project on Promoting Effective Communication and Decision Making in Diverse Populations, funded by the Agency for Healthcare Research and Quality and the National Cancer Institute. He has served as a member of many national and international advisory committees, including the Advisory Committee for the National Breast and Cervical Cancer Early Detection and Control Program, Department of Health and Human Services, and the Institute of Medicine's Committee on Clinical Research in the Public Interest. Currently, he serves on the Institutes of Medicine's Committee on Identifying Priority Areas for Quality Improvement.

KENNETH B. WELLS, MD, MPH [liaison], is professor-in-residence of Psychiatry and Biobehavioral Sciences at UCLA Neuropsychiatric Institute and Hospital and Senior Scientist at RAND. He is a psychiatrist and health services researcher. Dr. Wells directs the UCLA-NPI Health Services Research Center, which focuses on improving quality of care for psychiatric and neurologic disorders across the lifespan. He is the principal investigator of the NIMH-funded UCLA/RAND Center for Research on Managed Care for Psychiatric Disorders; the Robert Wood Johnson-funded Alcohol, Drug Abuse, and Mental Health Supplement to the Community Tracking Study; and of the Agency for Health Care Policy and Research (AHQPR) Patient Outcomes Research Team (PORT-II). Dr. Wells is chair of the Institute of Medicine's Neuroscience and Behavioral Health Board.

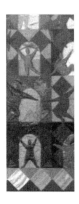

Index